Praise for *Understanding H*

"Comprehensive and well-written ... will quickly become a go-to, must-read resource for healthcare delivery science. Thoughtfully details the value of investment in improving health delivery at a time when vast amounts of data are being generated on a minute by minute basis. These 21 chapters with easy to digest visuals and key points provide the tools to move to a modern value-based, population-centered delivery model ... provides the tools and techniques to analyze and utilize the zettabytes of data being generated in healthcare delivery and research and helps maximize the opportunities where clinical operations intersect with research questions ... advances our knowledge and practice for years to come."

—David H. Roberts, MD, Steven P. Simcox, Patrick A. Clifford, and
James H. Higby Associate Professor of Medicine, Harvard Medical School

"Arguably the biggest contribution that this generation has made to the future of the healing professions is care delivery science. It's not just about knowing what works, but how to make it work consistently for every person we serve. This new science is the foundation upon which the present generation's contributions primarily will rest. You hold in your hands 35 years of investigation and learning, condensed into understandable principles and applications. It is a guidebook for effective care delivery leadership, practice, and success. Learn from it, enjoy it, then go forth and create a new profession that defines a new and better world!"

—Brent C. James, MD, MStat, Clinical Professor,
Stanford University School of Medicine

"Today's disjointed and complex systems of care too often fail to address the multiple health and social needs of individuals and communities. We can no longer accept the disconnect between research on what works in healthcare and its application to improving the reliable delivery of high value care to all. Howell and colleagues have given us an expertly curated volume that brings together the issues, frameworks, methods and tools used in healthcare delivery science as well as practical suggestions on how to embed healthcare delivery science into health systems. This is a must read for anyone who, like me, is frustrated with the pace of our progress and is committed to creating a learning health system for all."

—Lisa Simpson, MB, BCh, MPH, FAAP, President and CEO, AcademyHealth

Understanding Healthcare Delivery Science

NOTICE

Medicine is an ever-changing science. As new research and clinical experience broaden our knowledge, changes in treatment and drug therapy are required. The author and the publisher of this work have checked with sources believed to be reliable in their efforts to provide information that is complete and generally in accord with the standards accepted at the time of publication. However, in view of the possibility of human error or changes in medical sciences, neither the authors nor the publisher, nor any other party who has been involved in the preparation or publication of this work, warrants that the information contained herein is in every respect accurate or complete, and they disclaim all responsibility for any errors or omissions, or for the results obtained from use of the information contained in this work. Readers are encouraged to confirm the information contained herein with other sources. For example, and in particular, readers are advised to check the product information sheet included in the package of each drug they plan to administer to be certain that the information contained in this work is accurate and that changes have not been made in the recommended dose or in the contraindications for administration. This recommendation is of particular importance in connection with new or infrequently used drugs.

Understanding Healthcare Delivery Science

Michael D. Howell, MD, MPH
Principal Scientist and Chief Clinical Strategist
Google Health
Google, LLC
Palo Alto, California

Jennifer P. Stevens, MD, MS
Director, Center for Healthcare Delivery Science
Beth Israel Deaconess Medical Center
Assistant Professor of Medicine
Harvard Medical School
Boston, Massachusetts

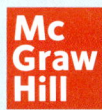

New York   Chicago   San Francisco   Athens   London   Madrid
Mexico City   New Delhi   Milan   Singapore   Sydney   Toronto

Understanding Healthcare Delivery Science

Copyright © 2020 by McGraw Hill Education. All rights reserved. Printed in China. Except as permitted under the United States Copyright Act of 1976, no part of this publication may be reproduced or distributed in any form or by any means, or stored in a database or retrieval system, without the prior written permission of the publisher.

1 2 3 4 5 6 7 8 9 DSS 24 23 22 21 20 19

ISBN 978-1-260-02648-1
MHID 1-260-02648-5

This book was set in Times NR MT Std by MPS Limited.
The editors were James Shanahan and Kim J. Davis.
The production supervisor was Catherine Saggese.
Project management was provided by Touseen Qadri, Jyoti Shaw, and Ishan Chaudhary of MPS Limited.

Library of Congress Cataloging-in-Publication Data

Names: Howell, Michael D., author. | Stevens, Jennifer P., author.
  Title: Understanding healthcare delivery science / Michael D. Howell, Jennifer P. Stevens.
  Description: New York : McGraw-Hill Education, [2020] | Includes bibliographical references and index. |
  Identifiers: LCCN 2019017647 (print) | LCCN 2019021789 (ebook) | ISBN 9781260026498 (ebook) | ISBN 1260026493 (ebook) | ISBN 9781260026481 (paperback) | ISBN 1260026485 (paperback)
  Subjects: LCSH: Medical care—Quality control. | Health planning. | Patients—Safety measures. | Patient satisfaction. | BISAC: MEDICAL / Dentistry / General.
  Classification: LCC RA399.A1 (ebook) | LCC RA399.A1 H69 2020 (print) | DDC 362.1—dc23
  LC record available at https://lccn.loc.gov/2019017647

McGraw Hill Education Professional books are available at special quantity discounts to use as premiums and sales promotions, or for use in corporate training programs. To contact a representative, please visit the Contact Us pages at www.mhprofessional.com.

Contents

Contributors .... *xiii*
Preface .... *xv*
Dedication .... *xvii*
Introduction .... *xix*

PART I: WHAT IS HEALTHCARE DELIVERY SCIENCE, AND WHY DO WE NEED IT?

Chapter 1
Introduction... 3

The Problem: How Research and Operations Are Organized
 in Healthcare Today 3
Historical Context: How Did It Get This Way? 4
Why Now Is Different: Two Key Changes in Context 5
Why It Matters: Problems with Thinking Too Simply About Healthcare 12
Healthcare Delivery Science 17
References 19

Chapter 2
Complexity 23

What Happens When We View Healthcare as Complicated? 23
What Is a Complex Adaptive System? 26
Why It Matters: Fitting the Right Measurement Tool to the Question 31
Healthcare Delivery Science: A Field of Research Where
 Healthcare Itself Is the Organism Under Study 34
References 35

Chapter 3
Quality and Safety in Healthcare 37

The Best the World Has Ever Seen 37
Three Critical Papers to Know 37
An Inflection Point: To Err Is Human and Crossing the Quality Chasm 39
More Recent Estimates About Deaths from Medical Error 41
International Comparisons 42
Have Improvement Efforts Worked? 45
How We Put It All Together 46
References 49

Chapter 4
What Does the Future Hold? 51

Introduction 51
Value Drives Change 53
The "Postsafety" Era 55
Healthcare Delivery That Delivers Health 56
Consumerism Versus Personalization 60
The Doctor Will See You Now? 62
Informed Healthcare Information Technology (IT) 64
Conclusions 66
References 68

PART II: MAKING CHANGE IN THE REAL WORLD—TOOLS FOR HEALTHCARE IMPROVEMENT

Chapter 5
Human Factors 73

Human Factors: An Introduction 74
Cognitive Reasoning, Errors, and Biases in Healthcare ... 77
Hierarchy: What Is It, How Do We Measure It, and
   Why Does It Matter? 86
Tools for Understanding Complex Systems 91
Conclusions 96
References 97

Chapter 6
How Teams Work 104

Types of Teams 105
What Do Teams Need to Succeed? 107
Poorly Functioning Teams in Healthcare 108
Teams in Aviation and the Birth of Crew Resource Management
   (CRM) 110
CRM in Healthcare 111
Leading Teams Through Change 112
References 114

Chapter 7
Leadership and Culture Change 117

Leading Change Is Difficult 117
Where to Start 121

What Is Implementation Science? 123
Implementation Science Frameworks 123
Integrating Implementation Science Frameworks for
    the Purpose of Change Management 132
References 133

Chapter 8
Standard Quality Improvement Tools and Techniques ... 137

Introduction 137
Preventing Adverse Events and Improving Patient Safety 137
Identifying Patient Safety Events 139
Root Cause Analysis (RCA) 142
Failure Mode Effects (and Criticality) Analysis
    (FMEA and FMECA) 151
Safety I and Safety II 154
Process Improvement and Quality Improvement 155
References 159

Chapter 9
Lean Improvement Techniques in Healthcare ... 162

A Brief History of Lean 163
The Rules of Lean 165
A Concrete Definition of the Ideal 166
The 8 Wastes 167
Tools from Lean 170
Summary 175
References 176

Chapter 10
Partnering with Community, Professional, and Policy Organizations ... 178

Introduction 178
How Health Is Created 179
Key Stakeholders in Shaping Health 181
Engaging with Local Public Health Agencies 186
Approaches to Successful Partnerships 194
Concluding Thoughts 195
Acknowledgments 196
References 196

PART III: SEEING THE TRUTH—ANALYTICS IN HEALTHCARE

Chapter 11
Data in Healthcare........................203

Part 1: Fundamental Issues in Healthcare Data.. 203
Part 2: The Importance of Understanding Data Lineage, and
 How This Leads Mature Organizations to Both Informal
 and Formal Data Governance.. 206
Part 3: Basic Understanding of Relational Database Structures 211
Part 4: Review of Common Approaches to Actually Accessing
 Healthcare Data... 212
Conclusion 214
References 214

Chapter 12
Measuring Quality and Safety.....................216

Quality Measurement Frameworks 216
What Are You Trying to Achieve? Improvement, Comparison, or
 Accountability... 221
What Makes a Good Measure?... 222
Challenges 223
Common Measure Sets and Major Pay-For-Performance Programs 225
References 230

Chapter 13
Overview of Analytic Techniques and Common Pitfalls 233

Dinosaur Footprints and What They Tell Us
 About Data Analysis in Healthcare 233
The Four Horsemen of Mistaken Conclusions 235
The Critical Importance of Missing Data... 243
The Shape of Data: Categories of Data and Why They Matter 245
Overview of Analytic Methods 251
References 254

Chapter 14
Everyday Analytics........................256

Summarizing Your Data 257
Displaying Data.. 261
Outcomes Over Time, Part I – Run Charts 268
How to Tell if Two Groups Are Different: Univariable Tests of Difference
 and Measures of Comparison.. 270

Outcomes Over Time, Part 2—Statistical Process Control
    (SPC) Charts 279
Everyday Analytics.. 282
References 288

Chapter 15
Survey-Based Data 289

Introduction... 289
Perhaps the Most Important Thing You'll Learn in This Chapter 289
What Are Some of the Main Purposes of Surveys? 290
Overview of Conducting a Survey 293
Some Pitfalls.. 303
References 308

Chapter 16
Predictive Modeling 1.0 and 2.0 312

What to Expect in This Chapter 312
Predictive Modeling 1.0 313
Predictive Modeling 2.0 333
Taking Predictions to the Next Level... 338
References 339

Chapter 17
Predictive Modeling 3.0: Machine Learning 341

Definitions: What Is Artificial Intelligence? Machine Learning?.................. 341
A Brief History of Artificial Intelligence 344
Translating Epidemiology to Machine Learning 346
Categories of Machine Learning Used in Healthcare 347
Pitfalls in Using Machine Learning in Healthcare........................... 369
The Future 372
References 373

Chapter 18
What Everyone Should Know About Risk
    Adjustment................................... 377

What Is Risk Adjustment, and Why We Should Care? 377
What Risk Adjustments Are Available, and How Should We
    Assess Them?.. 381
Examples of Risk Adjustment Gone Awry 384
Using Risk Adjustment in Local Healthcare Delivery Science...... 385
References 387

Chapter 19
Modeling Patient Flow: Understanding Throughput and Census 390

Why Does Understanding Patient Flow Matter? 391
Understanding Patient Flow Conceptually 393
Analytical Approaches to Understanding Patient Flow............................397
Summary...412
References..413

Chapter 20
Program Evaluation............................416

Causal Methods...417
Quasi-Experimental Designs—Causal Inference in Observational Data..422
Evaluations in the Real World 430
References..431

Chapter 21
How to Embed Healthcare Delivery Science Into Your Health System 434

Introduction...434
How Do I Join (or Build) a Community of Healthcare Delivery Science? 434
How to Embed Healthcare Delivery Science in Your Health System 439
Summary..444
Reference 445

Index..*447*

Contributors

Sonia Y. Angell, MD, MPH
Division of General Medicine, Department of Medicine, Columbia University Irving Medical Center, New York, NY
Office of Deputy Commissioner, Division of Prevention & Primary Care, New York City Department of Health & Mental Hygiene, New York, NY
Chapter 10. Partnering with Community, Professional, and Policy Organizations

Joseph Dudas, MBA
Vice Chair, Supply Chain Management
Mayo Clinic
Rochester, Minnesota
Chapter 11. Data in Healthcare: Where It Comes From, How It Is Structured, How to Govern It, and How to Get Your Hands on It

Michael D. Howell, MD, MPH
Principal Scientist and Chief Clinical Strategist
Google, LLC
Palo Alto, California

Cullen D. Jackson, PhD
Director of Innovation, Department of Anesthesia, Critical Care, and Pain Medicine
Beth Israel Deaconess Medical Center
Instructor in Anesthesia
Harvard Medical School
Boston, Massachusetts
Chapter 5. Human Factors: Considerations for Healthcare Delivery

Anna Johansson, PhD
Instructor in Medicine
Harvard Medical School Director of Social Science Research, Division of Translational Research Program Director, IRB Navigation and Scientific Review
Vice Chair, Committee on Clinical Investigations Beth Israel Deaconess Medical Center Boston, Massachusetts
Chapter 5. Human Factors: Considerations for Healthcare Delivery

Sarah C. Shih, MPH
Assistant Commissioner, Bureau of the Primary Care Information Project
Division of Prevention and Primary Care
New York City Department of Health and Mental Hygiene
Long Island City, New York
Chapter 10. Partnering with Community, Professional, and Policy Organizations

Jennifer P. Stevens, MD, MS
Director, Center for Healthcare Delivery Science
Beth Israel Deaconess Medical Center
Assistant Professor of Medicine
Harvard Medical School
Boston, Massachusetts

Michael J. Wall, PharmD, MBA
Chief Analytics Officer
UChicago Medicine
Chicago, Illinois
Chapter 11. Data in Healthcare: Where It Comes From, How It Is Structured, How to Govern It, and How to Get Your Hands on It

Stephen Weber, MD, ScM
Professor of Medicine, Section of Infectious Diseases and Global Health
Chief Medical Officer and Senior Vice President for Clinical Effectiveness
University of Chicago Medicine
Chicago, Illinois
Chapter 4. What Does the Future Hold? The Kind of Healthcare Our Children's Children Will Receive

Preface

We are excited you're here. You have decided that you are interested in a field that challenges the type of healthcare we deliver. That asks, "Why aren't things better?" That says, "Didn't we already learn the best practices in this field? Why aren't we using them?" We hope that you, the new healthcare delivery scientists, will find this book useful as you begin to fundamentally change the healthcare we provide to our patients.

Healthcare delivery science is a new entity to address an old problem—one that hasn't been solved with discipline that have come before. In health services research, the insights we glean are largely separated from healthcare operations. In healthcare operations, we largely learn from the business literature and, perhaps, the field of industrial design … but not from advances in the quantitative healthcare sciences. For quality improvement, we have made important strides in understanding the risks to our patients and developed methods to try to combat them, but sometimes our analyses should reflect the fact that systems of care are profoundly complex. We hope this book brings a new perspective.

A major theme of this book is that, to be healthcare delivery scientist, you need to be a generalist. The right way to answer a question and really strive to improve the care we deliver to patients may require a new statistical method, a new survey, a new technique. We need to build ourselves a toolbox of tools to deliver better, safer, higher-value care; we can't always look to apply our reliable, comfortable technique to whatever problem lies before us. We have sought out experts in several different fields to expose you to these ideas, and their authorship is noted by chapter; all other chapters were written by Dr. Howell or Dr. Stevens.

How should you read this book? Part I defines this new field of healthcare delivery science. Chapter 1 explains how we got here. Chapter 2 explains the concept of complexity. Together, we can see that some methods will work for complicated problems (e.g., a reliable system that is the sum of its parts) while others will work only for complex systems, like the complex physiology and pathophysiology of the healthcare system. Chapter 3 opens the door to the urgency of the unsafe and low-quality care in our current system, while Chapter 4 suggests where we need to be in the future.

Part II focuses on several new disciplines that are rarely taught in most healthcare professional schools, including human factors (Chapter 5), teams (Chapter 6), implementation science and healthcare leadership (Chapter 7), quality improvement methodology and Lean thinking (Chapters 8 and 9), and the intersection of our healthcare system with our community, state, and federal partners (Chapter 10). We're excited to have these disciplines all in one place.

Finally, Part III gets to the meat of many of these methods. Chapter 11 serves as a revealing opportunity to look "under the hood" of how data architecture is (and should) be designed for a health system. This chapter alone should fundamentally make you look at your dataset from your health institution with skepticism and concern, which will make you a much better scientist. Chapters 12 to 14 should help you begin to poke at your data, consider how to present data, and understand why it matters, while Chapters 16 and 17 should lead you into new fields. Meanwhile, Chapter 15, on surveys, should give you a new, healthy respect for survey design; we hope that you will leave this text with a newfound respect for the sophistication of surveys and a view of the rocky shoals that call to those with poor survey designs. Finally, Chapters 19 and 20 should arm you with unexpected techniques from new fields to answer questions in healthcare that you didn't know you could ask.

We're thankful you're here. As the future of healthcare delivery science, the integration of many old and many new techniques, we know that you will ask the difficult, generalizable, and optimistic questions that fundamentally will challenge all of us to make healthcare better and safer for our patients. And you will be armed with the tools you'll need to do it.

Dedication

First, we'd like to thank Joe, Lucy, Shala, and Bridget. Writing a book turns out to be a ton of work, and you gave us the time, space, and support to do it.

Our brilliant guest authors have contributed tremendous expertise, time, and skills. (Writing a chapter also turns out to be a ton of work!). Thank you, Sonia Angell, Joseph Dudas, Cullen Jackson, Anna Johansson, Sarah Shih, Michael Wall, and Stephen Weber.

We were also amazingly fortunate to have several individuals who gave us truly helpful feedback on specific aspects of the book. Deena, Ashley, Alvin, Nissan, Iz, and Greg—thank you! Any errors that remain are ours, not theirs. We're also grateful to Shala Howell and Joe Wright, who are the writers we aspire to be—and who were great reviewers of the whole work.

We would also like to thank Kim Davis and Jim Shanahan from McGraw-Hill, whose unfailingly upbeat optimism about this text was infectious. We've been in great hands from the very beginning. Karla Pollick and Katie Annas were also instrumental to keeping us on track, making much of this book possible.

Finally, we realize that we've been profoundly fortunate throughout our careers—fortunate to have people whom we learned from, people who looked out for us, people who took a gamble on us. The risk of any list like this is that we will invariably leave some people out. But, nonetheless, Anne, Jane, Dan, Frank, Woody, Bruce, Ed, Eric, Phillip, Paul, Stephen, Pat, Krista, Nate, Eileen, Ken, Tom, and Danny—thank you. Topping this list are our parents.

From Michael: Thank you to my mom, Barbara, and my dad, Dwight, who taught me how to work hard, how to think critically, and how to keep family at the center.

From Jennifer: Thank you to my mother, Maxine, who reliably sends me reminders that she still thinks I'm the bee's knees, and who brings grace and brilliance to all that she does; and my father, David, my senior colleague, in whose footsteps I'm very lucky to follow both in medicine and publishing.

Introduction: How to Use This Book

THE GAP

Today, a widening chasm exists between those who actually deliver healthcare and those who study it and how it is delivered. Although rooted in understandable historical tradition, this gap results in tens of thousands of needless deaths and billions of dollars of wasted costs in healthcare every year.

Healthcare delivery science is an emerging field that attempts to bridge this gap. It brings research-quality methods to bear at the speed that real-world healthcare delivery requires, both by improving care and making discoveries.

WHO THIS BOOK IS FOR

Until very recently, no training programs in healthcare delivery science existed. Today, these programs are being created at an accelerating rate. If you are enrolled in one, or considering doing so, *Understanding Healthcare Delivery Science* will serve as a framework for this burgeoning field and its critical elements.

But chances are that you are someone else:

- Maybe you are a health services researcher or epidemiologist who is frustrated that discoveries don't reach patients, and you want to affect the care that patients actually receive.
- Perhaps you're a healthcare administrator who is tired of not truly *knowing* if a new program worked, and you sense the opportunity to do something better for your patients, staff, and providers.
- You might be a student in a master's program in a health-related field, and you want to bridge scholarship and real-world practice.
- Or maybe you are earlier in your career, studying business in college or university, and you want to focus on the future of healthcare.

This book is designed to fill that gap that all of you sense—to help bridge the divide between real-world healthcare operations and research-quality methods.

HOW TO USE THIS BOOK

This book focuses on what emerging practitioners and leaders of healthcare delivery science need to know to be successful. It is divided into four parts:

- Part I: What Is Healthcare Delivery Science, and Why Do We Need It?
- Part II: Making Change in the Real World—Tools for Healthcare Improvement
- Part III: Seeing the Truth—Analytics in Healthcare
- Part IV: How to Embed Healthcare Delivery Science into Your Health System

While the book is a coherent whole and progresses logically, each part and chapter is also designed to stand on its own. That makes it fine to skip around to meet your needs. Each of you will have a different background, with different strengths and different areas that you're trying to strengthen. For example, if you're a researcher or epidemiologist, Part II focuses on real-world tools for improvement and may represent new tools and techniques for you. Or if you're an operator/administrator, you may want to move directly from Part I to Part III, which introduces research-quality analytic methods.

There are several features of this book to be aware of:

Symbol	What It Means
	Case: As doctors, we know that we learn best from individual, realistic cases. Throughout the book, we will introduce you to Arbitrary Regional General Hospital, a hypothetical healthcare center facing a consistent, evolving case.
	Key Point: This symbol highlights particularly critical points throughout the text.
	Caution: It is surprisingly easy to make a mistake with healthcare data and in healthcare improvement. Like land mines, these traps can sometimes be invisible until you step on them—and they can result in real harm to patients. Throughout the text, we flag such vital points with this symbol.
	External Resource: Throughout the text, we provide references and links to important external agencies, organizations, and resources.

PART I

What Is Healthcare Delivery Science, and Why Do We Need It?

INTRODUCTION
The Paradox of Keeping Healthcare Operations and Research Apart

1

THE PROBLEM: HOW RESEARCH AND OPERATIONS ARE ORGANIZED IN HEALTHCARE TODAY

Healthcare operations and research are systematically separate in most of healthcare today. Although more than $100 billion is spent in the United States on medical research annually, and the National Institutes of Health (NIH) budget allocates more than $30 billion a year to identifying novel biologic pathways and new therapeutics, very little is spent on understanding or improving how current patient care is delivered. In fact, only 0.2%–0.3% of U.S. healthcare expenditures support health services research, the very broad category of study that focuses on how healthcare is delivered, its quality, and its cost. Instead, most research dollars focus on basic science, pharmaceutical research, and medical device development.[1]

But even this perhaps understates the problem. The vast majority of hospitals and healthcare systems simply do not have a research and development (R&D) department as it would be understood in most other industries, where the aims of R&D are aligned with the needs of the enterprise. Most hospitals and health systems do not have any research department at all. Even in the epicenters of academic medicine, almost all research is focused on basic science or clinical trials. This is reflected in total spending on R&D in healthcare delivery systems compared to other industries (Figure 1-1). To put this in perspective, the automobile industry spends 2000% more than the healthcare delivery system on R&D; even the food and beverage industry spends more than 500% more on R&D than the healthcare delivery system does. We see this at the local level, too: If you are responsible for healthcare operations, how often have you used research-quality methods to understand if a project *really* worked? If you are a researcher, how often have you engaged in the annual or strategic planning process for how care would be delivered at your health system? The chances are that the answer to both questions is the same: never.

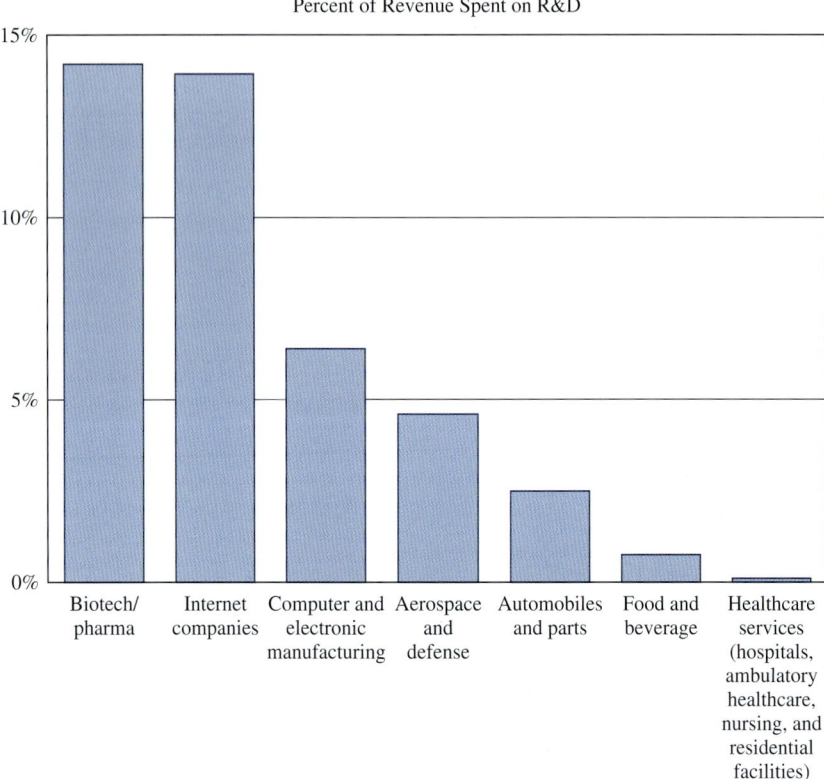

Figure 1-1 • R&D spending in U.S. industries. Although pharmaceutical, biotech, and medical device companies spend substantial amounts on R&D, the healthcare delivery system (hospitals, ambulatory care, nursing, and residential facilities) spend only about 0.1% of revenue on R&D. (Adapted from Moses et al, 2015)

Joe Biden, the 47th vice president of the United States, once said, "Don't tell me what you value. Show me your budget, and I'll tell you what you value."[2] The evidence is overwhelming that we have fundamentally undervalued R&D for the healthcare delivery system. But that is beginning to change.

HISTORICAL CONTEXT: HOW DID IT GET THIS WAY?

Healthcare changed almost unimaginably in the 20th century. Harvard professor Lawrence Henderson called 1912 the Great Divide:

> *For the first time in human history, a random patient with a random disease consulting a doctor chosen at random stands a better than 50/50 chance of benefiting from the encounter.*[3]

Key Point

Research and operations are kept remarkably separate in healthcare today. The healthcare delivery system spends much less than 1% of revenue on R&D.

Antibiotics were developed and tested, transforming pneumonia from a disease that William Osler called the "captain of the men of death"[4] to the paragon of a treatable disease. Surgical and anesthetic techniques advanced tremendously in complexity, while becoming safer by orders of magnitude. Physicians and surgeons discovered things as fundamental to modern practice as the clinical chemistry of the human body.[5] The impact of the Flexner report transformed medical education, healthcare developed into an industry, and physicians became a true profession.[6]

The Physician's Workshop

As medicine evolved and the complexity of care increased, hospitals became central to the delivery of care. No longer was a hospital a place where people went to die—rather, it was a place they went for healing. However, the hospital (and, by extension, the healthcare delivery system) became viewed as nothing more than the so-called physician's workshop[7]— rather than as a critical, complex, and intrinsic part of how care was actually delivered. Physicians viewed autonomy from hospitals as both an ethical and a financial imperative. The goal was that physicians could practice medicine without interference from non-physician managers and administrators. In some states, this was even enshrined into legislation that prevented non-physician-controlled corporations from directly employing physicians.[8]

Although this model perhaps made sense at one time, it also created tremendous complexity and difficulty by intentionally, methodically, and systematically separating physicians and researchers from the healthcare delivery system.

Key Point

For a century, the hospital and healthcare system were thought of only as the "physician's workshop." This model is no longer adequate for today's needs.

WHY NOW IS DIFFERENT: TWO KEY CHANGES IN CONTEXT

Healthcare delivery science wouldn't have made sense until recent decades. Even in the latter half of the 20th century, a significant amount of care was simply delivered in one-to-one doctor/patient interactions, and data generated by the encounter were almost all in the form of difficult-to-decipher, handwritten notes on paper. What has changed?

Complexity—of Both Healthcare and How it is Delivered

Two key developments over the past quarter-century drive today's need for healthcare delivery science: (1) dramatic increases in the complexity of care itself, and of the delivery system; and (2) marked growth in the amount of data that patients generate even in routine healthcare encounters.

Complexity of the Care Itself

The complexity of the actual care that we deliver increases on an almost-daily basis. Whether considered as novel pharmacological therapies for previously untreatable diseases, technological advances for minimally invasive treatment, or the longitudinal management of multiple complex conditions, medical care today is increasingly complex.

The first percutaneous transluminal coronary angioplasty (PTCA) was not performed until September 1977. By 2007, 30 years later, PTCA had become such a standard of care that how soon you got the artery open when patients arrived at the emergency department (door-to-balloon time) became a national core quality measure for the Joint Commission and the Centers for Medicare and Medicaid Services (CMS). By 2015, more than 95% of Americans with acute myocardial infarction received coronary angioplasty within 90 minutes of emergency department (ED) arrival.[9] In 2017, percutaneous replacement of aortic valves has become routine;[10] this procedure was not even performed in pigs until the 1990s, with the first human attempt made only in 2002.[11]

Chemotherapy, radiation, and surgery served as the mainstays of treatment for cancer for decades. Bone marrow and stem cell transplantation brought new hope, but also complexity. Between 1990 and 2016, their use more than tripled.[12] In the late 1990s and 2000s, molecularly targeted therapies reached the mainstream with drugs like rituximab, trastuzumab, imatinib, and others. Today, chimeric antigen receptor (CAR) T-cell therapy has been approved by the U.S. Food and Drug Administration (FDA).[13] In this therapy, T cells are removed from a patient with cancer. They are then genetically edited and engineered to specifically identify an antigen expressed on the patient's cancer. The cells are grown and expanded, and then reinfused into the patient. This means that every treatment is tailored uniquely for every patient. This would have seemed like science fiction just a few years ago.

But complexity in care is not just limited to esoteric, leading-edge treatments for life-threatening conditions. As care has improved, patients survive with more and more chronic conditions: diabetes, hypertension, chronic kidney disease, and on and on. Multimorbidity, the presence of multiple chronic, comorbid conditions, increased by 40% between 2003 and 2009. The majority of elderly adults have multiple chronic conditions; 15% of those over 65 years old have five or more.[14] Reflecting their underlying medical complexity, the average 65-year-old takes 5 medications,

Key Point

The actual, technical medical care that we provide has become increasingly complex over a comparatively short time span. Not restricted to acute, lifesaving technologies, this complexity also applies to the care of patients with multiple chronic conditions across the care continuum.

and this increases as we age; 13% of Americans take 10 or more medications at the same time.[15]

Although many other examples exist, these illustrations, taken together, paint a picture of just how much the complexity of the care that we provide has truly increased. And, as care has become more complex, so has its delivery system.

Complexity of How Healthcare is Delivered

Delivering care today requires a healthcare delivery system that may now be as complex as a living organism. On the occasion of his induction into the Royal College of General Practitioners, patient-safety pioneer Don Berwick reflected on how his father, also a physician, would have seen today's healthcare system and its complexity:

> *The tasks of healing have simply passed the capacity of any single human mind, no matter how skilled or altruistic or self-surveillant. You—and your patients—have now become irrevocably part of something far larger than yourself, and the craft of care has transformed into the machinery of care ... The terms are these: complexity, interdependence, pervasive hazard, a changing distribution of power and control, and, borne on the back of technology, distributed, democratised capacities that my father could not ever have even imagined.*[16]

Key Point

The healthcare delivery system may now be as complex as a living organism, and this complexity is often underappreciated.

Today's level of patient complexity has become more than a single physician can care for. Even in the early 2000s, each Medicare patient saw a median of seven physicians in a year.[17] Each physician was accompanied by nurses, pharmacists, and other clinicians who helped deliver care. This extends to the inpatient setting: according to a 2015 study, when hospitalized, 90% of Medicare patients required at least one specialist consultation, with an average of 2.6 specialty consultations per hospitalization.[18]

But focusing just on these numbers—as daunting as they are—dramatically underestimates the true complexity of how the healthcare system contributes to patient outcomes, independent of physician decision-making and action. Take as an example a single national health priority, the reduction of *Clostridium difficile* infection (known as "*C. diff*" for short). This infection is common, lethal, expensive—and increasing in incidence. It is important enough that its rates are publicly reported and influence hospitals' payments by Medicare. We now know that environmental cleaning is absolutely critical to preventing *C. diff*. This bacterium forms spores that survive a long time in the environment and are not killed by the usual cleaning methods (or by alcohol-based hand sanitizers). Guidelines now recommend that the rooms of patients with *C. diff* be cleaned with bleach.[19] The importance of environmental services (EVS) team members for protecting patients is being increasingly recognized: they are now sometimes called "secret weapons for preventing healthcare-associated infections."[20]

Think of all the individual people and individual systems that have to be in place for this supposedly "simple" cleaning to happen. Imagine that Mr. Smith was just discharged after treatment for *C. diff*. The ED is full of patients waiting for admission. It is so crowded that the waiting room is filling up with sick patients. There is a lot of pressure to fill every empty room with a new patient—as quickly as possible. An EVS worker is called to do the room cleaning. How many other people and systems are needed to ensure that the cleaning happens? A lot.

Before this, the hospital's infection control team would have created a protocol that required bleach-based room cleaning for *C. diff* patients. Someone with special expertise must have created the protocol, and in most states, the protocol usually has to be approved by an organized body with delegated authority from the medical staff. Many hospitals use contracted vendors to manage EVS functions: appropriate contractual requirements had to have been negotiated for this kind of cleaning. Was bleach available at the point of need? The hospital's supply chain team must have known of the need for bleach, identified a vendor, sent a purchase order, received it in the hospital dock, and delivered it to EVS supply. Was the right personal protective equipment available for the EVS worker?

Even if all these criteria have been satisfied, how would the EVS worker know to perform a special type of room cleaning for this patient? If the hospital has an electronic health record (EHR), it needs to integrate the microbiology results with the patient-flow system with the EVS dispatch system. If the hospital is non-electronic, then this function may fall to the nurse. And if all those items have worked correctly, the EVS worker must still have been trained to do the bleach-based cleaning in a safe, effective way, and must carry the procedure out reliably.

This example—even though it is simplified compared to reality—helps to highlight just how complex the healthcare delivery system must be to deliver what sounds like a simple intervention (cleaning a room with bleach). None of these depend on physician acumen or nursing competency: They are inherent characteristics of the system that determines whether you or your loved one will catch a potentially lethal infection. How many things could go wrong and reduce the safety of the next patient in that room? All of them—if any one item in the system fails, the next patient is at demonstrably higher risk of catching *C. diff*. And this is a really, really simple intervention. How much more complexity is required to harvest, genetically engineer, and then redeliver a T-cell population tailored to target a specific patient's cancer? Or to manage the outpatient care of an 85-year-old woman with congestive heart failure, stage III chronic kidney disease, type II diabetes, osteoporosis, and depression? The point is this: Today's healthcare delivery system may be as complex as a living organism, and this represents one of the key changes that drives the need for healthcare delivery science.

Big Data in the Everyday

The problem in healthcare used to be scarcity of data—both for taking care of patients and for making new discoveries. It was expensive and difficult to collect data from patients. Today, the problems have changed. Now, the problems are the logistical, computational, and statistical challenges of handling data sets at a scale that was unimaginable even 25 years ago. Moreover, these data sets are cluttered, siloed, and fragmented in ways that trick, trap, and deceive the unwary administrator or researcher.

The evidence for this critical contextual change is overwhelming. In 2008, only 1.5% of U.S. hospitals had a comprehensive EHR,[21] and only 4% of ambulatory physicians reported an extensive, fully functioning EHR system.[22] The Health Information Technology for Economic and Clinical Health (HITECH) Act became law in 2009 and created significant financial incentives to promote EHR adoption. The incentives worked. By 2015, 90% of U.S. hospitals had an EHR that was not just basic level, but offered more advanced functionality.[23] In the same year in the ambulatory setting, 86.9% of U.S. office-based physicians had an EHR, and 77.9% of those had a certified EHR.[24] These startling trends in adoption (Figure 1-2) represent a transformational change in the availability of data generated by routine healthcare.

How much data, then? One report estimated that the amount of healthcare data in 2013 was 153 exabytes and would grow to 2.314 zettabytes by 2020.[25] (An exabyte is 1 billion gigabytes, and a zettabyte is 1,000 exabytes.) How much information is 153 exabytes, the estimated amount of healthcare data in 2013? Let's think about it this way: An autobiography or memoir is a textual summary of someone's life. If an average autobiography is 300 pages long, then the amount of healthcare data in 2013 is equivalent to the same textual information as if we gave every human being on Earth about 40,000 autobiographies. The 2020 prediction (2.314 zettabytes)

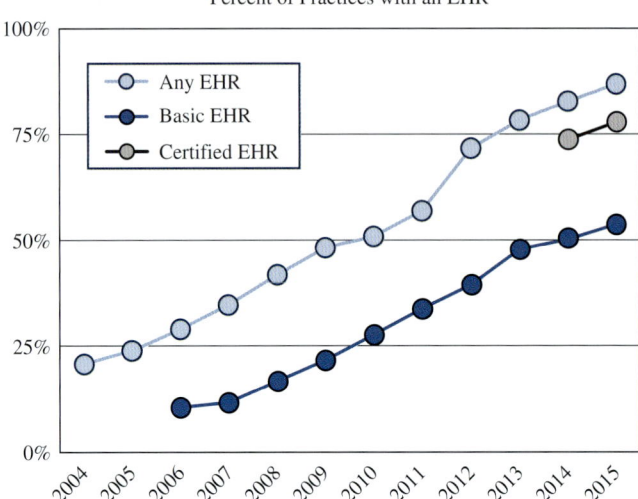

Figure 1-2 • Rapid adoption of EHRs in the United States. Rapid adoption of the EHR has transformed the availability of healthcare data for discovery, understanding, and improvement. EHR availability more than tripled in a single decade. (Adapted from Office of the National Coordinator for Health Information Technology (2016).)

would be the equivalent of almost 600,000 books for every man, woman, and child on the planet.*

It is almost impossible to think about this scale of data. One analogy that is sometimes helpful is to translate it to time. Instead of a kilobyte, imagine a kilosecond (~1000 seconds). How long ago was a kilosecond? A kilosecond was about 17 minutes ago. How about a megasecond? A megasecond was about 12 days ago. How much longer is an exasecond? An exasecond ago was before the Big Bang!

The term *big data* seems vastly overused in today's media, but it is probably appropriate here. Further indicating that this is a new factor in healthcare, the term *big data* did not even appear in PubMed as a noun until 2008. (PubMed is the standard database of medical literature

---

*Here are the math and the assumptions being used in this example. We assumed that an average book was 300 pages long, and that each page has 1,750 characters, including spaces. Each book would then have 525,000 characters. (An alternative approach is to assume that an average book is 80,000 words, and that each word consists of five letters followed by a space. That estimate amounts to 480,000 characters on average.) Without data compression, each letter requires 1 byte of information. We estimated that there are 7,373,761,000 people on Earth, using the World Population Clock from the Centers of Disease Control and Prevention (CDC). Then, it is just multiplication and division: 153 exabytes = 1.53×10^{17} kB = 1.53×10^{20} bytes. (1.53×10^{20} / 7,373,761,000 = 20,749,248,586 bytes for every person on the planet. At 525,000 bytes for an average book, that's 39,522 books for every man, woman, and child on the planet in 2013. Similar math gets you from 2.314 zettabytes to an estimate of 597,744 books per person on earth.

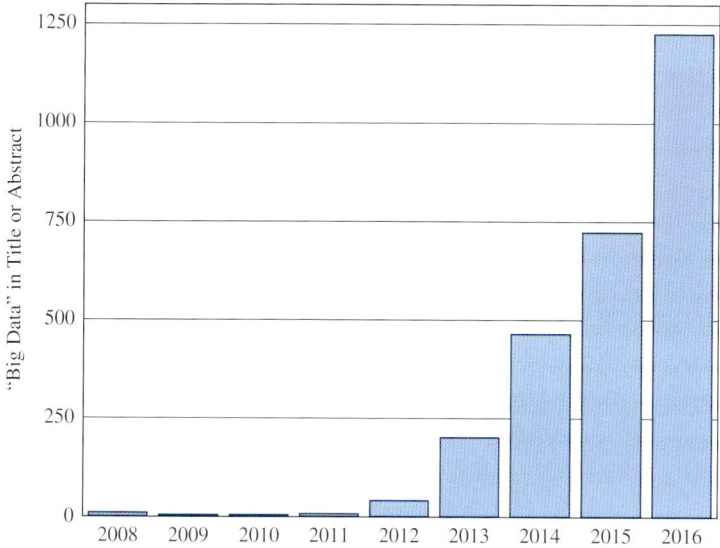

Figure 1-3 • Growth of the phrase *big data* in the titles or the abstracts of medical articles. That phrase did not appear in the medical literature as a noun until 2008. It now appears to be on an exponential growth curve. (Source: PubMed.)

maintained by the National Library of Medicine.) Big data, as a key term in the medical literature, is now growing at an almost precisely exponential rate (Figure 1-3).

A critical point is that we often think about big data in healthcare applying solely to genomics, bioinformatics, and other areas of complex basic science. This is no longer the case. In today's world, patients now leave behind dense electronic footprints as they pass through every healthcare encounter. During a single day, a moderately complex patient in an intensive care unit (ICU) may easily generate 100,000 points of data recorded in an EHR (and orders of magnitude more if waveforms from cardiac and respiratory monitoring are captured). Even the most routine of healthcare activities, hand hygiene, can create startling amounts of data. We know one hospital that installed electronic hand-hygiene monitoring and recorded more than 70 million observations in a single year—each individually time- and location-stamped.

Dealing with these data is not just a new problem; it's also a tremendously difficult one. We often hear physicians, administrators, and researchers drastically misjudge the amount of skill, technique, and effort required to join these data sets together and to transform data into information (and eventually into knowledge). On the other hand, it is surprisingly effortless to get the wrong answer out of these data sets and not

Key Point

Healthcare is now truly a "big data" field. By one estimate, there were 1.53 exabytes of healthcare data in 2013: the equivalent of about 40,000 300-page books for every man, woman, and child on Earth.

realize that you've made a mistake. We will delve deeply into this later in the book (see Chapters 11, 12, and 13), but for now, recognize that one of the greatest pitfalls in healthcare delivery science is assuming that using electronic healthcare data is easy. Instead, think of it like a basic science technique: even though DNA exists, no one would expect to be able to read a nucleotide sequence without training in polymerase chain reaction (PCR), high-throughput sequencing, and other tools of molecular biology. In fact, when we provide postdoctoral training for physicians who want to work directly with granular, raw healthcare data, we provide similar lengths and amounts of training as those moving into basic science labs to work with genomics and proteomics receive. You should treat healthcare data with the same respect, realizing that there are as many opportunities for error as there are for discovery.

WHY IT MATTERS: PROBLEMS WITH THINKING TOO SIMPLY ABOUT HEALTHCARE

It is almost impossible to resist the temptation to think simply about healthcare. "If only," we think: "If only we had more information about why this patient is in shock, we could save her." "If only the doctors would remember to give prophylactic medicine, no one would get blood clots." "If only we measured quality and made the results public, hospitals would kill fewer patients."

Is there any harm to thinking in this way? Absolutely. This natural human inclination to simplify leads us to act in ways that seem completely logical, but that turn out to waste billions of dollars and kill thousands of patients. The belief that the healthcare delivery system is just the physician's workshop is naïve, a mistake, and dangerous. Rather, we need to recognize that the healthcare delivery system is closer in complexity to a living organism than to a factory floor—and we need to treat it with that level of analytical and process-design respect. Instead, we often assume that we are smart enough to understand both a patient's physiology and the delivery system's response to intervention. If something is "obviously" correct, we act. This section will review three examples where we did just that—and where serious unintended consequences ensued.

Tight Blood Sugar Control in the Critically Ill

By the late 1990s, we knew that patients in the ICU who developed high blood sugar were more likely to die and more likely to get infections. We worried that maybe it was just that patients who were sick also got high blood sugar (and were also more likely to die), but it made perfect sense that high blood sugar *caused* bad outcomes in the ICU. After all, out-of-control diabetes was worse than in-control diabetes in the ambulatory setting, and high blood glucose impaired wound healing. A 1971 petri-dish study even showed that high glucose levels caused neutrophils, one of the body's key immune cells, to be worse at attacking and eating bacteria.[26] So, when a single-center, nonblinded randomized trial was published in 2001 in the *New England Journal of Medicine*, we were ready to act. This study showed that using insulin to keep blood sugar normal in ICU patients reduced mortality from 8.0% to 4.6%, with a P value of 0.04. (The *P value* is a statistical test. Traditionally, we say that something is "statistically significant" if its P value is <0.05.) In this case, "normal" blood sugar meant 80–110 mg/dL, rather than the 180–200 mg/dL that was a common target.

We would later come to recognize that there were red flags in this study—some things that should have led us to question its results more than we did. But we were primed, and the country and world reacted. "Tight glycemic control" protocols spread like wildfire and were implemented in truly massive numbers of ICUs across the world. Just three years after the trial was published, major national clinical guidelines recommended tight glycemic control for diseases like sepsis.[27] In 2004, the nationally impactful Joint Commission presented its most prestigious quality and patient safety award, the Ernest Amory Codman Award, to a hospital that had rigorously implemented a glycemic control protocol in its ICU.[28] Glycemic control for postcardiac-surgery patients became a core measure of quality as part of the Surgical Care Improvement Program, with both required reporting to CMS and pay-for-performance through CMS's Value-Based Purchasing Program.

The right study was eventually done and published in 2009. The cleverly named Normoglycemia in Intensive Care Evaluation–Survival Using Glucose Algorithm Regulation (NICE-SUGAR) study enrolled patients in 42 hospitals. NICE-SUGAR found that tight glycemic control *increased* the odds of death by 14%: 27.5% of patients receiving tight glycemic control died within 90 days, compared with 24.9% in the usual-care group. Put another way, for every 38 patients treated with tight glycemic control, 1 extra patient died.[29]

The internationally renowned critical care scholar Brian Kavanaugh summed up the potential amount of harm done by this naïve approach to glycemic control in a 2016 article:

If the multinational data are indeed broadly applicable to mechanically ventilated ICU patients, then implementation of protocols directing glucose normalization might potentially have been responsible for approximately 26,000 additional deaths per year in the United States alone (assuming approximately 1 million ventilated ICU patients per year in the United States). Ironically, in some health care systems, reimbursement had been made contingent on the use of such protocols.[30]

The actual number is probably substantially less than 26,000, but the number of attributable deaths is almost certainly substantial—all from rapid spread of an innovation intended to improve quality.

The Cleveland Health Quality Choice Program

In 1989, the country wanted healthcare reform—better outcomes for lower cost. A unique partnership in Cleveland took the lead, bringing together healthcare purchasers (businesses), physicians, and hospitals to launch the Cleveland Health Quality Choice Program. This profoundly innovative program set out to improve the health of residents of four counties with a straightforward and well-reasoned strategy: "[I]f Cleveland businesses can reliably identify the highest quality, cost-effective hospital services, then this information can be used to encourage their employees to choose these institutions for their hospital care."[31] For its time, the program used remarkably sophisticated risk adjustment to level the playing field based on patient characteristics. It had a laudable focus on both ensuring data integrity (which is often overlooked) and being attentive to presenting its risk adjustment and comparative tools in a way that was accessible for its users—whether they were chief executive officers (CEOs) or physicians.[32]

The Cleveland Health Quality Choice Program brought tremendous hope and was much lauded. The *Wall Street Journal*, for example, covered its birth in a story called "Pioneer Project Publishes First Rankings of Cleveland Hospitals."[33] An early report then suggested that the program's public reporting on hospital mortality data resulted in improved survival and decreased mortality rates.[34] When the program was shuttered a decade later, the *Wall Street Journal* lamented its passing with an article titled "Operation That Rated Hospitals Was a Success, but the Patience Died," attributing its closure largely to disagreements among participants and diminished financial pressure from medical inflation.[35] An article in the medical literature was even more hyperbolic: "This is the story of the martyrdom of an idea, an organization that embodied that idea, its director, and a group of staff and volunteers committed to making it work."[36]

The truth was remarkably different. The Cleveland Health Quality Choice Program in fact had no impact on whether patients lived or died, on how long they remained in the hospital, or where they chose to get their care.[37–39] The literature that emerged is maybe best summarized in one article's headline: "Cleveland Health Quality Choice Was a Failure, not a Martyr."[40]

What happened? How did the early reports get it so wrong? Put simply, they used analytical methods that failed to take into account the complexity of the healthcare delivery system. First, it turned out that mortality was improving everywhere at exactly the same rate as was happening in Cleveland—an effect that was ignored in early analyses, but that meant that the improvement had nothing to do with the program itself.[39] Second, and much more concerning, was the phenomenon of *death shifting*. Mortality in hospitals went down, but deaths immediately after discharge from hospital went up by the same amount. The hospitals looked better, but patients died at the same rate because they died just after discharge.[38] The reasons for this were less clear. There was some concern that patients may have been discharged in an unstable condition,[38] but there was also a signal of increased use of postacute care such as skilled nursing facilities.[41] Most analyses done by hospitals and healthcare systems in 2017 are easily susceptible to just these kinds of errors.

Caution

Thinking too simply about healthcare is dangerous and expensive. We need to respect the healthcare system's complexity, and this sometimes requires the use of sophisticated analytic methods, even for routine operations.

The Fifth Vital Sign

Anyone who has ever experienced unremitting pain understands that it creates tremendous suffering. Watching a loved one suffer may even be worse, especially if we think that treatments may exist that either eliminate the pain or disconnect the physical symptom of pain from the suffering that it engenders. Medical care has attempted to divorce pain-causing stimuli from the experience of pain and the suffering created by that pain. Pain is the enemy, and we have been victorious before: the development of general anesthesia represented a tremendous victory over the almost-unbelievable pain and suffering that accompanied surgery. The magnitude of this is hard to exaggerate. "Of all milestones and achievements in medicine," write Daniel Robinson and Alexander Toledo about the development of anesthesia, "conquering pain must be one of the very few that has potentially affected every human being in the world. It was in 1846 that one of mankind's greatest fears, the pain of surgery, was eliminated."[42]

In 1996, the evidence was overwhelming that pain was being undertreated.[43] But the scourge of chronic pain seemed conquerable—if only physicians would take it seriously. In that year's Presidential Address of the American Pain Society, a patient's rating of pain was linked to the concept of vital signs:

Vital signs are taken seriously. If pain were assessed with the same zeal as other vital signs are, it would have a much better chance of being treated properly. We need to train doctors and nurses to treat pain as a vital sign. Quality care means that pain is measured and treated.[44]

Guidelines from then on recommended treating pain like vital signs—and even recommended that they be charted on the same sheets of paper.[43] The Veterans Administration developed a toolkit called "Pain as the Fifth Vital Sign" and launched an improvement program to ensure that veterans' pain was being adequately treated.[44] By 2000, the Joint Commission on Accreditation of Healthcare Organizations released standards for pain assessment and management.[45] While Joint Commission standards are neither laws nor government regulations, they have a tremendous impact on hospitals' behavior.[46] Because the Joint Commission accredits more than 20,000 U.S. healthcare organizations, these standards affect the healthcare of millions of Americans.

Subsequently, Medicare also began requiring U.S. hospitals to submit data from patient experience surveys. Linked both to finances (via hospital Medicare reimbursement) and to brand (via public reporting of hospital quality), these surveys included a series of pain-focused questions, such as, "During this hospital stay, how often did the hospital staff do everything they could to help you with your pain?" Together, these all seemed like a virtuous cycle: researchers identify an important problem; experts develop a clinical guideline; the Joint Commission issues standards; policymakers begin paying and publicly reporting based on performance.

We recognize 20 years later that these well-intentioned efforts led to major unintended consequences. First, the measurement of pain did not improve the treatment of pain. When researchers studied the "Pain as the Fifth Vital Sign" program, they found that it had not improved the quality of pain management.[47] In other settings, the prescription of opioids increased, but patients' disability did not improve.[48] In 2013, there were enough opioid prescriptions written that every single American adult could have one.[49] Worse, between 1999 and 2010, deaths from prescription opiates more than tripled, far outpacing deaths from heroin (Figure 1-4). By 2007, nonmedical opioid use was costing the United States more than $50 billion a year.[50] In 2009, for the first time ever, more Americans died from drug overdose than from automobile accidents.[51] The opiate epidemic had arrived. Clearly, the epidemic has many causes, but none could argue that the outcome of Pain as the Fifth Vital Sign played out as intended.

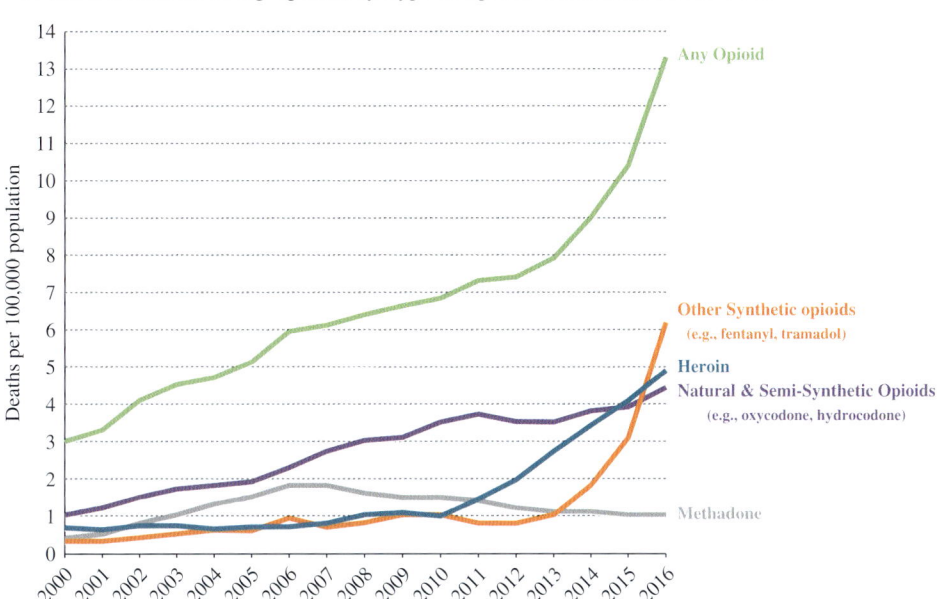

Overdose Deaths Involving Opioids, by Type of Opioid, United States, 2000–2016

Figure 1-4 • U.S. Deaths from the opioid epidemic. (Source: CDC. Centers for Disease Control. Opioid Data Analysis and Resources. December 19, 2018. https://www.cdc.gov/drugoverdose/data/analysis.html. Accessed 4 June 2019. From https://www.cdc.gov/drugoverdose/images/data/opioid_deaths_multicolor.gif.)

HEALTHCARE DELIVERY SCIENCE

Modern healthcare is a paradox. What would have seemed impossible or miraculous at the beginning of our lifetimes has become routine today—but we simultaneously understand that medical error results in tens or hundreds of thousands of deaths in the United States every year, and we provide low-value care that bankrupts tens or hundreds of thousands of Americans every year.

Healthcare delivery science is the emerging field that tries to resolve this paradox. We now know that the healthcare delivery system is profoundly complicated: In purely mathematical terms, it may well be as complex as a living organism. But until recently, we have treated it as simple—like the "physician's workshop" that hospitals were designed as in the early 20th century. Even when health services researchers and others have used sophisticated techniques to advance our understanding of healthcare delivery, these efforts have almost always been separate from the operational enterprise. Healthcare traditionally draws a bright line between research and healthcare operations, resulting in surprisingly distinct silos of people who do healthcare operations and people who study them. This is remarkably different than how we view the rest of medical

> **Key Point**
>
> Healthcare delivery science represents the overlap between operational innovation and research. The healthcare system itself is the organism under both study and treatment. Healthcare delivery science integrates research-quality methods into what we actually do in the real world.

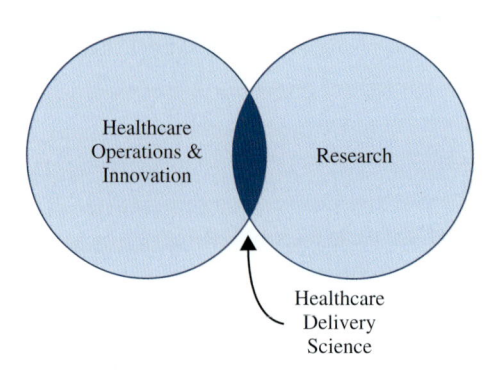

Figure 1-5 • Conceptual model of healthcare delivery science.

research, where we value investigators with expertise in the clinical field to which their work applies.

This leads to three significant problems that manifest themselves across the healthcare system:

- Wasting and ignoring discoveries every day—leaving tremendous amounts of knowledge on the table, undiscovered
- Failing to spread isolated successes across the system—or, even worse, spreading the wrong ones
- Focusing research only on the *what*, not the *how*—ignoring that the delivery system is itself a complex organism

Modern healthcare exhibits tremendous variation, both across and within systems. We make changes in how we care for patients on an almost-daily basis, but only rarely do we design research-quality analysis methods into operational improvements so that we can really understand if they worked … and so that other healthcare systems can learn, too. Because today's patients generate almost genomic-scale data as they pass through routine healthcare encounters, we now have the opportunity to use research-quality methods to understand real-world operational programs.

The emerging field of healthcare delivery science attempts to do exactly this—to glean knowledge that is otherwise lost in a sea of variation, passing by at real-world speeds. The field's definition and boundaries are still emerging, but at its heart, healthcare delivery science represents the overlap between operational innovation and research (Figure 1-5). The healthcare system itself is the organism under both study and treatment. These are not patient-level interventions and questions: Instead, they are the study of changes in the way in which patient-level interventions are delivered. Healthcare delivery science integrates research-quality methods into what we actually do in the real world.

KEY POINTS

- Research and operations are deeply separate in modern healthcare, but only for historical reasons. Today, even the food and beverage industry spends more than 500% more than the healthcare delivery system does on R&D.
- Two fundamental changes bring about the need for healthcare delivery science: (1) dramatic increases in the complexity of care itself and of the delivery system; and (2) marked growth in the amount of data that patients generate, even in routine healthcare encounters.
- The healthcare delivery system may now be as complex as a living organism. Using naïve methods to understand it leads to wasted effort and—when things go truly awry—the waste of billions of dollars and thousands of lives.
- Routine healthcare today generates quantities of data that were previously unimaginable. By one estimate, the amount of healthcare data in 2013 was equivalent to every man, woman, and child on Earth writing their autobiography… 40,000 times each.
- Healthcare delivery science represents the overlap between operational innovation and research. The healthcare system itself is the organism under both study and treatment. Healthcare delivery science integrates research-quality methods into what we actually do in the real world.

REFERENCES

1. Moses H 3rd, Matheson DH, Cairns-Smith S, George BP, Palisch C, Dorsey ER. The anatomy of medical research: US and international comparisons. *JAMA*. 2015;313(2):174–189.
2. Biden's remarks on McCain's policies. *The New York Times*, September 15, 2008. Accessed February 22, 2017, from https://www.nytimes.com/2008/09/15/us/politics/15text-biden.html.
3. Marmor TR. *The Politics of Medicare*. New York: Aldine de Gruyter; 1970.
4. Reynolds AR. Pneumonia: The new "captain of the men of death": its increasing prevalence and the necessity of methods for its restriction. *JAMA*. 1903;XL(9):583–586.
5. Gawande A. Desperate measures. Annals of medicine. *New Yorker*. 2003;79(10):70.
6. Cooke M, Irby DM, Sullivan W, Ludmerer KM. American medical education 100 years after the Flexner report. *N Engl J Med*. 2006;355(13):1339–1344.
7. Pauly MV. *Doctors and Their Workshops: Economic Models of Physician Behavior*. National Bureau of Economic Research; 1980.
8. Goldsmith J, Kaufman N, Burns L. Health Affairs blog: The Tangled Hospital-Physician Relationship. 2017. Accessed February 16, 2017, from http://healthaffairs.org/blog/2016/05/09/the-tangled-hospital-physician-relationship/.

9. National Quality Forum. Heart Race: How Timely Care Saves Lives. 2017. Accessed February 19, 2019, from http://www.qualityforum.org/Heart_Race.aspx.
10. Reinohl J, Kaier K, Reinecke H, et al. Effect of availability of transcatheter aortic-valve replacement on clinical practice. *N Engl J Med*. 2015;373(25):2438–2447.
11. Cribier A, Eltchaninoff H, Bash A, et al. Percutaneous transcatheter implantation of an aortic valve prosthesis for calcific aortic stenosis: first human case description. *Circulation*. 2002;106(24):3006–3008.
12. D'Souza A, Zhu X. Current Uses and Outcomes of Hematopoietic Cell Transplantation (IICT): CIBMTR Summary Slides. 2016. Accessed February 19, 2017, from https://www.cibmtr.org/referencecenter/slidesreports/summaryslides/pages/index.aspx.
13. FDA. *FDA Approves Axicabtagene Ciloleucel for Large B-cell Lymphoma*. Accessed June, 4, 2019, from https://www.fda.gov/drugs/resources-information-approved-drugs/fda-approves-axicabtagene-ciloleucel-large-b-cell-lymphoma.
14. Pefoyo AJ, Bronskill SE, Gruneir A, et al. The increasing burden and complexity of multimorbidity. *BMC Public Health*. 2015;15:415.
15. Aitken M, Valkova S. Avoidable costs in US healthcare. IMS Institute for Healthcare Informatics, Parsippany, NJ. 2013.
16. Berwick DM. The epitath of profession. *Br J Gen Pract*. 2008; advance online publication.
17. Pham HH, Schrag D, O'Malley AS, Wu B, Bach PB. Care patterns in Medicare and their implications for pay for performance. *N Engl J Med*. 2007;356(11): 1130–1139.
18. Stevens J, Nyweide D, Maresh S, et al. Variation in inpatient consultation among older adults in the United States. *J Gen Intern Med*. 2015:1–8.
19. Dubberke ER, Carling P, Carrico R, et al. Strategies to prevent Clostridium difficile infections in acute care hospitals: 2014 update. *Infect Control Hosp Epidemiol*. 2014;35(6):628–645.
20. Rodhe RE. A secret weapon for preventing HAIs: a scientist's message to hospitals trying to rid themselves of healthcare-associated infections. *Elsevier Connect Healthcare*: Elsevier; 2017.
21. Jha AK, DesRoches CM, Campbell EG, et al. Use of electronic health records in U.S. hospitals. *N Engl J Med*. 2009;360(16):1628–1638.
22. DesRoches CM, Campbell EG, Rao SR, et al. Electronic health records in ambulatory care--a national survey of physicians. *N Engl J Med*. 2008;359(1):50–60.
23. Office of the National Coordinator for Health Information. Hospital Selection of Public Health Measures in Medicare EHR Incentive Program, Health IT Quick-Stat #16. 2016. Accessed February 22, 2017, from http://quickstats/pages/FIG-MU-Hospitals-Public-Health-Measure-Attestations.php.
24. Office of the National Coordinator for Health Information. Office-Based Physician Electronic Health Record Adoption, Health IT Quick-Stat #50. 2016. Accessed February 22, 2017, from http://quickstats/pages/physician-ehr-adoption-trends.php.

25. IDC and EMC. Vertical Industry Brief: The Digital Universe: Driving Data Growth in Healthcare. 2014. Accessed February 23, 2017, from https://www.emc.com/analyst-report/digital-universe-healthcare-vertical-report-ar.pdf.
26. Van Oss CJ. Influence of glucose levels on the in vitro phagocytosis of bacteria by human neutrophils. *Infect Immun*. 1971;4(1):54–59.
27. Dellinger RP, Carlet JM, Masur H, et al. Surviving sepsis campaign guidelines for management of severe sepsis and septic shock. *Crit Care Med*. 2004;32(3):858–873.
28. Joint Commission. 2004 Ernest Amory Codman Award Winners. January 1, 2011. Accessed February 26, 2017, from https://www.jointcommission.org/2004_ernest_amory_codman_award_winners/.
29. NICE-SUGAR Study Investigators, Finfer S, Chittock DR, et al. Intensive versus conventional glucose control in critically ill patients. *N Engl J Med*. 2009;360(13):1283–1297.
30. Kavanagh BP, Nurok M. Standardized intensive care. Protocol misalignment and impact misattribution. *Am J Respir Crit Care Med*. 2016;193(1):17–22.
31. Summary report from the Cleveland Health Quality Choice Program. *Qual Manag Health Care*. 1995;3(3):78–90.
32. Rosenthal GE, Harper DL. Cleveland Health Quality Choice: a model for collaborative community-based outcomes assessment. *Jt Comm J Qual Improv*. 1994;20(8):425–442.
33. Winslow R. Pioneer project publishes first rankings of Cleveland hospitals. *Wall Street Journal*. April 29, 1993, B3.
34. Rosenthal GE, Quinn L, Harper DL. Declines in hospital mortality associated with a regional initiative to measure hospital performance. *Am J Med Qual*. 1997;12(2):103–112.
35. Burton TM. Operation that rated hospitals was a success, but the patience died. *Wall Street Journal*. 1999.
36. Neuhauser D, Harper DL. Too good to last: did Cleveland Health Quality Choice leave a legacy and lessons to be learned? *Qual Saf Health Care*. 2002;11(2):202–203.
37. Baker DW, Einstadter D, Thomas C, Husak S, Gordon NH, Cebul RD. The effect of publicly reporting hospital performance on market share and risk-adjusted mortality at high-mortality hospitals. *Med Care*. 2003;41(6):729–740.
38. Baker DW, Einstadter D, Thomas CL, Husak SS, Gordon NH, Cebul RD. Mortality trends during a program that publicly reported hospital performance. *Med Care*. 2002;40(10):879–890.
39. Clough JD, Engler D, Snow R, Canuto PE. Lack of relationship between the Cleveland Health Quality Choice project and decreased inpatient mortality in Cleveland. *Am J Med Qual*. 2002;17(2):47–55.
40. Clough JD, Engler D, Canuto PE. Cleveland Health Quality Choice was a failure, not a martyr. *Qual Saf Health Care*. 2002;11(4):391.
41. Sirio CA, Shepardson LB, Rotondi AJ, et al. Community-wide assessment of intensive care outcomes using a physiologically based prognostic measure: implications for critical care delivery from Cleveland Health Quality Choice. *Chest*. 1999;115(3):793–801.

42. Robinson DH, Toledo AH. Historical development of modern anesthesia. *J Invest Surg*. 2012;25(3):141–149.
43. Quality improvement guidelines for the treatment of acute pain and cancer pain. American Pain Society Quality of Care Committee. *JAMA*. 1995;274(23):1874–1880.
44. Department of Veterans Affairs. Pain as the 5th Vital Sign Toolkit. *Veterans Health Administration* 2000. Accessed March 5, 2017, from https://www.va.gov/painmanagement/docs/Pain_As_the_5th_Vital_Sign_Toolkit.pdf.
45. Baker DW. History of the Joint Commission's pain standards: lessons for today's prescription opioid epidemic. *JAMA*. 2017;317(11):1117–1118.
46. Devers KJ, Pham HH, Liu G. What is driving hospitals' patient-safety efforts? *Health Aff (Millwood)*. 2004;23(2):103–115.
47. Mularski RA, White-Chu F, Overbay D, Miller L, Asch SM, Ganzini L. Measuring pain as the 5th vital sign does not improve quality of pain management. *J Gen Intern Med*. 2006;21(6):607–612.
48. Sites BD, Beach ML, Davis MA. Increases in the use of prescription opioid analgesics and the lack of improvement in disability metrics among users. *Reg Anesth Pain Med*. 2014;39(1):6–12.
49. Centers for Disease Control and Prevention (CDC). Prescription Opioids. 2016. Accessed March 28, 2017, from https://www.cdc.gov/drugoverdose/opioids/prescribed.html.
50. Meyer R, Patel AM, Rattana SK, Quock TP, Mody SH. Prescription opioid abuse: a literature review of the clinical and economic burden in the United States. *Popul Health Manag*. 2014;17(6):372–387.
51. U.S. Department of Health and Human Services. Addressing Prescription Drug Abuse in the United States: Current Activities and Future Opportunities. 2013. Accessed March 6, 2017, from https://www.cdc.gov/drugoverdose/pdf/hhs_prescription_drug_abuse_report_09.2013.pdf.

COMPLEXITY
Thinking About the Healthcare System as a Living Organism

As a healthcare delivery scientist, you will ask fundamental questions about whether interventions in healthcare made a difference for your patients and your organization. But how can we evaluate these interventions? The examples in Chapter 1 demonstrated what happens when we make the fundamental and human mistake of taking an oversimplified approach to healthcare. Human beings look for patterns and metaphors to explain large, complex problems. Our very tendency to look for coincidence reflects our natural ability to anchor ourselves onto events that we can easily explain. However, these reductionist biases lead us to either assume the innate utility of our interventions without studying them, or when we do study these interventions, to use designs (such as *pre/post* comparisons) that may lead us to think that our interventions work when they don't.

Healthcare systems are complex adaptive systems (CASs). In this chapter, we will first look at the downside of oversimplifying healthcare. Second, we will dissect the concept of a complex adaptive system and learn why this is useful in healthcare delivery science. Third, we will look at the key features of a complex adaptive system to understand how this will structure our approach to understand healthcare delivery.

Key Point

A complex adaptive system describes a series of interconnected, heterogeneous components of a whole that change and alter in nonlinear ways.

WHAT HAPPENS WHEN WE VIEW HEALTHCARE AS COMPLICATED?

Complicated and complex systems are not the same thing.[1,2] A *complex system* is one that resembles a living organism. The more we examine that system under a microscope, the more we discover. In short, the whole of a complex system is greater than the sum of its parts. We will explore the elements of a complex system throughout this chapter. A *complicated system*, however, can be unwound into individual pieces that can be understood. The internal combustion engine appears impressive and has transformed human society. But it can be taken apart. An engine can be disassembled into small, understandable pieces. A complicated system is *exactly* the sum of its parts.

In healthcare, there are systems that are strictly complicated. Take as an example the process of inserting a central line, a large-diameter, venous catheter that is placed into a large, central vein in a patient to provide intravenous (IV) medication. We regularly perform this procedure, and if done incorrectly, it can lead to a high risk of infections and other life-threatening complications for a patient.[3] For a doctor in training, this appears to be a daunting task, not least because these types of catheters are usually placed in patients who are critically ill. But the procedure itself can be broken down into a series of very specific steps. First, we gather together the necessary supplies. Second, we get the patient into the right position and make sure that he or she is comfortable. Third, we take a certain type of quick-drying antiseptic and sterilize the area of the patient's body where the needle will go. And so on. When done reliably, life-threatening infections and other complications can be avoided.[4-6] The process is *deterministic*: the outcome is determined from the inputs in a predictable, linear way.

Recognizing when a healthcare delivery problem is complicated is very useful (even if healthcare delivery problems are usually complex rather than complicated—more on that later in this chapter). We can understand these types of problems by breaking them down into discrete subunits, improving the subunits, and putting the process back into action. More important, when we study changes in complicated processes, we can rely on more straightforward analytic methods that we will discuss in detail in Part III of this book. Consider our central-line example. Let's say we found that, in one hospital, the physician always had a mask for herself, but not for the nurse. The nurse routinely had to leave the room—slowing down the procedure and putting the patient at risk of harm—to go and get a mask. One proposed intervention could be to put two masks instead of one into prepackaged central-line supplies and our metric could be how many times a nurse had to leave the bedside for supplies during central-line procedures. We don't need to make complicated problems more complicated than they need to be.

However, humans are preprogrammed to see most problems as complicated, even when they are complex. We have a hard time imagining large numbers, anticipating future consequences beyond the immediate, and revisiting our assumptions.[7,8] The field of evolutionary psychology, and in some cases the business literature, have noted the selection for traits in the human mind that were likely beneficial in a prehistoric time of scarce resources and immediate decision-making. For example, a person's skill at solving short-term problems for her or his Stone Age tribe would be selected for, with major survival benefits. We have evolved to apply tools to complicated systems—solve the problem in front of us, assume direct

> **Key Point**
> Complicated systems can be broken into smaller, understandable pieces. A complicated system is *exactly* the sum of its parts.

cause-and-effect relationships, and think in the short term, not the long term—with every system we encounter. But in healthcare, and in other settings, these assumptions can fail.

Overreliance on History

Humans have fundamental limitations in dealing with complex (as opposed to complicated) ideas. Dorner and his team of researchers studied these innate limitations and the bad outcomes that can result.[8] In one study, participants were given total dictatorial control for 10 years over a computer-generated rural society and had to make decisions about healthcare, food supply management (including pest control), and housing. All the participants made benevolent choices—better medical care, greater pest control, and increased food supply, all leading to increased life expectancy for the electronic inhabitants—over the six prescribed planning sessions, during which the participants could interact with the society. But in all but one case, these artificial societies fell into ruin in just 7 computer years. In each case, why did the participants not anticipate the predictable famine that came from overpopulation, or fail to react to it in a timely way?

In this and subsequent experiments, the research team identified several important characteristics about the unsuccessful management of complex systems, in contrast to the rare successful manager. Initial interactions with the computer-generated society were filled with questions, reflections, and hypothesis generation, but during subsequent planning sessions, decisions rapidly became the most common actions. In several cases, the disconnect between decision-making and actual data became extreme. Some participants developed large-scale projects that they pushed forward despite increasing accounts of the arrival of famine and rising fatalities. The few successful participants coupled generation of hypotheses with the actual *testing* of these hypotheses.[8]

The sessions during which participants could interact with the program got shorter and shorter as participants relied on the assumptions they had derived in their initial interactions with the computer program. Once they had drawn their conclusions, they continued to rely on these conclusions despite sometimes-conflicting data. Finally, at the end, when more and more imaginary members of their society were dying of famine, the participants became increasingly sarcastic, describing the ways in which the outcome was inevitable and out of their control.[8]

It is tempting to look back on the failure of the participants in these experiments and imagine that we could do better. Of course an increasing life expectancy would lead to a growing population, which would eventually outpace the food supply if we didn't pay enough attention. Of course we would ask more questions and test more hypotheses.

But recent history suggests otherwise. Let's revisit the example of the opioid epidemic, the "Fifth Vital Sign," described in the previous chapter. From the beginning, providers and patient groups agreed that treating pain was fundamental to providing patient-focused care, leading to national efforts to create a set of best practices to require all physicians to hold themselves to the same standard of pain management. But what happened? We saw that pain and disability remained unchanged but opioid prescriptions rose rapidly, leading to a large nonprescription opioid economy and a subsequent rapidly evolving heroin, fentanyl, and carfentanil market.[9–12]

In retrospect, providing a highly addictive substance to huge numbers of people seems to have been a bad idea. But the individual agents, including the physicians, clinicians, and patients, would not have characterized their interest in achieving adequate pain control as nefarious. The overlap with the computer-generated society described earlier is notable. At the outset, there was substantial collaboration and decision-making, followed by a persistence of these hypotheses, even in the face of growing, concerning data, leading to a feeling of helplessness and frustration with a terrible outcome.

The moral here is not to criticize the troubling outcomes that occurred in both of these cases. Instead, this highlights the urgency of understanding and building the tools for healthcare delivery science. How can we continue to generate and test our hypotheses? How else should we characterize the health system, if not as an industrial, deterministic process?

WHAT IS A COMPLEX ADAPTIVE SYSTEM?

The Definition

A *complex adaptive system* describes a series of interconnected, heterogeneous components of a whole that change in nonlinear ways. Each word in the phrase itself helps clarify the meaning. Each component of a CAS is not identical to other components, nor is it connected in routine, predictable ways—*complex*. The system itself is interconnected, rather than arranged in a linear, easily reducible way. The *adaptability* of this system is particularly challenging, creating a system that responds to perturbations and evolutionary pressures in a dynamic way.[13,14]

Complex adaptive systems do not operate with careful specifications and grand, overarching designs, but instead with a limited number of simple rules. Zimmerman and coauthors described the experiment called the "Boids," originally described by Craig Reynolds.[2] They explained that with three simple rules—avoid others, match direction with neighbors, and move toward the center of mass—the boids fly in flocks in a lifelike way.

They explained that "while this does not prove that birds actually use these simple rules, it does show that simple rules—minimum specifications—can lead to complex behaviors."[2] Another example for review are the series of patterns that emerge from John Horton Conway's Game of Life, a type of mathematical model termed a "cellular automaton", which also generates complex interactions and patterns derived from four simple rules.[15]

We are surrounded by complex adaptive systems in life. Each living organism functions as a complex adaptive system, with individual cells connected by a range of cell signals, multiple loci of control, and unpredictable outcomes from straightforward perturbations. Human societies throughout history have functioned in similar ways, with each individual person and his or her motivations, hopes, and desires interacting with other individuals, larger social conditions and rules, novel perturbations, and seemingly unpredictable outcomes. Other structures are also complex adaptive systems, such as beehives and the Internet.

Healthcare systems and our methods of delivering healthcare are fundamentally complex adaptive systems. Each healthcare professional interacts with other providers within the larger structure of his or her department, the hospital, the state, professional societies, and any political context. The larger hospital or clinic that houses those providers has its own purpose (e.g., providing healthcare to the underserved), but other competing constraints (e.g., remaining fiscally solvent), while interacting with larger external forces such as the insurance market and state and federal politics. At the same time, the providers care for individual patients, each of whom has his or her own individual pressures, demands, hopes, and views of his or her health. The patients themselves are part of larger communities and social trends, which influence how they view the healthcare system and what they hope for or fear about it.

Key Point
Healthcare delivery systems function as complex adaptive systems.

Consider the system of an emergency department (ED) within a large urban hospital as a concrete example of a complex adaptive system in healthcare. Each physician works a set of shifts. In any given shift, that physician must interact with a range of patients, other providers in the ED, and other providers throughout the hospital. On either side of each interaction are ranges of motivation, personal needs, professionalism, and emotion, producing any one of a number of outcomes. The context of each of these interactions includes the overall census of the ED, and the hospital at large, during that shift. The clinical context, separate from the physical context, may include evidence-based medicine recommendations (e.g., whether a patient should receive invasive revascularization for ischemic cardiac disease, and if so, how quickly).

It is easy to see how, when confronted with the true complexity of a system, we might fall back on our natural tendency to look for patterns.

How should we challenge ourselves to measure the current state of healthcare and develop testable interventions of a complex adaptive system within that context?

The Key Features of a Complex Adaptive System

A complex adaptive system has several features that represent significant departures from deterministic systems. In deterministic systems, the outcome is predictable. In complex systems, the outcome *may* be predictable, with at least some degree of confidence. Of greatest importance, however, is recognizing healthcare as an evolving, multilayered organism that lives in the space between deterministic systems and chaotic ones.[16,17]

The following features of complex adaptive systems provide guidance in understanding them:

1. ***Connections.*** A complex adaptive system is driven in large part by the connections between the individual agents that the systems contain. The connections evolve over time, are dependent on history, and can be quite layered. As an example, take a connection between a single physician and a single nurse in a clinic. This relationship is informed by the history of those two professions and by the approach of the clinic to the two groups. More important, however, the connection between these two people fluctuates daily based on their personal and professional lives and yesterday's patients and workflow. The interaction between two individuals is somewhat independent of the system as a whole but occasionally collides with it.
2. ***Evolution and emergence.*** A complex adaptive system evolves over time. The system itself sets up its own independent hierarchies and builds an organic structure for the organization, based on daily patterns and self-organizing structures. Managers may interject hierarchical systems of control within the system, and leaders may create guideposts for the organization as a whole, but these actually are largely external to the evolving structure that the complex adaptive system creates for itself.

   Part of the reason for internal organic structures that emerge within a complex adaptive system is the inability of the individual actors to truly see the whole. Said another way, as Dorner explained, "[W]hat we really want to see may not be visible."[8] Healthcare providers, patients, and managers do not possess some overarching view of the delivery system itself, including where it has come from and where it is going. Instead, they must make the decision in front of them. All of these decisions and choices, each informed by the local interconnectedness of the actors, move the larger system over time.

3. *Nondeterministic*. A complex adaptive system is nondeterministic, which is to say it has a system trajectory that is fundamentally unknowable. Put another way, the same inputs into the system may not generate the same output every time. Retrospectively, there may be a narrative that can be constructed—a "How did we get here?" story—but from the vantage point of the start of the story, we cannot reliably predict the outcome.

There are, however, "attractors" in complexity theory, or underlying principles that guide the larger group and can be used to both understand and guide the system.[18,19] An understanding of the attractors of a system does not allow us to predict a series of outcomes, but rather to understand the simple rules under which the system operates. For example, we may not know where our flock of birds—or boids—will fly, but we can know how far apart they will be from each other. Understanding these rules is critical for understanding healthcare. For example, for physicians, one attractor may be autonomy. Clinical guidelines that are viewed as restraining an individual physician's autonomy may be largely ignored by a group of doctors, despite substantial evidence for the individual components of the guidelines.[19,20] For the staff of a busy pediatrics clinic, another attractor might be the desire to feel involved in decision-making. By engaging frontline office staff, a clinic could generate innovative ideas about patient flow that lead to substantially decreased wait times for patients, but the success of the ideas would largely come from the degree to which staff felt that they had participated in the final decisions.

Key Point

When either leading or studying healthcare systems, understanding attractors is essential.

A Non-healthcare Example: Wikipedia as a Complex Adaptive System

Wikipedia is a free-content, web-based encyclopedia project created in 2001, written in multiple languages by users, and organized by volunteer editors. It has rapidly grown into one of the largest references on the Internet, with 5,772,600 English-language articles as of January 1, 2019, and approximately 800 new articles added each day. If the entirety of the English-language project was printed in *Encyclopedia Britannica*-sized volumes, the English Wikipedia alone would contain over 2,443 books (the 2010 *Encyclopedia Britannica* was 32 volumes). All of Wikipedia contains over 43 million articles in 265 languages.[21]

The entire process is designed around a limited number of guidelines, including that the content is free, it maintains a neutral point of view, and that users behave civilly to each other and in the spirit of the project. Behind the project, there is a limited management structure. While there are over 6 million editors as of 2008, there are far fewer administrators, and even fewer stewards, who are elected. Overarching the entire structure is a seven-member board.

Wikipedia successfully meets all the definitions of a complex adaptive system.[22] A small number of rules have generated this enormous resource. Connections among the individual actors generate the content and move the larger entity. The larger organization has evolved over time in a largely unpredictable pattern—but with guiding attractors. Beyond the simple principles guiding the project, the individual content of the pages evolves in nondeterministic ways, with open boundaries, and requiring multiple levels of feedback as the overall project evolves.

Bringing It Together: Using Complicated Solutions for Complex Systems

When Medicare was created in 1965, the federal health insurer mandated that only patients who have been cared for in an acute care hospital for 3 consecutive days would be eligible to have Medicare also cover skilled nursing facility (SNF) admission and care. This arbitrary cutoff was intended to help manage the scare resource of rehabilitation beds in an era when most hospitalizations extended well beyond 3 days (the average hospital length of stay in 1965 was 7.5 days). Healthcare organizations at the time were worried that SNFs would be overrun and bankrupt the system. If patients needed to stay beyond the 3-day minimum, they could still be admitted to a SNF, but they would need to pay out of pocket for the additional costs.[23]

If we consider the 3-day rule as the pebble that was dropped in the pond over 50 years ago, what has happened to the complex system of healthcare provided to Medicare patients? First, SNFs have a financial incentive to send patients back and forth to the hospital because patients sent into the hospital will return to the SNF with an additional rehabilitation benefit, which Medicare has estimated may have cost as much as $2.6 billion in 2005.[23] Second, the 3-day rule has continued to evolve as the rest of the healthcare system evolved, with rules layered upon rules. Third, depending on the individual interactions among patients, physicians, nurses, families, and administrative staff designed to move patients through the system, some patients are likely staying longer in the hospital, even if they do not need it (and incurring both greater cost to the system and higher risk of hospital-acquired infections and errant medical procedures), to avoid the high daily out-of-pocket SNF costs. One study of total knee arthroplasty patients found a higher average length of stay for patients with Medicare than those with other insurance coverage, even after adjustment for patient demographics and comorbidities, suggesting these patients were intentionally kept in the hospital longer.[24]

The 3-day rule functions much like the original participants in Dorner's experiments: they assessed the situation, made a decision, and acted on it. The larger healthcare system had responded to this simple rule as an evolutionary pressure. Efforts to remove the 3-day rule, despite policy consensus that it no longer serves its intended purpose, have been unsuccessful.

WHY IT MATTERS: FITTING THE RIGHT MEASUREMENT TOOL TO THE QUESTION

How, then, do we move forward to develop hypotheses about healthcare delivery, perturb the system in meaningful ways, measure change, and move to a better understanding of healthcare delivery? As healthcare delivery scientists, we can no longer view the healthcare system as solely an industrial process but as the organism of study. This means that we must evaluate the aspect of the organism we are interested in and arrive at the right method for gaining a greater understanding of it.

Throughout Part II of this book, we will describe multiple parametric and nonparametric strategies for studying healthcare delivery. Some methods, such as methods to compare measures of central tendency or linear predictive modeling, will be immediately familiar from studying other biological processes. Other methods, such as discrete event simulation and agent-based modeling, may be less familiar. But all employ techniques well tested in other fields dedicated to complex adaptive systems.

Fortunately, several aspects of complex adaptive systems open the door to investigative methods used in different fields of research, including health services research, econometrics, biological sciences, engineering, and others.

Key Point

Understanding how healthcare functions as a complex adaptive system guides us toward the right method to study healthcare innovations.

- Variation is everywhere in complex adaptive systems.

  Crucial to understanding healthcare as a complex adaptive system is to understand the role of variation. The individual actions and behaviors of providers delivering care in this environment are not only subject to patient care needs, but also the larger environment around them.[25] Some of this variation is derived from the variation in patients for whom the healthcare system cares, but much of it is derived from nonpatient sources such as the providers, the physical plant of the system, the payor mix, and the reimbursement strategies.

We will come to find that variation in healthcare may not be desirable, but it is very useful for creating understanding and discovery. The ability to measure and understand variation, both patient- and nonpatient-derived, is fundamental to many statistical methods described in this book. For example, if a provider refers some but not all of his or her patients with asthma to a pulmonologist, we can use the heterogeneity of that exposure to look at the usefulness of involving a specialist in asthma management. By taking advantage of the randomness of how this variation is distributed across healthcare delivery, we can conduct the necessary studies to understand the success of our delivery innovations.

- In a complex adaptive system, all individual actors are not the same.

Critical to our interpretation of much of the biological literature is our ability to assume that we can summarize data in terms of averages and consider effects of interventions as averaged across an entire population. For example, we think in terms of the benefit of screening for lung cancer or the incremental benefit of a new cancer treatment in terms of the average benefit among the population. However, in a complex adaptive system, all components of that population are not the same, nor do they all behave in similar ways or have the same motivations.[25] Studying healthcare delivery only on the scale of average treatment effects may fail to accurately characterize the true benefit (or harm) among subpopulations.[26]

In healthcare operations, we often smooth over this kind of variation with averages, medians, and other simple measures of central tendency. But this heterogeneity is actually the source of rich information about how we can consider the benefits and harms of our interventions. One solution here is to make use of a broad set of methods that consider both the summary of treatment effects, but also the subgroups and clusters of the population in question in the analysis.[25] All nurses are not the same, even within the same institution. Can we instead consider our analyses with more finely defined clusters, such as years of training, years at the hospital, number of day and night shifts, or even network analyses that allow us to see social clusters and patterns of behavior?

Another solution is to examine our outliers. As we seek average treatment effects and look for opportunities to establish external validity, outliers in data may be given short shrift. However, outliers in a complex adaptive system may provide useful information about how people in the healthcare delivery system think and function. Is that data point an outlier because the data were recorded incorrectly?

Or is the diversity of our populations of study leading to a more heterogeneous set of outcomes than we were expecting?

Take as an example the question of whether it is beneficial to employ critical care-trained physicians 24 hours a day, rather than just during the daytime. Prior to a national trend toward having so-called overnight intensivists available to patients, most attending physicians were available by phone and could be called in from home. However, the intensive care units (ICUs) and the rest of the hospital were either staffed by advanced practice providers, doctors in training, or hospitalists. Based on the face validity that sicker patients needed critical care-trained physicians at all hours, business leaders required that hospitals make this change.[27,28] However, researchers at the University of Pittsburgh found no benefit of having intensivists at night at hospitals that already staff their ICUs with intensivists during the day.[29] This group asked an important question of healthcare delivery, by recognizing that all ICUs were not the same. We could ask further: Are there still more subtle differences in how healthcare delivery environments use intensivists that have been lost in the details of this study?

- The parts of a complex adaptive system learn and adapt.

Many current methods for measuring and understanding healthcare assume that the various participants in healthcare are static actors, and any specific trait or knowledge at that point in history will remain true for all time. Methods that fall prey to this assumption include cross-sectional analyses, surveys, and in-depth qualitative analyses conducted at a single time. Even studies that consider time often fail to use methods that explore how the penetrance of an exposure might change over time.[25]

The Hawthorne effect, where people who are observed in a study change their behavior because they are being observed, was one of the first descriptions of changing actors in a complex system. In particular, the researchers observed how the individual agents under study might change during the course of the investigation. During the 1920s, sociologists studying worker productivity at Western Electric sought to study the impact of better lighting on productivity. During the time of the research, however, other changes were also taking place, all of which increased the productivity of both the poorly lit group and the well-lit group.[30] The Hawthorne effect has been quantified in healthcare: In one study that looked whether clinicians completed good hand hygiene when observed versus not observed found a threefold difference when the participants were in line of sight of an auditor.[31] But despite this early understanding of the complex ways that individuals interact with one another and evolve during an experiment, we often leave this element of complex systems out of our experimental designs.

Analytic designs for healthcare delivery science can accommodate the learning nature of the healthcare system. Time remains an important variable, and longitudinal designs that allow researchers to explore variation in action over time may yield the most robust results. At the very least, researchers must understand the shortcomings of data that fail to build in learning elements.

HEALTHCARE DELIVERY SCIENCE: A FIELD OF RESEARCH WHERE HEALTHCARE ITSELF IS THE ORGANISM UNDER STUDY

Healthcare delivery itself is multilayered and interconnected. But all of us quickly fall prey to relying on our assumptions, failing to generate and test hypotheses, and rapidly making decisions based on the immediate problems surrounding us. When we understand healthcare itself as having complexity similar to that of a living organism, we can begin to identify how best to study and routinely test and challenge our assumptions.

KEY POINTS

- Healthcare delivery systems function as complex adaptive systems.
- Complicated and complex systems are not the same. Complicated systems are the sum of their parts; they are deterministic. Complex systems, on the other hand, are more than the sum of their parts; they are emergent, nonlinear, and nondeterministic.
- Our natural tendencies are to make rapid assumptions about our immediate environment and look for solutions without continuing to test our hypotheses. These natural tendencies often fail in the face of complex systems.
- Complex adaptive systems have several common features: (1) they are driven by connections among individual actors, (2) they evolve over time, and (3) they are nondeterministic.
- Fortunately, complex adaptive systems also have features that create opportunities for evaluation, such as variations over time and space. Using methods that have evolved in other fields such as biology, economics, and health services research, we can capitalize on these features to study healthcare delivery systems as living organisms.

REFERENCES

1. Rouse WB. Health Care as a complex adaptive system: implications for design and management. *The Bridge*. 2008:17–25.
2. Zimmerman B, Lindberg C, Plsek P. *Edgeware: Insights from Complexity Science for Health Care Leaders*. Irving, TX: VHA Inc.; 1998.
3. Centers for Disease Control and Prevention (CDC). Vital signs: central line-associated blood stream infections—United States, 2001, 2008, and 2009. *MMWR Morb Mortal Wkly Rep*. 2011;60(8):243–248.
4. Goeschel CA, Holzmueller CG, Pronovost PJ. Hospital Board Checklist to improve culture and reduce central line-associated bloodstream infections. *Jt Comm J Qual Patient Saf*. 2010;36(11):525–528.
5. Institute for Healthcare Improvement. *Prevent Central Line Infections*. 2011. Accessed July 28, 2011, from http://www.ihi.org/explore/CentralLineInfection/Pages/default.aspx.
6. Pronovost PJ, Watson SR, Goeschel CA, Hyzy RC, Berenholtz SM. Sustaining reductions in central line-associated bloodstream infections in Michigan intensive care units: A 10-year analysis. *Am J Med Qual*. 2016;31(3):197-202.
7. Nicholson N. How hardwired is human behavior? *Harv Bus Rev*. 1998;76(4):134-147.
8. Dorner D. The logic of failure. *Philos Trans R Soc Lond B Biol Sci*. 1990; 327(1241):463–473.
9. Mularski RA, White-Chu F, Overbay D, Miller L, Asch SM, Ganzini L. Measuring pain as the 5th vital sign does not improve quality of pain management. *J Gen Intern Med*. 2006;21(6):607–612.
10. Cicero TJ, Ellis MS, Harney J. Shifting patterns of prescription opioid and heroin abuse in the United States. *N Engl J Med*. 2015;373(18):1789–1790.
11. Dart RC, Severtson SG, Bucher-Bartelson B. Trends in opioid analgesic abuse and mortality in the United States. *N Engl J Med*. 2015;372(16):1573–1574.
12. Rudd RA, Aleshire N, Zibbell JE, Gladden RM. Increases in drug and opioid overdose deaths—United States, 2000–2014. *MMWR Morb Mortal Wkly Rep*. 2016;64(50–51):1378–1382.
13. Coffey DS. Self-organization, complexity, and chaos: the new biology for medicine. *Nat Med*. 1998;4(8):882–885.
14. Institute of Medicine Committee on Quality of Health Care in America. *Crossing the Quality Chasm: A New Health System for the 21st Century*. Washington, DC: National Academies Press; 2001.
15. Gardner M. Mathematical games: the fantastic combinations of John Conway's new solitaire game "life." *Scientific American*. 1970;223:120–123.
16. Plsek PE, Greenhalgh T. Complexity science: The challenge of complexity in health care. *BMJ*. 2001;323(7313):625–628.
17. Wilson T, Holt T, Greenhalgh T. Complexity science: complexity and clinical care. *BMJ*. 2001;323(7314):685–688.
18. Plsek PE. Paul E. Plsek on creativity and innovation in organizational change. Interview by Paul L. Green. *J Healthc Qual*. 2000;22(4):20–23, 30.

19. Cabana MD, Rand CS, Powe NR, et al. Why don't physicians follow clinical practice guidelines? A framework for improvement. *JAMA*. 1999;282(15):1458–1465.
20. Timmermans S. From autonomy to accountability: the role of clinical practice guidelines in professional power. *Perspect Biol Med*. 2005;48(4):490–501.
21. Wikipedia: statistics. 2017. Accessed April 14, 2017, from https://en.wikipedia.org/wiki/Wikipedia:Statistics.
22. Faucher JPL, Everett AM, Lawson R. A Complex Adaptive Organization Under the Lens of the LIFE Model: The Case of Wikipedia. The Fourth Organization Studies Summer Workshop: Advancing Ecological Understanding in Organization Studies, Pissouri, Cyprus, June 5–8, 2008. Accessed April 14, 2019, from https://www.academia.edu/497009/A_Complex_Adaptive_Organization_Under_the_Lens_of_the_LIFE_Model_The_Case_of_Wikipedia.
23. Lipsitz LA. The 3-night hospital stay and Medicare coverage for skilled nursing care. *JAMA*. 2013;310(14):1441–1442.
24. Hernandez VH, Ong A, Post Z, Orozco F. Does the Medicare 3-Day rule increase length of stay? *J Arthroplasty*. 2015;30(9 Suppl):34–35.
25. Litaker D, Tomolo A, Liberatore V, Stange KC, Aron D. Using complexity theory to build interventions that improve health care delivery in primary care. *J Gen Intern Med*. 2006;21(Suppl 2):S30–S34.
26. McDaniel RR Jr, Lanham HJ, Anderson RA. Implications of complex adaptive systems theory for the design of research on health care organizations. *Health Care Manage Rev*. 2009;34(2):191–199.
27. Chalfin DB. Implementation of standards for intensivist staffing: is it time to jump aboard the Leapfrog bandwagon? *Crit Care Med*. 2004;32(6):1406–1408.
28. Kahn JM, Matthews FA, Angus DC, Barnato AE, Rubenfeld GD. Barriers to implementing the Leapfrog Group recommendations for intensivist physician staffing: a survey of intensive care unit directors. *J Crit Care*. 2007;22(2):97–103.
29. Wallace DJ, Angus DC, Barnato AE, Kramer AA, Kahn JM. Nighttime intensivist staffing and mortality among critically ill patients. *N Engl J Med*. 2012;366(22):2093–2101.
30. The Hawthorne effect. *The Economist*. November 3, 2008: Online extra. Accessed May 31, 2019, from https://www.economist.com/news/2008/11/03/the-hawthorne-effect.
31. Srigley JA, Furness CD, Baker GR, Gardam M. Quantification of the Hawthorne effect in hand hygiene compliance monitoring using an electronic monitoring system: a retrospective cohort study. *BMJ Qual Saf*. 2014;23(12):974–980.

QUALITY AND SAFETY IN HEALTHCARE
The Evidence So Far 3

THE BEST THE WORLD HAS EVER SEEN

Much of this chapter will focus on sobering statistics about quality and safety and healthcare, but we start simply with this: Healthcare today is the best the world has ever seen. Just two centuries ago, the average life expectancy was only about 25 years. Today, it is more than 70. Infant mortality has fallen dramatically, not only in the United States (Figure 3-1), but also worldwide. And improvements haven't only been because of reduced infant mortality: life expectancy after the age of 65 has also risen. Diseases that used to be uniformly lethal have been converted to chronic, manageable conditions. Formerly experimental, esoteric treatments are now routine. For example, between 1990 and 2016, the use of bone marrow and stem cell transplantation more than tripled,[1] and today we use a patient's own reengineered T cells to target their cancer—something that would have seemed like science fiction only a few years ago. Healthcare today is the best the world has ever seen.

THREE CRITICAL PAPERS TO KNOW

In spite of this, the overwhelming evidence is that healthcare today is neither safe nor high quality. There are a few landmark papers that every healthcare delivery scientist should know about because they help form the bedrock of the field. These studies, and ones that followed from them, helped launch the modern quality and safety movements.

The Harvard Medical Practice Study: Incidence of Adverse Events and Negligence in Hospitalized Patients (1991)

The Harvard Medical Practice Study[2] reported the results of an analysis of 51 randomly selected hospitals in New York State. In this seminal piece of research, the authors reviewed the medical records of 30,121

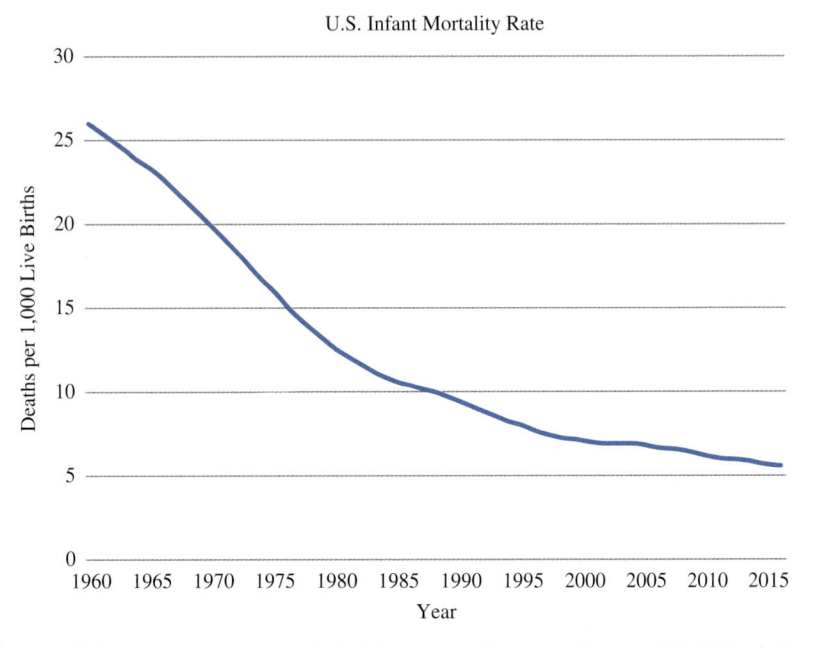

Figure 3-1 • Improvements in U.S. infant mortality rate. (*Source: World Bank Data https://data.worldbank.org/indicator/SP.DYN.IMRT.IN?locations=US.*)

randomly selected patients from 1984. Each chart was screened by a nurse and a medical record analyst; those patients who screened positive had their records reviewed by two separate board-certified physicians. They assessed whether (1) adverse events were due to medical management and (2) if adverse events were related to "negligence," which the study defined as substandard care.

The researchers found that 3.7% of hospitalizations included adverse events. Of these, 13.6% led to death. Just over a quarter of these adverse events were judged to be related to negligence, and both the number of adverse events and the rate of negligence rose with patient age. When this study was weighted to account for all of New York State, the authors estimated that there were 98,609 adverse events and 27,179 adverse events involving negligence in the 2.7 million hospitalizations in the state that year.

Utah-Colorado Study: Incidence and Types of Adverse Events and Negligent Care (2000)

Together with the Harvard Medical Practice Study, the Utah-Colorado study of adverse events in hospitalized patients[3] formed the underpinnings of the Institute of Medicine's profoundly impactful report, *To Err Is Human: Building a Safer Health System*.[4] This study randomly

Key Point

The Harvard Medical Practice Study, published in 1991, found that 3.7% of hospitalizations had adverse events, of which 13.6% were fatal. When this study was weighted to account for all of New York State, the authors estimated that there were 98,609 adverse events and 27,179 adverse events involving negligence in the 2.7 million hospitalizations in the state that year.

selected representative hospitals from Utah and Colorado and then randomly sampled 15,000 patients who stayed at these hospitals in 1992. The researchers then used methods similar to those of the Harvard Medical Practice Study, screening charts for signals of adverse events, followed by physician review. This study found that 2.9% of hospitalizations resulted in an adverse event, and that 6.6% of these resulted in death. Additionally, they found that 27.4% (Colorado) and 32.6% (Utah) of adverse events were due to negligence. This study also found that adverse drug reactions were the most common cause of nonoperative adverse events.

The Quality of Health Care Delivered to Adults in the United States (2003)

The two preceding studies focused on adverse patient safety events in hospitalized patients. In 2003, a linchpin study for understanding the quality of care delivered to Americans, especially in ambulatory settings, was published in the *New England Journal of Medicine*.[5] This study is well known enough that it is often referred to simply as "the McGlynn study" after its first author, Elizabeth McGlynn. It enrolled participants from 12 metropolitan communities via random-digit dialing and obtained both a telephone survey and medical records from 6,712 patients. The researchers created quality indicators for the most common acute and chronic health conditions, as well as preventive care measures, by reviewing established national guidelines and literature and then presenting them to multispecialty expert panels using the Delphi method of consensus. Participants in the study received only 54.9% of recommended care. A striking finding was that this held for preventive care (54.9% of recommended care), chronic care (56.1%), and acute care (53.5%). The authors concluded that "[t]he deficits we have identified in adherence to recommended processes for basic care pose serious threats to the health of the American public."

Key Point

The McGlynn study (2003) showed that Americans receive only about half the recommended care—regardless of whether it is acute, chronic, or preventative care.

AN INFLECTION POINT: TO ERR IS HUMAN AND CROSSING THE QUALITY CHASM

Two reports published by the Institute of Medicine helped change the face of quality and safety work, starting its transformation from being a rare pursuit of a few scholars to a national priority.

To Err Is Human (1999)

Many observers credit the Institute of Medicine's 1999 report, *To Err Is Human*,[4] as a turning point in how the United States thought about patient safety. (Note: The Institute of Medicine was renamed the National Academy of Medicine in 2015 to reflect its status as part of the National Academies.) Although the studies cited in this report had been known for years, it extrapolated their estimates of patient harms to national levels for the United States, estimating that between 44,000 and 98,000 Americans die each year as a result of medical error. This finding captured the public's attention more, perhaps, than any Institute of Medicine report either before or since. The report's language was honest—and stark. It may be hard to believe today, but at the time, patient safety was infrequently discussed—and when it was, it usually happened behind closed doors.[6] Seeing such an august body write the following was startling and helped move the national and international conversation forward:

> **Key Point**
>
> *To Err Is Human* was a 1999 report from the Institute of Medicine that many regard as a turning point in the quality and safety movement in healthcare.

When extrapolated to the over 33.6 million admissions to U.S. hospitals in 1997, the results of the study in Colorado and Utah imply that at least 44,000 Americans die each year as a result of medical errors. The results of the New York Study suggest the number may be as high as 98,000. Even when using the lower estimate, deaths due to medical errors exceed the number attributable to the 8th-leading cause of death. More people die in a given year as a result of medical errors than from motor vehicle accidents (43,458), breast cancer (42,297), or AIDS (16,516).[4]

Crossing the Quality Chasm: A New Health System for the 21st Century (2001)

If *To Err Is Human* was a wake-up call, the Institute of Medicine's next report laid out an approach to beginning to improve the health system. *Crossing the Quality Chasm* was released in 2001.[7] Although our understanding of quality and safety has evolved significantly since this report came out, several concepts from *Crossing the Quality Chasm* permeate how we think of quality and safety today.

Quality as a System Property

Problems with patient care are often viewed today—as they were at the time of this report—as individual failures of physicians, nurses, and other clinicians. You can see this, for example, in the Harvard Medical Practice Study's conceptualization of adverse events as negligence. *Crossing the Quality Chasm* made a national statement that helped change the conversation: "Poor designs set the workforce up to fail, regardless of how hard they try. If we want safer, higher-quality care, we will need to have redesigned systems of care."[7] While our understanding of system science and complex adaptive systems has evolved substantially since then (see Chapter 2), *Crossing the Quality Chasm*'s recognition of the importance of systems in generating high-quality care helped move both scholarship and practice forward.

The Six Aims for Improvement

Defining quality and measuring high-quality care are both conceptually challenging and operationally difficult tasks (see Chapter 12). The Institute of Medicine laid out a way of thinking about high-quality care that was broad enough to be conceptually attractive, but specific enough to be practical. High-quality healthcare should be safe, effective, efficient, timely, patient-centered, and equitable (Table 3-1). Today, these aims are often used in developing quality improvement programs and performance measurement approaches, as well as in physician training about quality. They should be part of the lexicon of any healthcare delivery scientist.

Table 3-1 SIX AIMS OF A HIGH-QUALITY HEALTHCARE SYSTEM

Aim	Description in Crossing the Quality Chasm[7]
Safe	Avoiding injuries to patients from the care that is intended to help them
Effective	Providing services based on scientific knowledge to all who could benefit, and refraining from providing services to those not likely to benefit
Efficient	Avoiding waste, including waste of equipment, supplies, ideas, and energy
Timely	Reducing waits and sometimes-harmful delays for both those who receive and those who give care
Patient-centered	Providing care that is respectful of and responsive to individual patient preferences, needs, and values, and ensuring that patient values guide all clinical decisions
Equitable	Providing care that does not vary in quality because of personal characteristics such as gender, ethnicity, geographic location, and socioeconomic status

MORE RECENT ESTIMATES ABOUT DEATHS FROM MEDICAL ERROR

It has been decades since some of the studies described previously were published, and in the intervening years, researchers have spent a lot of effort trying to quantify exactly how many people are hurt by medical care and exactly how likely patients are to get the right (or wrong) care.

For example, one study used the Global Trigger Tool and found a 10-fold increase in adverse events compared to voluntary reporting and billing-based methods.[8] Another study of North Carolina hospitals found that one of four hospital admissions had an adverse event, with little change over a five-year period.[9]

We can safely conclude that patient safety remains an important problem, and significant numbers of deaths continue to occur because of problems with care. However, some studies over the past few years have produced extremely high estimates of deaths from medical care. For example, one study estimated that instead of 100,000 deaths per year from error in the United States, there are 400,000, with seriously harmful events being 10–20 times more common (i.e. 2 million to 4 million per year).[10] Since according to the Centers for Disease Control and Prevention (CDC), there were 715,000 deaths in U.S. hospitals in 2010 (and about 25% of these cases occurred in patients 85 years or older), the implication from this study is that more than half of deaths in U.S. hospitals are caused by medical care. This seems implausible on its face, particularly when combined with the fact that overall hospital death rates fell by 20% (from 2.5% to 2.0%) between 2000 and 2010.[11]

Another 2016 publication grabbed headlines with its eye-catching title ("Medical Error—The Third-Leading Cause of Death in the US").[12] We agree with Shojania and Dixon-Woods (the editors of *BMJ Quality and Safety* and profoundly well-regarded patient safety researchers) that this estimate is implausible, methodologically problematic, and likely to be wrong.[13] We appreciate the need to call attention to the issue of patient safety, but we also recognize potential harms from overestimates of deaths from care, which may lead clinicians to avoid changes and improvements. In the end, one preventable death is too many, and the lack of a precise estimate does not obviate the need for improvement.

Caution

More recent papers may overstate the number of patients who die as a result of medical error, although whatever estimate one believes is true is obviously far too high.

INTERNATIONAL COMPARISONS

Comparing healthcare systems across national boundaries is complicated. A few measures are commonly used for this purpose: infant mortality, maternal mortality, life expectancy, and cost [usually expressed as a percentage of gross domestic product (GDP) spent on healthcare]. One way to represent value in healthcare is to compare healthcare expenditures to life expectancy at birth. In this regard, the United States lags significantly behind other countries (Figure 3-2). We achieve midrange life expectancy compared to other similar countries but have markedly higher expenditures on both a total and a per-capita basis.

Key Point

The United States spends more on healthcare than any other country, but it does not achieve similar gains in life expectancy.

CHAPTER 3 | QUALITY AND SAFETY IN HEALTHCARE

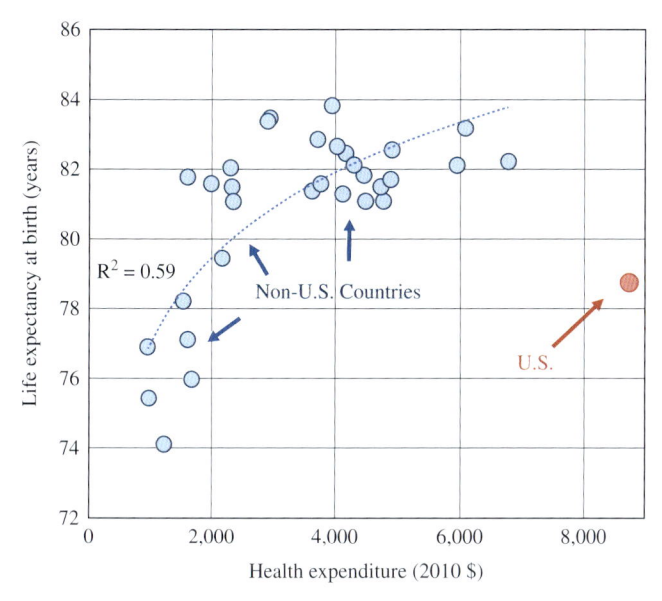

Figure 3-2 • Value in Health (U.S. and international comparisons). This chart compares national healthcare expenditures to life expectancy at birth—one approach to representing value in health and healthcare systems. The countries represented include Australia, Austria, Belgium, Canada, Chile, the Czech Republic, Denmark, Estonia, Finland, France, Germany, Greece, Hungary, Iceland, Ireland, Israel, Italy, Japan, Latvia, Luxembourg, Mexico, the Netherlands, New Zealand, Norway, Poland, Portugal, Slovenia, Spain, Sweden, Switzerland, Turkey, the United Kingdom, and the United States. (*Source: Data are from World Bank—World Development Indicators (http://data.worldbank.org/data-catalog/world-development-indicators) and the Organisation of Economic Co-operation and Development (OECD; https://stats.oecd.org/) via Esteban Ortiz-Ospina and Max Roser (2018), "Financing Healthcare"; https://ourworldindata.org/financing-healthcare with a Creative Commons CC BY-SA 3.0 AU license.*)

How many of these differences are due to healthcare remains uncertain, and these results point out important differences between health and healthcare. Most experts agree that the vast majority of health is influenced by forces outside of healthcare: genetics, environment, and behavior (though changing behavior is an important goal of the healthcare system). Some of the most obvious examples include improving health are public sanitation, mosquito control, and large-scale vaccination programs. But less obvious factors also play a role. For example, wealth is directly related to longevity, and "wealth shocks," where a person experiences acute financial difficulty, appear to result in increased mortality from all causes.[14] Factors in the built environment (such as the presence or absence of sidewalks) strongly affect physical activity,[15] an important determinant of cardiovascular health. Further, early childhood education

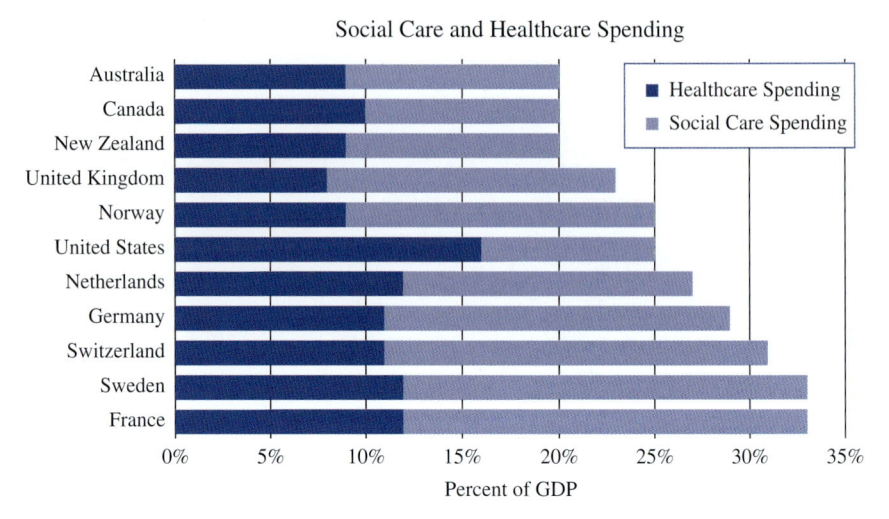

Figure 3-3 • Social care and healthcare spending in various countries. When spending on social care and healthcare is combined, United States spending is much more in the middle of the pack compared to numerous other countries. Total GDP numbers vary because these are slightly older data. (*Source: Bradley EH, Taylor LA. The American Health Care Paradox: Why Spending More Is Getting Us Less. New York: Public Affairs, 2013. Adapted from the Commonwealth Fund https://www.commonwealthfund.org/chart/2015/health-and-social-care-spending-percentage-gdp and OECD, Health Data 2009, Social Expenditure Dataset (Paris, France: OECD, 2009).*)

interventions such as full-day kindergarten result in lasting improvements in health outcomes.[16] These facts led researchers to study the question of how the *combination* of healthcare and social care spending compared across countries. As shown in Figure 3-3, the United States is much more in line with numerous other countries in this regard. This implies that at a national policy level, there are potentially significant tradeoffs between social care spending and healthcare spending. To a practicing clinician, this seems obvious: People are whole people, and all of us have seen many examples where healthcare issues are made markedly worse by poverty, homelessness, hunger, and inequity.

However, there is no doubt or disagreement that the United States has the most expensive healthcare of any country on the planet. The reasons for this, though, are the subject of significant debate. Until recently, the conventional wisdom was almost unequivocal that it was because of overutilization in the United States. Part of this overutilization was attributed to a less robust social safety net, but it was mostly attributed to the dominant payment model in this country—the fee-for-service system. There is no doubt that being paid for every service that one provides leads to the desire to provide more services, and that this increases utilization beyond what a patient might ideally need. This has been demonstrated in studies of supplier-induced demand, where (breaking one of the fundamental tenets of conventional economics) adding more supply increases demand for the service. This has been known since the 1970s, when it was discovered that adding 10% more surgeons to an area resulted in a 3% increase in per-capita utilization.[17] Because there is no mechanism to control overall costs, and instead there is an incentive to do more procedures and provide more services, fee-for-service has been strongly believed to be the central problem underlying U.S. healthcare spending—via the mechanism of inappropriately increased utilization. Here is a typical point of view (from "Healthcare's Dangerous Fee-for-Service Addiction," an article published in *Forbes*):

> *For its many users, healthcare's fee-for-service reimbursement methodology is like an addiction, similar to gambling, cigarette smoking and pain pill abuse. Doctors and hospitals in the clutches of this flawed payment model have grown dependent on providing more and more healthcare services, regardless of whether the additional care adds value.*[18]

This viewpoint is almost certainly correct, but research in 2018 suggested that it isn't the whole story—that the critical driver of overall healthcare spending in the United States may be prices, not overutilization. This study, published in *JAMA* and using 2016 data, compared U.S. spending and utilization to 10 other high-income countries. The authors found that utilization of most healthcare services such as hospital admission was similar between the United States and other countries, but that costs per service were higher. Specifically, administrative costs (such as insurance handling) were much higher in the United States, as were pharmaceutical costs. In addition, physician salaries were much higher: $218,173 for generalist physicians in the United States, as opposed to $86,607–$154,126 in the other high-income countries studied.[19] There are some subtleties in the interpretation of this study, but it provides compelling evidence that the healthcare cost story in the United States is even more complicated than we might have believed.

Key Point

The reasons for the high cost of U.S. healthcare are not due solely to overutilization, as was believed for many years. Low social care spending and high prices also contribute, perhaps dominantly so.

HAVE IMPROVEMENT EFFORTS WORKED?

Measuring patient safety and healthcare quality is a complicated, difficult topic (see Chapter 12), so any conclusions about whether quality and patient safety have improved need to keep that in mind. The *National Healthcare Quality and Disparities Report* concludes that the answer is a fairly unequivocal "yes:"

Quality of health care improved overall from 2000 through 2014–2015 but the pace of improvement varied by priority area:

- *Person-Centered Care: About 80% of person-centered care measures improved overall.*
- *Patient Safety: Almost two-thirds of patient safety measures improved overall.*
- *Healthy Living: About 60% of healthy living measures improved overall.*
- *Effective Treatment: More than half of effective treatment measures improved overall.*
- *Care Coordination: About half of care coordination measures improved overall.*
- *Care Affordability: About 70% of care affordability measures did not change overall.*[20]

Other views into this question have not been so positive. The National Patient Safety Foundation concluded that safety improvements have been slow and limited in scope and scale.[6] A study of North Carolina hospitals found that one of four hospital admissions had an adverse event, with little change over a five-year period.[9] A major effort to improve hospital quality, the Hospital Value-Based Purchasing Program, showed no discernible effect in mortality improvements.[21] More recently, a 2018 *NEJM* study found that Medicare's Bundled Payments Initiative for Medical Conditions program—an ambitious national approach to improve quality and reduce cost for common conditions—failed to improve mortality, readmission, or cost.[22]

HOW WE PUT IT ALL TOGETHER

How can we reconcile these seemingly contradictory findings? First, it is worth recognizing that Goodhart's Law may be at play here. This rule, attributed to economist Charles Goodhart, has been summarized as follows: When any measure becomes a target, it stops being a good measure.[23] This means that quality measures that become targets for reimbursement or a public rating may cease to actually measure underlying quality and outcomes. Improvements on these measures, then, become decoupled from meaningful improvements in patient outcomes, something that we have seen empirically demonstrated in numerous cases in healthcare.

Our view, though, is more positive, and at least somewhat more hopeful. We do believe that healthcare today is the best the world has ever seen. Infant mortality has fallen. Life expectancy has increased by decades. Diseases that used to be uniformly lethal have been converted

CAUSES OF DEATH.

Abridged Int. List No.	CAUSE OF DEATH.[1]	DEATHS IN REGISTRATION AREA: 1912.			Abridged Int. List No.	CAUSE OF DEATH.[1]	DEATHS IN REGISTRATION AREA: 1912.		
		Number.	Rate per 100,000 population.	Per cent.			Number.	Rate per 100,000 population.	Per cent.
	All causes [2]	838,251	1,387.2	100.0	24	Diseases of the stomach (cancer excepted) (102, 103)	11,346	18.8	1.4
1	Typhoid fever (1)	9,987	16.5	1.2	25	Diarrhea and enteritis (under 2 years) (104)	42,482	70.3	5.1
2	Typhus fever (2)	6	([3])	([4])	26	Appendicitis and typhlitis (108)	7,022	11.6	0.8
3	Malaria (4)	1,848	3.1	0.2	27	Hernia, intestinal obstruction (109)	7,192	11.9	0.9
4	Smallpox (5)	165	0.3	([4])	28	Cirrhosis of the liver (113)	8,176	13.5	1.0
5	Measles (6)	4,240	7.0	0.5	29	Acute nephritis and Bright's disease (119, 120)	62,267	103.0	7.4
6	Scarlet fever (7)	4,038	6.7	0.5	30	Noncancerous tumors and other diseases of the female genital organs (128, 129, 130, 131, 132)	3,658	6.1	0.4
7	Whooping cough (8)	5,619	9.3	0.7	31	Puerperal septicemia (puerperal fever, peritonitis) (137)	3,905	6.5	0.5
8	Diphtheria and croup (9)	11,013	18.2	1.3	32	Other puerperal accidents of pregnancy and labor (134, 135, 136, 138, 139, 140, 141)	5,130	8.5	0.6
9	Influenza (10)	6,237	10.3	0.7	33	Congenital debility and malformations (150, 151)	48,596	80.4	5.8
10	Asiatic cholera (12)		([3])	([4])	34	Senility (154)	14,362	23.8	1.7
11	Cholera nostras (13)	245	0.4	([4])	35	Violent deaths (suicide excepted) (164, 165, 166, 167, 168, 169, 170, 171, 172, 173, 174, 175, 176, 177, 178, 179, 180, 181, 182, 183, 184, 185, 186)	53,729	88.9	6.4
12	Other epidemic diseases (3, 11, 14, 15, 16, 17, 18, 19)	5,175	8.6	0.6	36	Suicide (155, 156, 157, 158, 159, 160, 161, 162, 163)	9,656	16.0	1.2
13	Tuberculosis of the lungs (28, 29)	78,465	129.9	9.4	37	Other diseases (20, 21, 22, 23, 24, 25, 26, 27, 36, 37, 38, 46, 47, 48, 49, 50, 51, 52, 53, 54, 55, 56, 57, 58, 59, 60, 62, 63, 66, 67, 68, 69, 70, 71, 72, 73, 74, 75, 76, 77, 78, 80, 81, 82, 83, 84, 85, 99, 100, 101, 105, 106, 107, 110, 111, 112, 114, 115, 116, 117, 118, 121, 122, 123, 124, 125, 126, 127, 133, 142, 143, 144, 145, 146, 147, 148, 149, 152, 153)	128,206	212.2	15.3
14	Tuberculous meningitis (30)	5,098	8.4	0.6	38	Unknown or ill-defined diseases (187, 188, 189)	6,946	11.5	0.8
15	Other forms of tuberculosis (31, 32, 33, 34, 35)	6,797	11.2	0.8					
16	Cancer and other malignant tumors (39, 40, 41, 42, 43, 44, 45)	46,531	77.0	5.6					
17	Simple meningitis (61)	6,928	11.5	0.8					
18	Cerebral hemorrhage and softening (64, 65)	46,797	77.4	5.6					
19	Organic diseases of the heart (79)	86,179	142.6	10.3					
20	Acute bronchitis (89)	6,723	11.1	0.8					
21	Chronic bronchitis (90)	4,907	8.1	0.6					
22	Pneumonia (92)	51,495	85.2	6.1					
23	Other diseases of the respiratory system (tuberculosis excepted) (86, 87, 88, 91, 93, 94, 95, 96, 97, 93)	37,085	61.4	4.4					

[1] Abridged International List of Causes of Death. The title or titles of the detailed International List that are included under each heading are shown by numbers in parentheses.
[2] Exclusive of stillbirths.
[3] Less than one-tenth of 1 per 100,000 population.
[4] Less than one-tenth of 1 per cent.

Figure 3-4 • Causes of death in the United States in the early 20th century. Healthcare has changed dramatically in just a century, as even a cursory glance at the leading causes of death in 1912 reveals. (*Source: Mortality Statistics 1912, Department of Commerce, https://www.cdc.gov/nchs/data/vsushistorical/mortstatsh_1912.pdf.*)

into chronic, manageable conditions. Treatments that were once purely hypothetical are now routine: In just two decades, bone marrow and stem cell transplantation more than tripled, and today patients receive their own reengineered T cells to target their specific cancer—something that would have seemed like science fiction only a few years ago.

It is easy to lose sight of the dramatic changes that have occurred in a comparatively short period of time. Figure 3-4 shows the leading causes of death in the United States in the early 20th century, from the U.S. Department of Commerce's 1912 Mortality Statistics. Typhoid fever, smallpox, malaria, whooping cough, diphtheria, and cholera all were among the top causes of death. But this situation has markedly improved, and not just for diseases that have been targeted by antimosquito measures and vaccines: The death rate from pneumonia was 85 per 100,000 then; today, it is 16 per 100,000[24]—more than an 80% decrease. It is hard to overstate the magnitude of these changes.

As medicine and healthcare have advanced, though, complexity has increased. Today, medical professionals are taking care of sicker patients, with more complicated therapies, at a faster pace than ever before. Patients who would have died 15 years ago are saved today, but they have residual chronic health conditions that wouldn't have been seen before. Patients who would have been in the ICU are now in the general ward. And patients who would previously have been hospitalized are increasingly cared for as outpatients. This means that there are many more opportunities for problems than there were in the past, in new venues—opportunities for failure of safety, for lapses in quality. For those of us who work in the field, it is obvious that we have a tremendously long way to go to achieve a safe and high-quality health system ... but it is simultaneously obvious that we have come a long way.

KEY POINTS

- Healthcare today is the best the world has ever seen, with profound reductions in infant mortality rates and improvements in life expectancy.
- But, healthcare today is neither safe nor high quality.
- Three important studies helped create our modern understanding of quality and safety: the Harvard Medical Practice Study, the Utah/Colorado adverse event study, and the McGlynn study of the quality of care in the United States.
- Two Institute of Medicine reports helped galvanize today's patient safety movement: *To Err Is Human* and *Crossing the Quality Chasm*.
- High-quality healthcare should be safe, effective, efficient, timely, patient-centered, and equitable (a goal called "the Six Aims").

REFERENCES

1. D'Souza A, Zhu X. *Current Uses and Outcomes of Hematopoietic Cell Transplantation (HCT): CIBMTR Summary Slides.* 2016. Accessed February 19, 2017, from https://www.cibmtr.org/referencecenter/slidesreports/summaryslides/pages/index.aspx.
2. Brennan TA, Leape LL, Laird NM, et al. Incidence of adverse events and negligence in hospitalized patients. Results of the Harvard Medical Practice Study I. *N Engl J Med.* 1991;324(6):370–376.
3. Thomas EJ, Studdert DM, Burstin HR, et al. Incidence and types of adverse events and negligent care in Utah and Colorado. *Med Care.* 2000;38(3):261–271.
4. Institute of Medicine. *To Err Is Human: Building a Safer Health System.* Washington, DC: National Academies Press; 2000.
5. McGlynn EA, Asch SM, Adams J, et al. The quality of health care delivered to adults in the United States. *N Engl J Med.* 2003;348(26):2635–2645.
6. Berwick D, Shojania K. Free from harm: accelerating patient safety improvement fifteen years after *To Err Is Human*. Boston: National Patient Safety Foundation; 2015.
7. Institute of Medicine. *Crossing the Quality Chasm: A New Health System for the 21st Century.* Washington, DC: National Academy Press; 2001:4.
8. Classen DC, Resar R, Griffin F, et al. "Global trigger tool" shows that adverse events in hospitals may be ten times greater than previously measured. *Health Aff (Millwood).* 2011;30(4):581–589.
9. Landrigan CP, Parry GJ, Bones CB, Hackbarth AD, Goldmann DA, Sharek PJ. Temporal trends in rates of patient harm resulting from medical care. *N Engl J Med.* 2010;363(22):2124–2134.
10. James JT. A new, evidence-based estimate of patient harms associated with hospital care. *J Patient Saf.* 2013;9(3):122–128.
11. Centers for Disease Control and Prevention (CDC). *Trends in Inpatient Hospital Deaths: National Hospital Discharge Survey, 2000–2010.* NCHS Data Brief No. 118, March 2013. Accessed May 11, 2018, from https://www.cdc.gov/nchs/products/databriefs/db118.htm.
12. Makary MA, Daniel M. Medical error—the third leading cause of death in the US. *BMJ.* 2016;353:i2139.
13. Shojania KG, Dixon-Woods M. Re: Medical error—the third leading cause of death in the US. *BMJ.* 2016;353.
14. Pool LR, Burgard SA, Needham BL, Elliott MR, Langa KM, Mendes de Leon CF. Association of a negative wealth shock with all-cause mortality in middle-aged and older adults in the United States. *JAMA.* 2018;319(13):1341–1350.
15. Guo JY, Gandavarapu S. An economic evaluation of health-promotive built environment changes. *Prev Med.* 2010;50(Suppl 1):S44–S49.
16. Hahn RA, Rammohan V, Truman BI, et al. Effects of full-day kindergarten on the long-term health prospects of children in low-income and racial/ethnic-minority populations: a community guide systematic review. *Am J Prev Med.* 2014;46(3):312–323.

17. Fuchs VR. *The Supply of Surgeons and the Demand for Operations.* In: National Bureau of Economic Research Cambridge, Mass., USA; 1978. Accessed May 24, 2019, from https://www.nber.org/papers/w0236/.
18. Pearl R. Healthcare's dangerous fee-for-service addiction. *Forbes.* September 25, 2017. Accessed August 15, 2018, from https://www.forbes.com/sites/robertpearl/2017/09/25/fee-for-service-addiction/.
19. Papanicolas I, Woskie LR, Jha AK. Health care spending in the United States and other high-income countries. *JAMA.* 2018;319(10):1024–1039.
20. Agency for Healthcare Research and Quality. *2016 National Healthcare Quality & Disparities Report (AHRQ Pub. No. 17-0001).* 2017. Accessed May 24, 2019, from https://www.ahrq.gov/research/findings/nhqrdr/nhqdr16/index.html.
21. Figueroa JF, Tsugawa Y, Zheng J, Orav EJ, Jha AK. Association between the Value-Based Purchasing pay-for-performance program and patient mortality in US hospitals: observational study. *BMJ.* 2016;353:i2214.
22. Joynt Maddox KE, Orav EJ, Zheng J, Epstein AM. Evaluation of Medicare's Bundled Payments Initiative for Medical Conditions. *N Engl J Med.* 2018;379(3):260–269.
23. Strathern M. "Improving ratings": audit in the British University system. *Eur Review.* 1997;5(3):305–321.
24. Centers for Disease Control and Prevention (CDC). *National Center for Health Statistics: Pneumonia FastFacts.* 2017. Accessed August 15, 2018, from https://www.cdc.gov/nchs/fastats/pneumonia.htm.

WHAT DOES THE FUTURE HOLD?
The Kind of Healthcare Our Children's Children Will Receive

Stephen Weber

INTRODUCTION

There is no shortage of speculation about the future of the U.S. health system. The mainstream media, bloggers, futurists, and pundits are fast and eager to not only predict the system's future, but also to fit today's unfolding events to their own narrative of the subject. Decisions made and policies deployed now, often with incomplete information and understanding, could have outsized and dramatic effects on our future health and economy. However, how sure can we really be of what the future will hold for patients and providers?

Healthcare delivery and policy have already sustained several recent cataclysmic changes. First, in 2003, Congress passed the Medicare Prescription Drug, Improvement, and Modernization Act. This act created Medicare Advantage, a program of tremendous importance to today's healthcare environment. Medicare Advantage, or Part C, represented an important evolution of non-fee-for-service options for Medicare beneficiaries. Then came the Affordable Care Act (ACA). The ACA, or the Patient Protection and Affordable Care Act, was landmark legislation passed on March 23, 2010, and it largely came into effect in 2014. The law was the first major expansion of healthcare coverage in the United States since the creation of Medicare and Medicaid in 1965. Largely due to expansions in Medicaid eligibility and the creation of insurance markets, the numbers of uninsured Americans rapidly fell.[1,2] While many of the great gains in insurance coverage were made due to Medicaid expansion, the law also created insurance markets in order to make available insurance premiums with a standardized list of essential health benefits to all, regardless of preexisting health conditions. The law also made several major changes to healthcare delivery, including:

- incentives and penalties for hospital readmissions among Medicare beneficiaries.
- penalties for hospitals for hospital-acquired conditions and patient harms
- pay-for-performance payment incentives for hospitals and physician practices.
- an experiment around bundling payments for care across hospitals, physician organizations, and posthospital care.
- a new type of care organization, the Accountable Care Organization (ACO), that integrated care and payment across outpatient, inpatient, and post-hospitalization services. Groups that formed ACOs could share in savings incurred by better-coordinated and higher-value care through participation in the Medicare Shared Savings Program (MSSP). Organizations willing to incur some of the risk could also participate as Pioneer ACOs.
- increased funding to the National Health Services Corps.
- the Center for Medicare and Medicaid Innovation, to further put in place experiments in healthcare payments to increase value for beneficiaries of Medicare and Medicaid.
- the Patient-Centered Outcomes Research Trust Fund, which supports the Patient-Centered Outcomes Research Institute, a grant-giving and research organization.

Key Point

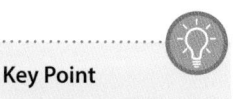

Healthcare is moving toward value-based care, even though most U.S. healthcare remains fee-for-service in 2019.

What do these transformative laws mean for the care that our children will receive? Themes are evolving both within and outside healthcare that are a prelude, if not a preview, to what will come in the near and distant future. Some of these drivers are internal to the care system: increased accountability for safety and outcomes, greater engagement of patients and families, and increased appreciation of the economic toll of an inefficient system. Equally important, though, are influences from outside healthcare, many of which mirror trends in other industries, including the rise of technology both in business intelligence and as a platform for service. But what principles, values, and structures will ultimately sort these influences toward a coherent and rational final product?

This inflection point in healthcare is not entirely unique. A look back to 50 years ago reveals a period of equally dramatic change. The demographic and cultural shifts that surfaced across American society after World War II and through the 1950s and 1960s dramatically influenced medical care, as did the stunning breakthroughs in clinical knowledge and practice. During that period, numerous institutions and organizations, ranging from a strengthened National Institutes of Health (NIH) to the Centers for Medicare and Medicaid Services to multinational pharmaceutical firms, had an influence on how care is delivered. What has emerged is an imperfect product, but one that has delivered remarkable advances in the care and management of diseases such as cancer and heart disease. If there has been an organizing principle in U.S. healthcare over the past half-century, it has been the focus on improving outcomes through the application of evidence derived from clinical trials and other controlled studies.

So what principles and values will ultimately be reflected in the health system of the future? This chapter will discuss the powerful forces that will shape American medicine by the year 2069. It will examine the principal drivers of change and look to cultural and technological influences that will need to be both embraced and distilled every bit as much as those of the past 50 years. In this context, we will discuss the role that the new science of healthcare delivery will play in the next 50 years in preparing an imperfect system to meet the needs of a population that expects and deserves better.

VALUE DRIVES CHANGE

The singular force that will drive the future of American healthcare is the urgent need to extract value from a system that is (at least for now) both inefficient and insufficiently effective. Figure 4-1 summarizes the unsustainable reality of medical care in the United States, highlighting not only the enormous financial investment, expressed as a proportion of gross domestic product (GDP), but also surprising underperformance in terms of the ultimate outcome of care—mortality. This uncoupling of outcome from investment not only underserves patients in need, but also places an intolerable drag on the economy at all levels: rising costs that threaten the solvency of the Medicare trust, employers burdened by the expense of sponsored health insurance, and the risk of excessive costs and even bankruptcy faced by underinsured families confronting catastrophic illness or injury. As a result, there is the cold calculation that without fundamental change in how we deliver and pay for medical care, the risk to our economy and society extends well beyond the walls of hospitals and clinics. Indeed, this motivation is so powerful, urgent, and all-encompassing that it serves as the underpinning of all the trends that are discussed in the rest of this chapter.

But what is meant when we discuss "value" in healthcare? Value in this context can be expressed mathematically as the quotient derived from clinical outcomes (quality) divided by expense (costs). This is an approach

I | UNDERSTANDING HEALTHCARE DELIVERY SCIENCE

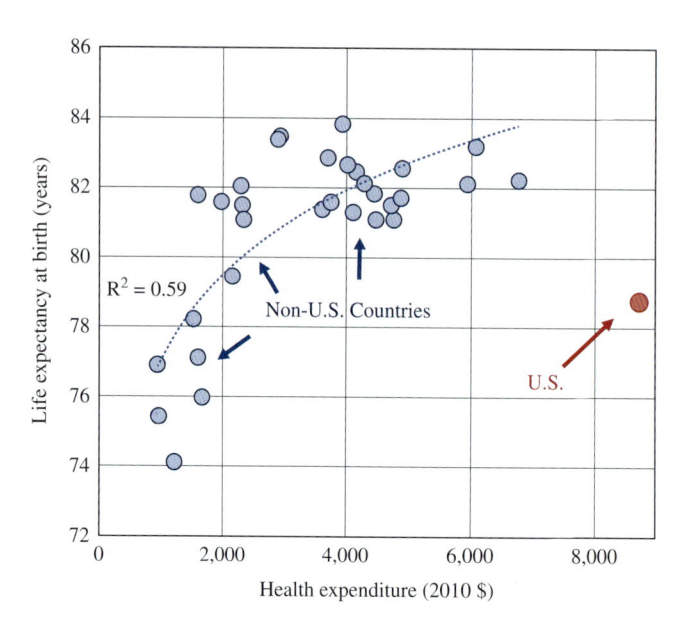

Figure 4-1 • Value in health (US and international comparisons). This chart compares national healthcare expenditures to life expectancy at birth, one approach to representing value in health and healthcare systems. Countries represented include Australia, Austria, Belgium, Canada, Chile, the Czech Republic, Denmark, Estonia, Finland, France, Germany, Greece, Hungary, Iceland, Ireland, Israel, Italy, Japan, Latvia, Luxembourg, Mexico, the Netherlands, New Zealand, Norway, Poland, Portugal, Slovenia, Spain, Sweden, Switzerland, Turkey, United Kingdom, and the United States. (Source: Data are from World Bank – World Development Indicators (http://data.worldbank.org/data-catalog/world-development-indicators) and OECD (https://stats.oecd.org/) via Esteban Ortiz-Ospina and Max Roser (2018) – "Financing Healthcare". https://ourworldindata.org/financing-healthcare with a Creative Commons CC BY-SA 3.0 AU license.)

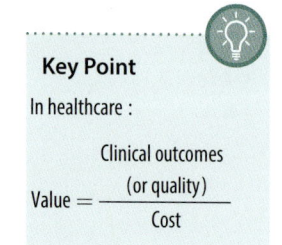

> **Key Point**
>
> In healthcare :
>
> $$\text{Value} = \frac{\text{Clinical outcomes (or quality)}}{\text{Cost}}$$

championed by scholars such as Michael Porter.[3] Therefore, practices and policy that either improve clinical quality or reduce expense will maximize value. Optimal value is assigned to interventions that do both. This framing is simple but not dogmatic. Reasonable questions and debates can be raised about perspective ("value to whom?"), as well as the appropriateness of embedding additional terms and refinements (such as patient satisfaction). But for our purposes, recognizing that the U.S. healthcare system inarguably underperforms in both the numerator and denominator of the value equation is sufficient to drive the discussion.

No matter one's politics, the ACA went a long way toward focusing on the importance of value in healthcare. However, by no means should one conclude that the move to value was inspired by or a consequence of the ACA, or any partisan policymaking for that matter. There were rumblings for the past several decades (under national legislative and executive leadership from both political parties) that sought to promote improved outcomes and cost control. However, the ACA was the first U.S. public policy measure that broadly and comprehensively aimed to address the issue of value in healthcare. Driving improved outcomes, bending the proverbial cost curve, and expanding access for the uninsured are the central pillars of the ACA. Even with subsequent modifications and inconsistency in application, the legislation stands as the most aggressive policy to address the underperformance of the healthcare system. However, the ACA is ultimately flawed in both conception and execution, especially in a partisan political environment. Achieving even basic quality performance has been a struggle, and the cost curve appears difficult to change.

So, while policy and practice to date have acknowledged the importance of value to American medicine, the interventions have been inadequate and insufficiently impactful. Rather than abandon this effort, though, it appears that a more studied understanding of the policies and practice of medicine is essential. More specifically, a rigorous and intensive examination of clinical operations and care delivery is a necessity. As is the case for our clinical advances, this will require the application of precise, research-quality methods—an uncompromising approach to meticulous design and execution, as well as the contribution of experts and expertise from other domains, clinical and nonclinical.

In short, it is healthcare delivery science (HDS) that stands at the center of a brighter future for American healthcare. The sections that follow will examine specific trends in care delivery that are likely to play out over the next half-century. For each, we will discuss in the context of maximizing value while simultaneously pointing to the contribution to be made by the science of healthcare delivery.

THE "POSTSAFETY" ERA

One of the most significant trends in American healthcare over the past 25 years has been the emergence and embrace of the patient safety movement (see also Chapter 3). An appreciation of the human toll associated with medical errors has prompted thorough introspection and regulation—a sea change in how medicine is taught, practiced, and reimbursed. So, how will this deep and relatively newfound commitment to patient safety play out over the next 50 years?

Comparisons between healthcare and aviation have served well in the history of patient safety and potentially point to a way forward. High-reliability practices such as checklists and team training had their roots in aviation and were later applied with considerable fanfare and some measure of success in clinical practice. Going forward, it is reasonable to expect that continued study, particularly in the domain of human factors analysis, will play a role in further strengthening the culture, practice, and safety outcomes in healthcare. At the same time, as has been true in aviation, there is an inflection point at which timely delivery of safe care does not become a distinguishing feature of medicine, but in fact is a baseline expectation of everyone who is served by the system. Put another way: When booking travel recently, to what extent did you make your selection of airline and flight based on the likelihood of harm, or even death?

We should expect (and hope) that in the next half-century, healthcare will enter its own postsafety era, as is essentially the case for the domestic airlines of today. Ensuring safety will still be critical and demand investment and attention on the part of practitioners and provider organizations. However, we should expect a level of reliability that allows safety concerns to pass out of the consciousness of the patients. In this context, harm events, rare as they should be, will not serve as the basis for distinction in the market or a data point for provider rankings. Rather, one anticipates a future in which mistakes and errors in clinical care are dealt with in much the same way that airline incidents (both near-misses and actual events) are presently managed. Investigations become the basis of shared learning and industrywide response and improvement, such as is driven by the National Transportation Safety Board (NTSB) and Federal Aviation Administration (FAA) for airlines today.

HDS will undoubtedly play a critical role in reaching this ambitious future state. As harm events become progressively more rare, the quantitative and expert demands for analysis and understanding necessary to drive innovation will become more rigorous. Happily, the days of reporting a single institution observational study of a series of harm events should become all but impossible, owing to the infrequency of such events. Expert attention will be essential to manage confounding and bias and to execute investigations across multiple sites of care. Novel applications of knowledge about team dynamics and human factors will be essential. Perhaps most significantly, continued integration of methods, including tools from manufacturing (e.g., lean production), will be essential to bring us to a state in which medical errors become as rare as defects in the manufacturing of precision products.

HEALTHCARE DELIVERY THAT DELIVERS HEALTH

But if safety can one day be taken for granted by a patient in the same way that it is for an airline passenger, on what basis will the most effective providers and healthcare systems be distinguished? How can outcomes be further optimized? Once again, let's return to the value equation. Maximizing clinical outcomes while reducing expense is difficult under any circumstance. However, this endeavor is especially challenging in the context of a patient hospitalized for advanced disease with complications as a consequence of poorly managed chronic health issues. Much has been written about the disproportionate economic impact of end-of-life care, where enormous expenditures in critical care and salvage therapies often prove fruitless in averting the inexorable onset of loss of function and even death.[4-6]

However, for all but a few exceptional cases, there are innumerable upstream factors that brought the patient to this moment of extraordinary need. With critical and honest review, we appreciate that for these patients, there were opportunities to avoid this end game: preventative measures not applied, therapeutic relationships never forged, appointments cancelled, medications doses missed, referrals to resources and expertise not provided, and risks and vulnerabilities not identified.

If the American healthcare system is to deliver value as a means of sustaining itself over the next 50 years, the greatest impact and the wisest investment will be in early and sustained efforts to promote wellness and health. As has been articulated in many settings and contexts, not only is this the most dramatic shift needed in our health system, but it will also require foundational changes in practice and incentives in medicine. Even with the more recent ventures into capitated care and value-based reimbursement, Americans still receive their care largely in a fee-for-service environment.[7] In this context, there is a perverse but strong economic incentive to concentrate resources, investment, and innovation in service to the most acutely ill and complicated patients. Reimbursement predicated on volume of services promotes not only aggressive care, but more of it. There is an arms race between health systems large and small, academic and nonteaching, to offer more and more complex and intensive services for a relatively small set of patients in need, such as positron emission tomography (PET) scans, proton therapy, and robotic surgery. From the perspective of value, this deployment of assets is neither efficient nor rational. Outcomes are not enhanced at the population level, nor are expenses reduced. In short, value is not added.

To some extent, the historical focus of HDS mirrors these peculiar incentives of modern American healthcare. Preeminent centers and experts in the field have built their reputations on avoiding harm and improving the management of hospitalized patients, often the most critically ill. Major contributions have been made in preventing sepsis, predicting cardiac arrests, and avoiding healthcare-associated infections among

Key Point

If the American healthcare system is to deliver value, the greatest impact will be in early and sustained efforts to promote wellness and health.

critically ill patients. Part of this focus is understandable owing to the visible consequences of harm and risk events in hospitals. As one chief quality officer at a major academic medical center responded when asked why initial attention was focused on inpatient improvements: "Because that's where the bodies are accumulating." But if we accept the conclusions given previously and recognize that some of the biggest gains in safety have been or will be achieved, how will HDS redeploy to meet the real needs of the patients we serve, and in doing so, more meaningfully drive value in healthcare?

The simplest option is to say that the same tools, skills, and methods that have been so effective and impactful in reducing harm can be equally viewed as promoting health and wellness. Healthy individuals in the community can be stratified using objective data in much the same way as critically ill patients in an intensive care unit (ICU). Prediction models should be available (and in many cases already are) to identify at the time of a routine visit those people who are at highest risk for developing hypertension or diabetes in the next several years. Big data and machine learning could be applied to determine pathways to ensure that children at risk for accidents and trauma are identified and protected long in advance of an event.

To date, however, even where there has been innovative and potentially impactful work in these spaces, meant to answer these questions, the same kind of systematic efforts at implementation have not yet been applied. A big part of this gap likely relates to the complexity of the work and methodological complications encompassed in community-based research and practice. Outcomes in promoting wellness are much more challenging to define than in circumstances where we endeavor to prevent harm. In the latter case, death, disability, and loss of function are defined in a manner that is fairly well accepted. In terms of wellness, the outcomes are considered less precise by some, often relying on self-reported outcomes and survey instruments that themselves need to be created and validated. Even where investigators in this space might label this characterization oversimplified and unfair, the fact remains that such measures have not yet been fully adopted and embraced to drive system-level performance and accountability.

The advent of the electronic health record (EHR) and the integration of multiple clinical monitoring systems in the management of hospital patients have buoyed the work of HDS in acute care and hospital harm reduction. These systems and connections provide a wealth of data that become the fodder for deep analysis in predicting and improving hospital outcomes. In contrast, some of the most important inputs for predicting health and wellness in the community are not so well quantified and often exist well outside the sphere of even a comprehensive primary care setting. Data from consumer behavior, personal health habits, access to resources and social determinants of health are increasingly recognized as critical predictors and influencers of health and wellness. However, as discussed later in this chapter, their integration into a fuller vision of the patient remains aspirational.

But even apart from methodological considerations and challenges, there is a fundamental structural gap that to date has contributed to the failure to adopt this more global view of health and wellness at the level of provider organizations. Specifically, efforts in hospital harm reduction, while often originating as original research by independent investigators, have increasingly been adopted and disseminated by provider organizations and hospital leaders. Mindful of the potential impact of pay-for-performance schemes, public reporting, and national rankings, the time from innovation to deployment has been progressively shortened over the past two decades for interventions such as checklists for the prevention of central-line bloodstream infections and sepsis bundles and pathways. Pay-for-performance and related reimbursement schemes have heightened a sense of accountability around these measures.

Such is not the case for many outpatient and wellness-oriented programs and opportunities. In this context, the absence of central coordination (except in the case of large, ambulatory networks) has left the dissemination of such approaches to individual providers and practices motivated only by self-improvement. But the gap is not just a product of a lack of coordination, but also one of motivation. Put simply, there has not only been little economic incentive to promote wellness, but as noted earlier, there has actually been a reimbursement incentive to focus on illness and complex care through volume-based contracting.

Happily, this circumstance appears to be changing, and again the motivation emanates from the need to enhance value in American healthcare. Going forward, provider organizations, as well as individually incentivized practices and physicians are tasked with delivering improved outcomes at reduced cost. To the extent that the value equation is skewed toward ensuring that patients stay well (improve outcomes) and don't consume expensive resources (reduce costs), we should have every expectation that the same vigor previously applied in hospitals and acute care is soon to be applied to the promotion of wellness and health.

It seems a safe bet to predict that over the next several years, health-system quality programs will take a more active approach to turning their attention from inpatient harm reduction toward prevention and wellness activities. When assigning improvement resources, this can be a matter of assessing diminishing returns: Is it better to devote the effectiveness of an infection-prevention program to reduce the central-line-associated bloodstream infection (CLABSI) rate from 0.6 to 0.5 infections per 1000 central line-days, or to increase vaccination rates for pneumococcus from 80% to 90%?

But this change isn't just a simple matter of resource allocation on the front lines. Rather, this represents a fundamental philosophical shift. Health-system board members might ask management: "Wait—we don't get paid if a patient doesn't take her medicine?" The answer is a resounding "yes." As a consequence, the reach of provider organizations is apt to change. Having a population under care, such as in an ACO, Medicare Advantage plan, or other risk arrangement, comes to connote real accountability—not just as a passive service provider when the patient seeks care, but to ensure that patients are actively directed to tools, resources, and expertise that keeps them well.

If provider organizations are at the center, it will be essential to ensure that they have invested in HDS as a means of ensuring effectiveness, even if only from a business perspective. HDS offers the rigor and understanding to deploy resources and expertise to not only apply that which has already been developed through the methods of implementation science, but also to pioneer new innovations and tools.

CONSUMERISM VERSUS PERSONALIZATION

As uncertain as the future of American healthcare may seem, one certainty is that any discussion of the subject will eventually address the emergence of consumerism as a key influence. The recognition of the patient as a meaningful contributor to medical decision-making is an important foundation to any future state of American healthcare. Today, forward-thinking organizations and providers are embracing the rudiments of patient-centered care, although sometimes grudgingly.

From these important roots has emerged a much more assertive and far more influential movement, in which patients are not just included in questions of management, but also are the primary instigators of care, expect expanded and real-time access to providers, freely access their own healthcare data and information, and enjoy amenities of convenience and access, often supported by mobile technology and tools. This more expansive role for the patient in healthcare is informed by larger secular trends in consumerism across diverse industries. The American consumer has come to enjoy goods and services in essence tailored to his or her personal preferences and desires. We seek news from sources catering to our personal political persuasion, binge-watch entertainment at times of our

Key Point

Consumerism is an important force shaping the future of healthcare.

choosing, and select products from a global catalog of online selections rather than being constrained by the purchasing agents of local stores.

In healthcare, these changes have been further accelerated by the fact that many patients now experience the economic impact of their decisions and actions, having been previously insulated through the complex buffer of federal or employer-sponsored insurance. As insurance plans have come to place greater financial responsibility on patients through high deductibles and out-of-network surcharges, patients are directly exposed to the price of the services they receive. In this context, they are insisting on more say about and more convenience in their care. Patients increasingly expect an experience with healthcare that is more akin to their interactions with other industries and services: Hospitals should feel more like hotels, providers should offer appointments with the same convenience as a hairstylist, and information about performance should be as available for a health provider as it is for the purchase of a new car.

Recognizing these expectations, provider organizations have responded with an array of services and supports, especially for the coveted population of commercially insured patients. Branded mobile applications, 24/7 urgent care clinics, and amenities unheard of by the patients of two decades ago are now in abundance across the care landscape. The availability of these features is promoted aggressively by competing health systems in an effort to win the business of the quality-seeking healthcare consumer.

But is this the final state of consumerism in healthcare? Unchecked and irrational escalation is likely unsustainable as the expense of providing amenities and perks grows. The portfolio of amenities offered by providers in a market could become all but indistinguishable to consumers, no longer a distinctive feature in attracting and retaining patient business. The cost of developing and deploying such features, where they do not drive the numerator of the value equation (outcomes), ultimately could bankrupt a system that fails to deliver true value.

Is there a path forward, in which the appeal to individual patients actually supports value—a world in which assets are deployed and investments made that patients don't just enjoy, but that actually improve outcomes and reduce expense? The term *personalized medicine* has emerged in the lexicon to denote therapeutic approaches that are specifically customized for the needs of individual patients. In the case of oncology care, tumor cells can be examined from an individual patient and characterized such that responsiveness to an array of chemotherapy agents or other treatment options can be quantified and predicted. With this information, a regimen will be customized to the specific demands of a patient's disease, maximizing outcomes while eliminating the expense associated with trials of inferior and potentially toxic alternative treatments.

But for all the accomplishments in cancer genetics and pharmacogenomics, the wealth of information available about patients and their state of wellness or diseases is not "just" limited to the sequence of nucleotides in their genetic material. For all patients, there is an array of data points, equally rich, that describe not only their organic self (the biology and chemistry of body and cells), but also the environment in which they live and the lifestyle they pursue. Data regarding an individual's sociodemographics, preferences, and values are at least as rich as her or his genetic information. Embedded in this code of patient and environmental characteristics is the answer to which customized and targeted therapeutic and management tools will be most effective and whose deployment will improve the efficiency and reduce the cost of care.

Integration of this wealth of information will require precisely the tools and knowledge provided by expertise in HDS. In this domain, the importance of big data and machine learning cannot be overstated. Data sources ranging from patient-reported surveys, purchasing histories, and social media activity, as well as the conventional electronic health record (EHR) may help patients to customize and understand their health and care needs, but will need to be sorted, examined, and analyzed to best understand the needs of an individual patient. In the process, healthcare-delivery scientists and practitioners will be challenged to better and more meaningfully understand the personal values and preferences of the populations they serve.

This framework not only will dictate how we understand the needs and desires of individual patients, but will also compel us to change how we evaluate the effectiveness of our interventions. Medications, procedures, and other therapeutics will need to be examined to determine not just whether they outperform standard treatment or usual practice for the population as a whole, but also whether a given intervention—new or old—might actually be especially effective or valued for even exceptionally narrow segments of the patient population. HDS will be central to this ambitious effort.

THE DOCTOR WILL SEE YOU NOW?

In care that is truly value-based, the model of how it is delivered (not just the therapy offered) must be designed and deployed to maximize outcomes and to reduce costs. This has important implications for the roles and responsibilities for every member of the care team. Given both their expertise and the expense of physician time and activity, the care system of the future will almost certainly evolve to encompass a very different role for the physician.

CHAPTER 4 | WHAT DOES THE FUTURE HOLD?

If care teams are designed intelligently and deployed rationally, providers are expected to assume those roles and responsibilities that they alone can uniquely provide. For many doctors today, such a prospect might sound exceptionally attractive. The opportunity to be relieved of the responsibilities of documentation, regulatory compliance, interactions with payers, and other mundane, time-consuming, and non-value-added tasks appeals to an expert workforce at the nadir of professional fulfillment and resiliency. At the same time, however, the prospect of ceding some traditional responsibilities and expectations is likely to challenge these same physicians in terms of their professional identity and autonomy. As the role of the physician becomes more focused, by necessity the scope of practice for other care team members (not to mention technology) will only grow.

Advanced practice providers (APPs), most commonly physician assistants and nurse practitioners, have already assumed an important and valuable place in American healthcare and provide a useful framing to discuss these issues. APPs practice alongside physicians and other professionals in innumerable ambulatory and inpatient practices across the country, filling an important niche in care delivery, promoting safe practice and continuity of care and access.[8] At the same time, some physicians see this proliferation of alternative providers as an implicit threat to their livelihood. In this argument, where payment aligns with the volume of care delivered, APPs will both pull business from physicians and dilute the value of professional care by providing additional supply without changing demand. Some patients also are hesitant about their interactions with APPs, feeling as though they are being provided a different (or even lesser) level of service than they expect from a traditional, physician-based model. Perhaps most telling, many APPs continue to struggle with the uneven degree of autonomy and respect they get, sometimes even within the same group practices.

Ultimately, though, in the value-based environment of the future American health system, these dynamics will change. Where priority and reimbursement is placed not on the volume of services provided, but the outcomes delivered while managing expense, the only rational arrangement is to ensure that clinicians at all levels are working at their highest scope of practice. To ask a clinician to take on more than she or he can provide is apt to compromise outcomes. To ask him or her to engage in activities that someone else can do (at a lower level of compensation) will compromise costs.

However, getting to this rational alignment will take careful study and analysis. HDS should be at the center of these deliberations. The ability to dissect the impact of care model redesign and to truly understand both

Key Point

In value-driven care, all clinicians should operate at their highest scope of practice.

outcomes and the costs of care will require meticulous testing and examination of practice that go well beyond the positioning of professional societies and other interest and advocacy groups advancing a particular professional agenda.

A more intriguing, and potentially more threatening prospect to many, is the extent to which some of the functions of today's physicians and care team might be assumed not by other professionals, but by technology. Advances in artificial intelligence (AI) and machine learning, frequently championed by experts and leaders in HDS, will certainly play an increasing role in the future of patient diagnosis and management. Especially when incorporating data about patient preferences and personalization not otherwise available to doctors, the AI of the future could even outperform many physicians, particularly in the management of common conditions. Contemporary efforts to supplement physician judgment and knowledge with AI have been quite limited to date. However, current algorithms may simply lack the sophistication and breadth of information and data inputs needed to identify and follow the right and most precise course for a given patient.

A fuller discussion of the current status of machine learning and healthcare is in chapter 17, but the determination of the most appropriate role for AI in this context will not be resolved for many years. The next section starts to address some of the broader themes around digital health. For now, though, we need only acknowledge that this will be a critical area of focus for healthcare delivery scientists. However, their work must be both supplemented and challenged by collaborative expertise in fields as diverse as consumer science, mathematics, law, ethics, and philosophy, to name just a few. This is work that will be mirrored in industries across the spectrum, but arguably in none so important as medicine.

INFORMED HEALTHCARE INFORMATION TECHNOLOGY (IT)

How will technology be applied in healthcare in 50 years? It is interesting to ponder how a physician in 1969 might have answered this question. Would he or she have predicted the onset of mobile technology? Wearable apps? The promise of the EHR? This exercise alone points out the futility of anticipating the scope, impact, and capabilities of technology in healthcare a half-century into the future. But if the specific devices, programs, and functionality cannot be predicted, can we anticipate some trends with confidence? As we endeavor to do so, it will be useful to observe the contribution that HDS will make. That not only will help us and the industry respond to trends in technology and computing, but also will define demand for new technologies and capabilities. Seen in this light, we do well to match up the anticipated breakthroughs in computing and technology with the other trends already described in this chapter. In each case, we might better understand the role that HDS will play in managing and shaping these trends.

In the move toward wellness, more devices and technology will emerge that allow individuals to play a more active role in their own health. There are apt to be more tools that enable patients to make better decisions about their lifestyle, including (but not just limited to) diet and exercise, much as a number of commercial products do today. Ideally, these devices will be supported by the science of healthcare delivery, not driven simply by consumer preference and an attraction to the latest bells and whistles.

Technology is already a key driver in the emergence of consumerism in care delivery. The progression to personalized care will be informed by a progressively more refined and detailed understanding of a patient's lifestyle, health, wellness, and preferences; technology; and especially linkage to a patient's overall online presence. The comprehensive profile of a patient in the future will enable a degree of risk stratification and personalization of care that is currently unimaginable, and perhaps somewhat worrisome. HDS, and specifically work in machine learning and AI, will be essential to sort through this morass of personal data in a meaningful way. Of course, the linkage of this information creates new and ongoing issues about privacy and security. These are tremendously important to address carefully. Capabilities in encryption and data security will need to progress at a faster rate than the new technology and at least outpace advances in hacking and online predation.

As noted earlier, the role of the physician and the care team will change in the future. These changes will be influenced and accelerated by changes in technology. The availability of an incomprehensible amount and complexity of patient data will eventually outstrip the cognitive capabilities of individual physicians (if it has not already). In this context, the synthesis and interpretation of such information will need to be ceded either to decision support functions, or they will need to be processed, synthesized, and curated by experts and individuals apart from physicians. In either case, the physician of the future will no longer be solely responsible for digesting a tsunami of potentially critical data in support of the patient.[9]

As the role of the physician evolves so too will the expectations around physician practices. The capability for virtual visits and telemedicine will only expand as the fidelity and reliability of such supporting technology improves. But the capacity to link providers and patients meaningfully across geography could leave physicians finding themselves uncoupled from the overhead and challenge of hospital- or even office-based practices. The prospects are both daunting and energizing to many in the field. Optimizing these entirely new practices will require a deep understanding of both operations and research methods.

Finally: what comes of the EHR? The deployment of this powerful tool has been complicated and one can fairly ask whether the EHR has caused more harm than good to date. While the industry struggles with shortcomings in interoperability, physicians and providers struggle every day with the demands of documentation and access that are challenging the resilience and fulfillment of those in the profession. That being said, it is difficult to see these challenges as unresolvable or enduring, especially as the expertise of HDS and other contributors is brought to bear on the problems and opportunities.

The EHR of the future should be a shared platform accessed by both providers and patients through secure portals. Data are available to patients and providers wherever and whenever they need them, not retained on individual provider servers, together with information from other sources determined to affect health and wellness. HDS will provide important insights into the curation of these data, ensuring that relevant and related data are easily available with sufficient precision and in the appropriate context. In this future state, the EHR inarguably brings value to supporting a holistic view of the patient and her care, ensuring sufficient information capture to generate the best outcomes and avoiding the redundancy and hazards of fragmentation that come at great clinical and economic expense.

The EHR of the future also benefits from HDS through a radical redesign of how providers and others interact with the tool. The portals through which we examine the information about our patients will be reinvented with a greater understanding of human factors and behavior. Efficiency in documentation will not be predicated on faster typing or improved templates, but on entirely new interfaces between the patient, provider, and EHR at the time that care is delivered. Natural-language processing could be employed to capture raw communication at the time of an encounter. Discrete data can be catalogued and embedded in the record, even as the nuance of the conversation is captured and examined to better understand the needs of the patient and the expectations of the provider.

CONCLUSIONS

In this chapter, we have anticipated just a handful of the major trends and changes that are likely to come to the U.S. healthcare delivery system of 2069. We look forward to a system so free of unnecessary risk that personal safety from harm events can essentially be taken for granted. Instead, we will enjoy a system singularly focused on wellness and maximizing health, one in which acute illness and nonelective hospitalizations are not routine, but are seen as avoidable failures. In this future state, ideal or even perfect care will not be measured by adherence to a rote set of standards and best practices, but rather will embrace the uniqueness of each patient based on biology, environment, values, and preferences. To realize these ambitions, care teams will work with new expectations of established roles, but also deliver new capabilities and expertise to both individuals and technology.

As is the case for the metamorphosis unfolding in U.S. healthcare now, these longer-term trends will be driven and buoyed by the expectation and demand for value. This chapter has made the case that HDS can, should, and will play a central role in this trend, driving change and demonstrating value. HDS offers a holistic view paired with methodological rigor and an embrace of collaboration from other disciplines and expertise. But arguably the most important feature of HDS is its adaptability; it not only can respond to changes in the industry, but also can detect, anticipate, and drive those changes. HDS, when directed to solve the problem of value, is agnostic to reimbursement methods (even single-payer care), commercial interests, and political pressures. In essence, it is the fundamentally unpredictable nature of the future course of American healthcare that speaks to the importance of HDS.

Ultimately, the only certainty about the future of American healthcare is uncertainty. HDS offers the promise to not determine the future, but rather to ensure that no matter what the future brings, the healthcare delivery system that evolves is one that is not the product of random chance or ill-defined market forces, but rather is determined through careful consideration of evidence, science, and quantitative reasoning. HDS can help to ensure that the shifts in culture, values, and expectations of Americans will be reflected in our healthcare system.

Therefore, it is essential that HDS be embraced and embedded into not just clinical practice, but also healthcare management and policymaking. The science of healthcare delivery must be understood and appreciated by all stakeholders in the American health system of the future. Training will need to change not just in medical schools, but also in graduate schools dispensing masters of health administrations (MHA) and masters of business administration (MBA) degrees to America's future leaders. The interaction between healthcare operations and research must move from an abstract intersection in a Venn diagram to a way of business in healthcare delivery, practice, and policy.

With a huge portion of our economy at risk, and literally the lives of every American (present and future) on the line, can we really afford to continue to do business in a manner that is irrational and so lacking in logic and reason? The healthcare system of today is the product of shifting politics, uneven and burdensome regulations, a free market, and an economic model with perverse incentives that seemingly only punish the consumer (patient) consistently. Healthcare delivery science offers the opportunity to understand this system and to appreciate it as the living organism that it is—complex, fickle, and at times unpredictable.

It remains to be seen whether the many predictions made in this chapter will come true or not. However, one thing seems certain: If we are to have the healthcare system that we want for our children's children, it will be a consequence of making the smartest and most informed decisions, starting today.

KEY POINTS

- The singular force that will drive the future of American healthcare is the urgent need to improve value— where value is defined as clinical outcomes (quality), divided by expense (costs).
- If the American healthcare system is to deliver value as a means of sustaining itself over the next 50 years, the wisest investment will be in early and sustained efforts to promote wellness and health.
- Healthcare delivery scientists and practitioners will need to address consumerism in healthcare. We will be challenged to better and more meaningfully understand the personal values and preferences of the populations they serve.
- Healthcare delivery scientists can, should, and will play a central role in driving change and demonstrating value.
- Healthcare delivery science offers the promise not to determine the future, but rather to ensure that no matter what the future brings, the healthcare delivery system that evolves is determined through careful consideration of evidence, science, and quantitative reasoning.

REFERENCES

1. Blumenthal D, Abrams M, Nuzum R. The Affordable Care Act at 5 years. *N Engl J Med*. 2015;372(25):2451–2458.
2. Frean M, Gruber J, Sommers BD. Disentangling the ACA's coverage effects—lessons for policymakers. *N Engl J Med*. 2016;375(17):1605–1608.
3. Porter ME. What is value in health care? *N Engl J Med*. 2010;363(26):2477–2481.

4. Reid TR. How we spend $3,400,000,000,000. *The Atlantic*. June 15, 2017. Accessed May 24, 2019, from https://www.theatlantic.com/health/archive/2017/06/how-we-spend-3400000000000/530355/
5. French B, McCauley J, Aragon M, et al. End-of-life medical spending in last twelve months of life is lower than previously reported. *Health Affairs*. 2017;36(7):1211–1217.
6. Aldridge MD, Kelley AS. The myth regarding the high cost of end-of-life care. *Am J Public Health*. 2015;105(12):2411–2415.
7. Henry TA. *Despite APM participation, fee for service still dominates*. December 21, 2017. Accessed May 24, 2019, from https://www.ama-assn.org/practice-management/payment-delivery-models/despite-apm-participation-fee-service-still-dominates.
8. Auerbach I, Straiger DO, Buerhaus PI. Growing ranks of advanced practice clinicians-implications for the physician workforce. *N Eng J Med*. 2018;378(25):2358–2360.
9. Morris AH. Human cognitive limitations. Broad, consistent, clinical application of physiological principles will require decision support. *Ann Am Thorac Soc*. 2018;15(suppl 1):S53–S56.

PART II

Making Change in the Real World— Tools for Healthcare Improvement

HUMAN FACTORS
Considerations for Healthcare Delivery 5

Cullen D. Jackson and Anna Johansson

Cuiusvis hominis est errare, nullius nisi insipientis in errore perseverare. [To err is the nature of any man, to persist in error is of no one except a fool.]
—Marcus Tullius Cicero, 106 BCE–43 BCE, *Philippica XII*, ii, 5

Errare humanum est, perseverare diabolicum… [To err is human, to persist in error is diabolical…]
—Attributed to Lucius Annaeus Seneca ("the Younger"), c.4 BCE–65 CE

Human beings make mistakes—and have done so for millennia—and these quotes caution us to learn from these mistakes so as not to repeat them. In 1999, the Institute of Medicine (now the National Academy of Medicine) included a similar phrase in the title of its call to arms regarding patient safety—*To Err Is Human: Building a Safer Health System*. We discussed aspects of this report in Chapter 3. In this report, the authors take the idea a step further and outline the need for developing healthcare systems that plan for human error by "building safety into the processes of care";[1] that is, designing systems that support healthcare workers in providing high-quality and safe patient care and that reduce opportunities for making errors. In fact, they specifically state that "safety does not reside in a person, device, or department, but emerges from the interactions of components of a system."[1] Since the publication of this report, this philosophy has permeated the medical community, and the community now understands that errors are the result of a multifaceted and interconnected framework that includes humans *and* system features (e.g., organization, environment, tools, and teams) with which they interact. More strongly worded, it is not inherent human fallibility that causes errors, but the interactions between the elements of the system, of which humans are a part.

> **Key Point**
>
> It is not inherent human fallibility that causes errors, but the interactions between the elements of the system, of which humans are a part.

This line of thought also suggests that humans need to learn not just from their mistakes, but also about the overall system within which they work. Again, the Institute of Medicine's report highlights the need for learning systems: "Characteristics of highly reliable industries include an organizational commitment to safety, high levels of redundancy in personnel and safety measures, and a strong organizational culture for continuous learning and willingness to change."[1] While this was a new idea for healthcare, it was not a new idea in general. In fact, other high-reliability industries, such as commercial aviation, have already implemented these ideas into their operations and culture.

In the almost two decades following the publication of *To Err is Human*,[1] many initiatives have been started to create new models for providing healthcare, such as the Patient-Centered Medical Home (PCMH)[2] and the Perioperative Surgical Home (PSH)[3]—frameworks for providing more coordinated and focused care between members of a patient's clinical team and across healthcare systems—as well as new methods and tools for delivering care, such as electronic health records (EHRs), automated medication-dispensing systems (e.g., Pyxis, Omnicell), and patient portals. All these enterprises have had the same general goal—to improve healthcare quality and patient safety—and all of them can benefit from the application of human factors and ergonomics to their development. More specifically, these models of care—PCMH and PSH—deal greatly with the coordination of patient care across different providers and healthcare organizations or units, and the science of teams and organizations potentially could inform and improve the design of these coordinated-care models. In addition, the design and development of medical information systems, such as EHRs, could benefit from methods in user-centered design and usability testing.[4]

> **Key Point**
> The field of *human factors* focuses on how humans use their cognitive, physical, social, and psychological capabilities to interact with the systems around them—and how to design and develop methods and artifacts to optimize the fit between humans and other elements within these systems.

HUMAN FACTORS: AN INTRODUCTION

When the Institute of Medicine published *To Err is Human*, they specifically described the need to apply "human factors" to create a better healthcare system to reduce errors (patient safety) and improve reliability (healthcare quality). But what are these *human factors*?

The field of *human factors* concerns the scientific study of how humans use their cognitive, physical, social, and psychological capabilities (and are inhibited by their limitations) to interact with the systems around them, and then, using this knowledge, to design and develop methods and artifacts to optimize the fit between humans and other elements within these systems. The International Ergonomics Association (IEA) provides a more formal definition: "Ergonomics (or human factors) is the scientific discipline concerned with the understanding of interactions among humans and other elements of a system, and the profession that applies theory, principles, data, and methods to design in order to optimize human well-being and overall system performance."[5]

Complex systems are all around us; in fact, you encounter them all the time (and they're discussed in more detail in Chapter 2). When you commute to work in a car, train, or bus (or ride your bicycle), you're operating in a complex, dynamic system. At work, you are part of a multilayered organizational system, or maybe just on a small team operating in a complex context. Even at home, you likely use technology to interact with friends, colleagues, and people with shared interests over another complex system mediated by technology (e.g., Facebook). In all these contexts, the study of human factors and ergonomics is evident in the way that car dashboards are laid out so as not to steal a driver's attention from the road too long; through the ease with which commuter trains can be tracked via a smartphone app; in the design of a new operating room to ensure optimal workflow for staff and to minimize turnover time; and in the design of a countertop blender to make it easy to use and hard for the user to get injured.

If you have read *Cheaper by the Dozen*,[6] then you are familiar with some early work in human factors and ergonomics. Frank and Lillian Gilbreth are well-known for the advent of micromotion studies, which are designed to understand the movements that workers make during their tasks and then designing better methods for reducing the number of motions, making the movements more efficient, or both. The purpose of this method was not only to reduce the amount of time for completing a process, but also to *reduce worker fatigue*, which in turn would increase job satisfaction and allow workers to perform their tasks for longer periods of time. While much of their work focused on the human element in the work system, the Gilbreths also developed technology to fit the worker more readily, such as a bricklaying scaffold that further reduced motions and fatigue.[7]

Beyond industrial engineering and management in the early 20th century, human factors emerged on a larger stage during World Wars I and II. With the advent of mass production, the need for better weapons systems, and the high demand for combat-ready soldiers, sailors, and pilots, the traditional method of designing complex systems and rigorously training users to understand their complexity was no longer adequate.[8] Therefore, the U.S. military employed groups of experimental psychologists to conduct applied field research to solve these problems and help the military design systems to better fit the human.[8] After World War II,

Key Point

Beyond industrial engineering and management in the early 20th century, human factors emerged on a larger stage during World Wars I and II.

the military continued to expand its study of human factors, and each branch (the Army, Air Force, and Navy) developed its own research laboratory focused on studying how best to optimize the human-technology fit. Beyond the military, the discipline of human factors has reached into all aspects of our lives, including air and surface transportation, computer hardware and software, consumer products, medical devices and healthcare systems, and telecommunications, just to name a few.

Human Factors and Healthcare Delivery Science

So, how do we go from optimizing military lethality and survivability to healthcare delivery science, and what does human factors have to do with it? Human factors and ergonomics constitute the rigorous study of human interactions with other humans and other artifacts within a system and optimizing those interactions to support human performance (i.e., enhance capabilities and mitigate limitations) and overall system performance. Healthcare delivery science is the rigorous study of care delivery to the patient at multiple scales—community, institution, unit, and provider—to optimize the design of the care environment and medical technologies to fit the capabilities of caregivers and patients.

> **Key Point**
> The study and use of human factors can facilitate a better design of healthcare delivery systems.

The study and use of human factors can facilitate a better design of healthcare delivery systems. It can provide the healthcare delivery practitioner with the knowledge and tools to consider the system as a whole, with the human elements a primary focus (but not the only focus) for achieving quality and safety goals. By considering how healthcare delivery system design will influence, help, or hinder the human elements of the system, the practitioner is more likely to develop a system that is responsive to the needs of the people *working with the system* rather than forcing those people to *adapt to the system*. This should not be confused with the need to exhibit resilience in response to changes in the work environment; the adaptation should come from the human-system team working together, rather than the system forcing the humans to adapt in ways that either push the boundaries of their limitations or do not fully leverage their performance capabilities.

> **Key Point**
> Systems should be responsive to the needs of the people *working with the system* rather than forcing those people to *adapt to the system*.

Some examples of instances where the intersection of human factors and medicine have made a difference in the delivery of patient care include the following:

- Using high-fidelity simulation to understand the effects of label design on the safe delivery of medication in the operating room[9]
- Determining the usability and safety of multiple EHRs across multiple healthcare organizations[10]

- Understanding how the leadership style of surgeons (transactional or transformational) affects team behaviors in the operating room[11]
- Investigating the characteristics of a work system comprising ICU nurses working remotely with patient monitoring (i.e., telemedicine) and nurses at the monitored intensive care unit (ICU)[12]
- Building provider and patient safety into the healthcare environment[13,14]
- Using expertise from other industries to develop protocols to reduce errors and increase efficiencies in patient handoffs[15]
- Developing checklists to reduce cognitive bias and cognitive workload[16]

This chapter will not cover all the domains of human factors, as it is a vast discipline that touches on many facets of analysis and design of technology and complex systems. Instead, it will introduce you to some of the concepts and techniques in human factors that you may find useful in researching and developing solutions to challenges in healthcare delivery. These topics include the following:

- **Cognitive errors and biases**—What are they, and how do they influence decision-making and reasoning?
- **Social hierarchy**—How is it formed, and how do we measure its influence?
- **Tools for understanding complex systems**—What are they, and how do they help?

COGNITIVE REASONING, ERRORS, AND BIASES IN HEALTHCARE

If there's something you really want to believe, that's what you should question the most.

—Penn Jillette, illusionist

In this quote, Penn Jillette encourages us to question what we believe. He alludes to one method to debias the decision-making process—practicing thinking about your thinking, or practicing metacognition. *Metacognition is the process of critically evaluating your own thinking or decisions;*[17] it is sometimes referred to as *reflective thinking*.[18]

Key Point

Metacognition is the process of critically evaluating your own thinking or decisions.

To better understand decision-making, metacognition, and cognitive errors, let's start with an example. You're driving your car to an appointment, and you left the house a bit later than you had intended. You live in the Boston area, so despite the fact that your destination is only

15 miles away, it will still take 60 minutes to get there. You have your reliable global positioning system (GPS) active to help you navigate the best route, and it's updating the estimated time of arrival (ETA) in real time. Traffic is moderate, and your ETA is only 5 minutes before your scheduled appointment, so you're worried that you will be late. After 20 minutes of driving, you notice that your ETA has not changed, but you're still worried, so you start driving more assertively (i.e., increase your speed and proactively change lanes to get ahead of traffic). You make every light, and after another 20 minutes of driving in this assertive way, you notice that your ETA has decreased by only 1 minute. This minor success spurs you to drive even more aggressively, and 20 minutes later, you reach your destination *exactly* at the original estimated arrival time. And you're still 5 minutes early for your appointment.

So, what happened in this situation (taken from real life)? While no true errors (i.e., accidents) occurred, there likely were some near-misses (unreported in the example), given that you decided to use more aggressive and risky tactics to reach your destination. That is, you chose to accept more risk, which could have resulted in a much greater delay if an accident had occurred. But why did you make this decision? A couple of things drove this behavior (pun intended). You were anxious to arrive at your appointment on time, and given the vagaries of Boston traffic, this caused you to feel uncertainty with respect to when you might actually arrive, which created a perceived time pressure. However, you were using a very reliable GPS that usually reported an accurate arrival time even under dynamic traffic conditions, so what drove your decision-making behavior? You fell prey to the following cognitive biases:

- **Ascertainment bias/attribution error**—Living in the Boston area and being familiar with driving around the city, you assumed that traffic would be bad and that more assertive driving would be required.
- **Anchoring**—Despite the data presented by the GPS unit repeatedly indicating an on-time arrival, you persisted with your initial judgment that you would arrive late, based on your initial impressions of the traffic conditions.
- **Availability bias**—A recent bad outcome that you had in similar traffic conditions caused you to assume a bad outcome this time, given the saliency of your previous experience.
- **Commission bias**—Even though the GPS unit provided data based on normal driving behavior and showed an on-time arrival, you felt the need to "do something." So you chose to drive more aggressively, which increased the likelihood of an adverse event because it required you to push the boundaries of safe driving.

- **Confirmation bias**—When your more assertive driving was associated with a negligible improvement in arrival time, you chose to use this negligible improvement as confirmation of the correctness of your decision and persist with your more assertive behavior.

This example provides a starting point for understanding cognitive biases, so as to design tools, methods, and systems that mitigate their influence on the human decision-makers within a system. Next, we'll take a step back and discuss several frameworks of human error.

Some Theories of Human Decision-Making

So why do people not choose the most optimal strategy, or make errors in decision-making that often seem nonrational? Put another way, why don't humans use a more rational and statistical approach to making decisions by employing strategies suggested by statistical decision theory, Bayes' theorem, or subjective expected utility (SEU) theory?[19] In fact, researchers[20] have provided evidence suggesting that humans are "intuitive scientists."[19] However, it is clear that in real-world environments in which people are making high-stakes decisions under time pressure and uncertainty, as seen in operating rooms and emergency departments (EDs), decision-makers do not apply formal, statistical approaches to the situation. So, if humans are not using formal methods to make decisions—like defining the desired future outcomes, considering all strategies, considering outcomes based on each strategy, and choosing a strategy based on the most optimal outcome—then what are they doing?

There are several theories that try to explain human decision-making, particularly perceived lapses in rationality. William James, considered the father of American psychology, wrote that voluntary attention (which he also called "active attention") was effortful and difficult to sustain for more than brief periods of time,[21] although it could be extended if the material was interesting enough to the student or reader. He continued to state that "[t]he sustained attention of the genius…is for the most part of the passive sort,"[21] because geniuses will make many novel associations from what they read and sustain their attention using their own interest as a motivator. This thesis is at the heart of the concept of *reluctant rationality*—the idea that decision-making is influenced by the need to reduce cognitive workload, which is achieved by finding patterns in the regularity of our environment, and fails when new situations arise and more effortful analysis is required.[19]

Herbert Simon coined the term *bounded rationality* as a label for rational decision-making that takes into account the limitations of

Key Point

In real-world environments in which people are making high-stakes decisions under time pressure and uncertainty, humans do not apply formal, statistical approaches to decision-making.

Key Point

Reluctant rationality is the idea that decision-making is influenced by the need to reduce cognitive workload.

human cognition—specifically, limitations of knowledge and computational capacity.[22] That is, people cannot make pure, absolutely rational decisions because we cannot apply the rigor required to apply methods like SEU to problems encountered in the real world. Thus, we use the knowledge that we possess that is relevant to the situation, as well as our available cognitive capacity, to make decisions that may not be optimal, but provide satisfactory outcomes (i.e., satisficing);[19] that is, we're only able to consider a limited number of possibilities rather than all strategies or outcomes, as required by SEU theory. Gigerenzer and Goldstein[23] studied this concept by testing algorithms that used satisficing, based on the theory of probabilistic mental models,[24] against so-called "rational" algorithms using computational simulation. They found that the satisficing algorithms using limited knowledge (i.e., some relevant cues are missing from the data) performed as well as, or sometimes better than, the rational algorithms, which either conducted a complete search of all available information or integrated all the available information into one value.

Amos Tversky and Daniel Kahneman expanded on the concept of bounded rationality through their work explaining human judgment under uncertainty, for which Kahneman won the Nobel Prize in Economics in 2002 (Tversky passed away in 1996). Their seminal paper in *Science*[25] summarized several years of work[26–29] that centered on the idea that humans use heuristics to make subjective judgments of probability and these heuristics can lead to biases (i.e., the heuristics are processes that can lead to biases and fallacies in thought). The heuristics described in the paper are representativeness, availability, and anchoring.

The *representativeness heuristic*[27,28] deals with people interpreting probabilities based on the similarity of the current situation with previous observations, regardless of the base rate of those previous observations. Using this heuristic can lead to failures in decision-making under uncertainty, as similarities with previous experiences can increase the perceived likelihood of the outcomes of those experiences.

The *availability heuristic*[29] deals with people misestimating the frequency of events based on the ease of remembering them or with the salience of possible explanations (i.e., how easily they come to mind). Using this heuristic also can lead to biases related to the ease of imagining contingencies or consequences despite their actual frequency, or misestimating the frequency that two variables cooccur based on the strength of their perceived association, even when no relationship actually exists.

The *anchoring-and-adjustment heuristic* (also known as the *anchoring effect*)[25] occurs when people make estimates based on a chosen initial starting point (based on their perception of the problem or some

> **Key Point**
>
> Humans use heuristics (such as representativeness, availability, and anchoring) to make subjective judgments of probability. These heuristics can lead to biases in decision-making.

> **Key Point**
>
> The *representativeness heuristic* means that people interpret probabilities based on the similarity of the current situation to previous observations, regardless of the base rate of those previous observations.

> **Key Point**
>
> The *availability heuristic* deals with people misestimating the frequency of events based on the ease of remembering similar events.

known partial information that gives an initial perspective) and then have difficulty adjusting from that starting point given new data. Using this heuristic, different people working on the same problem might have different starting points based on their prior knowledge, and thus they will reach different estimates biased toward their particular anchor. While it is unclear why people stop the adjustment process, Epley and Gilovich[30] demonstrated that it generally ended when a plausible estimate was reached. Anchoring is thought to be related to the *hindsight bias* (or the *"knew-it-all-along" effect*), which occurs when people subsequently believe that an event was more predictable than it really was based on subsequent information (i.e., the anchor);[31,32] Fischhoff also calls the hindsight bias "creeping determinism."[33]

Bounded rationality and the associated heuristics previously described fit into a theoretical framework positing that there are two cognitive systems that mediate reasoning—System 1 and System 2.[34] Heuristics involve more intuitive processes (Type 1) and fit into System 1, and rule-based, purely statistical, and more analytical procedures (Type 2) fit into System 2; Kahneman introduced this idea into the public consciousness with his book *Thinking, Fast and Slow*.[35] Some features of the systems are as follows:

- System 1 (Fast)
  - Automatic, preconscious, heuristic, associative
  - Implicit, influenced by stereotypes
  - Contextualized, domain-specific
- System 2 (Slow)
  - Conscious, effortful, analytical, rule-based
  - Explicit, influenced by personal beliefs
  - Hypothetical, abstract, domain-agnostic

This framework is important to consider for a number of reasons. First, it enables us to better consider the underlying cognitive mechanisms that might contribute to errors and biases, which then allows mitigation strategies to be implemented. Second, a theory provides a basis for conducting studies to investigate its features, which in turn further informs the theory. For example, recent research has shown that some Type 1 processes may be consciously learned and automatized rather than linked to only evolutionary responses, and that some Type 2 processes may involve explicit associative learning (which can involve more heuristic-like behaviors) or selective attention.[36] Likewise, while it is assumed that the rule-based System 2 generally will provide normatively correct results, recent studies suggest that cognitive errors may result from omissions or errors in Type 2 processes[36] or from their becoming

Key Point

Anchoring bias, or the anchoring effect, occurs when people make estimates based on a chosen initial starting point and then have difficulty adjusting from that starting point given new data. In healthcare, this often plays out as *diagnostic anchoring*.

Key Point

System 1 thinking is fast, automatic, and implicit. Decisions are made based on heuristics, often in a preconscious way.

Key Point

System 2 thinking is *effortful* thinking – conscious, explicit, analytical, and slow automatized and shifted to a Type 1 process through repeated Type 2 error-free processing.[37] Finally, by couching human reasoning in this framework, we gain a better understanding of how the two systems might in fact work together.[34]

So, What Kind of Errors Do We Make in Healthcare?

There has been a considerable amount of research in healthcare about making decisions under uncertainty,[38–40] particularly diagnostic uncertainty.[41] To make the results more actionable and accessible to medical communities, much of this research has focused on clinical decision-making and reasoning in specific healthcare domains, such as primary care,[42] internal medicine,[43,44] emergency medicine,[45] anesthesia,[46,47] surgery,[48,49] dentistry and orthodontics,[50] and nursing.[51–53] In fact, so much work has been conducted on medical decision-making that Pat Croskerry listed 30 heuristics and biases in his 2002 paper[45] and then went on to state in 2013 that "[m]ore than 100 biases affecting clinical decision-making have been described, and many medical disciplines now acknowledge their pervasive influence on our thinking."[54]

> **Key Point**
>
> Numerous cognitive biases have been identified that can negatively impact the quality and safety of care.

Here is a list of some of the cognitive biases and heuristics that have been enumerated in the healthcare literature related to clinical reasoning and decision-making:

- Representativeness heuristic
    - Interpreting the current situation based on its similarity with previous observations (i.e., matching the current pattern with mental templates).
- Anchoring effect
    - Fixating on an initial assessment or estimate and insufficiently adjusting from it in the face of new data.
- Availability bias
    - Misestimating the frequency of events based on the ease of remembering, or salience of, possible explanations.
- Premature closure
    - Accepting an early feasible assessment (or diagnosis) before it has been verified or without fully considering alternatives (i.e., failure to acknowledge uncertainty in early estimates).
- Diagnostic momentum
    - Similar to premature closure, it involves a diagnosis being established without adequate verification and then passed on to others without further examination by them (e.g., colleagues, patients).

- Confirmation bias
  - Selecting data that favors early interpretations and ignoring data that do not, which can exacerbate anchoring.
- Ascertainment bias
  - Reasoning is shaped by expectations based on pseudoinformation (such as stereotypes or prejudices) rather than data.
- Fundamental attribution errors
  - Attributing performance to dispositional causes (i.e., blaming people) rather than looking for contextual or circumstantial factors.
- Omission
  - Tendency toward inaction rather than action out of fear of causing harm to self or others (i.e., "wait and see").
- Commission
  - Tendency toward action rather than inaction, even when the actions have no basis (i.e., "better safe than sorry").
- Feedback bias
  - The absence of feedback is misinterpreted as positive feedback with regard to the decision; this occurs when significant time passes between decision points and outcome data reporting.

While this is not an exhaustive list, it represents a subset of the heuristics and behaviors studied throughout the research literature on clinical decision-making. While many of these heuristics were discovered as a result of laboratory-based behavioral experiments to explain seemingly irrational performance when reasoning under uncertainty, they are still relevant to the healthcare delivery scientist because these same cognitive illusions can influence the execution of tasks in the field as well. For example, in reviewing and analyzing a data set, researchers might be inclined to go with an early interpretation of the data (e.g., the anchoring effect) or focus further analysis on features that support their initial hypothesis (e.g., confirmation bias). So, given that humans exhibit these heuristics and biases, how can we mitigate them to minimize errors that might occur when they are evoked?

How Do We Reduce the Influence of These Biases Within the System?

While the medical community believes strongly in the superiority of Type 2 processes for clinical decision-making,[37] it is still the case that in real-world settings with large patient volumes, time and resource constraints, reporting requirements, and other characteristics, clinicians will rely on the efficiency of Type 1 processes, which for the most part result in reasonable and relatively error-free decisions. Of course, because the two systems interact, System 2 can serve as a "surveillance system" for System 1 and help to mitigate some of the biases that can creep in when Type 1 processes are used. However, because System 2 is much more cognitively effortful to use, it can be affected by inattention, fatigue, and cognitive overload, which can result in errors as well.

One way to help mitigate potential errors is through *metacognition*—thinking about one's own thinking, as previously noted—which can help decision-makers decouple their reasoning from intuitive processes to engage in more analytical processes.[54] Metacognition is most apparent when one finds oneself pondering a particular choice or decision in hindsight, or when pausing in the process of deliberation to consider why a particular decision path is being taken or why a particular piece of data is more believable than another. This harkens back to the quote from Penn Jillette earlier in this chapter—the thing that you believe the most is the thing that you should question the most. That said, it can be difficult to consider if you're susceptible to, or using, more intuitive thinking because it functions on a more unconscious level, which can make it difficult to realize the need to use a debiasing strategy[55] in the moment.

Several specific strategies for debiasing decision-making have been suggested in the research literature. Croskerry[56] described a variety of strategies that he later classified into three categories—educational, workplace, and forcing functions:[57]

- **Educational:** Strategies to inoculate against future biased reasoning:
    - Develop awareness of possible cognitive biases.
    - Train oneself to take a reflective approach to problem-solving (i.e., metacognition).
    - Use mental rehearsal and simulation training of skills to overcome biases in specific contexts.
- **Workplace:** Strategies to use at the time of decision-making:
    - Minimize time pressure to allow more thoughtful reasoning.
    - Get more information.
    - Reflect deliberatively on initial diagnoses.
- **Forcing functions:** Strategies that help constrain the decision space
    - Force the consideration of alternatives (i.e., cognitive forcing strategies).
    - Use checklists.
    - Rule out the statistically rare, but significant diagnosis (ROWS, or Rule Out Worst-case Scenario).

While this list is not exhaustive, it provides a sample of the types of strategies that can be used to try to limit the influence of biases on decision-making through the use of Type 1 processes and heuristics. Some other specific examples of debiasing strategies were proposed by Stiegler and Tung[47] in consideration of cognitive processes used by anesthesiologists in their decision-making:

- Rule of Three
    - Consider three alternative explanations before making the diagnosis.
    - Reconsider the diagnosis if the first three treatments do not result in the desired outcome.
- Prospective hindsight
    - Imagine that the decision you made is wrong, resulting in an error, and consider what might have been missed.

Another way to help mitigate biases in reasoning is to externalize the decision-making process. One method to accomplish this is through communications with colleagues/team members or patients, which allow others to introduce information, insights, and opinions that may be unknown to the decision-maker into the process; Croskerry and colleagues[57] call this "group decision strategy." In fact, through this type of process, Bornstein and Yaniv[58] found that groups could make more rational decisions than individuals.

Cognition also can be externalized through the use of decision-support tools, such as electronic health records, decision-support systems, and cognitive aids (e.g., emergency manuals, checklists).[47,57] Furthermore, in the design and development of decision aids, the human factors practitioner can help mitigate some biases by the way that information is presented to the user (biases also can be inadvertently strengthened through the design of interfaces and interactions, so care must be taken). For example, tools can be designed to present information such that it enables the user to focus on relevant information without being distracted by other data (i.e., emphasize the signal and deemphasize the noise).

So far, we have focused this discussion on how the system influences decision-makers, but we also must consider how decision-makers influence the system. For example, when someone jaywalks across a street against the light, inevitably stopping traffic (no one wants to injure or kill a pedestrian), that person affects the broader traffic system. Of course, there may be reasons for jaywalking (the signals do not account for the pedestrian volume and don't give sufficient time for crossing; crosswalks are spread out too thinly; the person is rushed due to a malfunction on the subway; and so on), but that does not discount the fact that the individual decision influences other parts of the system. In the healthcare domain, one example of this is a surgeon's preferences for using particular tools for their procedures. These tools may be different than what other surgeons in the practice use, but they are effective, and the surgeon is quite proficient with them. However, this causes other issues within the system: These tools may require more training for scrub technicians and more equipment for processing, which adds operating and resource costs for the acquisition of the processing equipment and extra time for training. To mitigate these potential influences on the system, we enact rules, guidelines, and care pathways to try to reduce variations in practice that might affect the system. Of course, in turn, these types of guidelines also help manage complexity for the individual decision-maker (e.g., the surgeon)—a type of forcing function strategy, as described previously.

While this section has focused on human decision-making and cognitive error, it is a fallacy to conclude that failures in safety are due to "human error"; that is, failure purely due to the human making decisions at the effector end of a (potentially fallible) system.[33] In fact, the humans at the so-called sharp end are part of a complex system that strives to conduct high-quality, safe work in the face of complexity (see Chapter 2),[59] and it is an alignment of breakdowns at multiple levels of the system (the latent failure model) that leads to failures at the operator[19] (see Chapter 8). Woods and his colleagues argue that these breakdowns occur because the system cannot adapt to the complexity of the situation, and safety is really an emergent property of appropriate adaptations; they call this *resilience engineering*.[59] This is an important consideration in investigating and designing healthcare delivery systems because it emphasizes the need to focus on more than one level of the sociotechnical system to understand how decisions are made, who is making them, and how agents at various levels of the system adapt. Given that people rarely work alone within complex healthcare systems, the next part of this chapter will introduce and discuss the concept of social hierarchy, which represents another potential avenue for introducing bias, and thus influencing human reasoning and decision-making.

HIERARCHY: WHAT IS IT, HOW DO WE MEASURE IT, AND WHY DOES IT MATTER?

> *We have a culture in the FBI that there's a certain pecking order and it's pretty strong, and it's very rare that somebody picks up the phone and calls a rank or two above themselves.*
>
> —Coleen Rowley, special agent with the Federal Bureau of Investigation (FBI), in testimony to the Senate Judiciary Committee in June 2002 regarding FBI actions prior to the 9/11 terrorist attacks (Associated Press, January 2, 2005)

What Is Hierarchy?

Hierarchy is an enduring structural feature in modern, complex organizations. While hierarchies can function to establish order and coordination, research in corporate and educational settings has shown that they affect both the quantity and quality of information exchanged, thereby constraining or enabling group decision-making in critical ways.[60,61] Status is the fundamental basis for social hierarchy because those at the top are seen as more competent and legitimately owning their status, thereby granting legitimacy to the resulting hierarchy,[62] which is why status is one of the most powerful influences on hierarchy formation. Research in sociology has demonstrated that the information-exchange process in a decision-making group reflects the social hierarchy when the members of the group differ in important status characteristics.[63,64] Characteristics such as a person's organizational role, time in service, ethnicity, race, profession, rank, gender identity, and expertise (i.e., characteristics that commonly differentiate us)[65] can limit the potential positive impact of diversity within an organization or group because they are key to contributing to the group hierarchy. Therefore, while hierarchies can be efficient and functional for groups under certain conditions, they can have real, practical, and sometimes disastrous implications in the context of complex decision-making, which have been seen in many high-risk industries, including healthcare,[66,67] research and development,[61] and national defense.[68] And yet it is ironic that groups with diverse membership in terms of status characteristics can actually produce higher-quality decision outcomes in complex tasks than groups comprising primarily high-ability problem solvers.[69,70]

One sociological theory, referred to broadly as *expectation states theory,* explains the role of group member status in shaping group hierarchy. The theory describes the precise mechanisms by which the status characteristics that differentiate group members produce unequal patterns of interaction in face-to-face task groups.[63,65] More specifically, research in expectation states theory shows that people routinely use status characteristics to form performance expectations, which produce patterns of unequal contributions within the group. Humans use such factors as occupation, gender, race, and expertise to decide on others' competence because of the generalized stereotypes associated with these characteristics. In fact, experiments have created hierarchies to demonstrate the effect of status differentiation for occupation and institutional roles,[71] gender,[71–74] race,[75] and expertise.[76,77]

What makes status characteristics so powerful, and how precisely do they shape a group hierarchy? Status characteristics that differentiate us

Key Point

Research in sociology has demonstrated that the information-exchange process in a decision-making group reflects that group's social hierarchy.

Key Point

Diversity improves group decision making. Research shows that groups with diverse membership in terms of status characteristics produce higher-quality decision outcomes in complex tasks.

Key Point

Expectation states theory is a framework from sociology that explains how and why the status characteristics of members of groups (like gender, race, and organizational role) shape a group's hierarchy.

confer social advantage (or disadvantage) and estimations of social worth,[78] which often apply without limit to scope.[79] Furthermore, all members of the group—both low- and high-status members—hold the performance expectations they generate (e.g., not only do men believe that men are better in math and science, but women hold this belief as well). For example, if team members perceive one member to be especially qualified to perform a task, other team members will defer to that member—now considered the high-status member. Subsequently, lower-status group members become less likely to offer other (sometimes critical) information to the group to aid decision-making and task completion because they perceive the information they hold as less valuable. As such, high-status group members often enjoy more opportunities to contribute, have more influence, and have their contributions more positively evaluated, whereas low-status group members defer to high-status members and limit their contributions.[63,80]

The question often becomes: Is the quality of the decision contribution to a group better for high-status group members, or worse for low-status members? More recent research examining the neural mechanisms underlying hierarchy, status, and task performance have shown that these perceptions of status within the hierarchy, and the resulting performance expectations, are completely contrary to what might actually be happening. For example, Boksem and colleagues created a performance-based status ranking using a time estimation task, creating low, medium, and high status levels to examine the neural basis for approach versus inhibitory behavior.[81] Using continuous electroencephalography (EEG) monitoring, which captures neural activity noninvasively using a cap with embedded electrodes, they found that during execution of a task, a greater magnitude of EEG signal deflections was associated with medial frontal negativity (MFN) for the low-status group. MFN is an event-related potential (ERP) associated with the self-evaluation of performance outcomes, particularly in a social context.[81] Their results support their hypothesis that low-status subjects, in an effort to mitigate the social consequences of poor performance, exhibit greater inhibitory behavior. That is, low-status subjects were more likely to actively monitor their own performance and adjust their behavior to effectively improve performance, suggesting that cognitive function is not impaired for low-status subjects.

How Is Hierarchy Measured?

Expectation states theory also offers a measurement framework for precise, reproducible measures of group structure by allowing researchers to quantify behaviors. Known as the *observable power and prestige order (OPPO)*, it captures observable inequalities during face-to-face interactions using four conceptual categories of behavior. These categories are quantity of opportunities to participate ("action opportunities"), contributions to the task ("performance outputs" or "action rates"), positive and negative evaluations, and how much influence group members have, as indicated by acceptance or disagreement with contributions.[64,80] Researchers use this framework by capturing the communications and interactions between group members during face-to-face discussions, typically via video for later viewing to more accurately code (or assign) the group members' behaviors to each category.

> **Key Point**
> A group's hierarchy can be quantitatively, reproducibly measured using tools like *observable power and prestige order (OPPO)*.

To be used effectively, the OPPO categories must be made observable, or operationalized, so that the group's behaviors can be assigned to an appropriate conceptual category. The OPPO categories are commonly operationalized as speaking time, directives or commanding statements, statements of compliance or agreement, disagreements, and questions. *Speaking time* is a general measure of hierarchy in which high-status group members are expected to have higher rates, and directives are more typical of high-status members, as they are meant to control the course of the discussion.[73,82–84] Statements of compliance or agreement indicate acceptance and are made in response to statements by other group members.[72] Questions are considered passive, and therefore are characteristic of low-status members' interactions in task groups;[72] that is, low-status group members are more likely to ask for suggestions, information, or opinions rather than give them. Finally, disagreements suggest influence because they indicate that the speaker has a differing opinion concerning the discussion and perceives no risk to their status from sharing it with the group. Once operationalized in these ways, researchers count the number of each statement-type spoken by each individual[80] based on the recorded discussion. The proportion of statements contributed by each group member then reflects the unequal distribution of interaction, which therefore describes the group status hierarchy.

In addition to categorizing the types of statements that each group member makes according to the OPPO framework, it is important to consider the content of the statements as they can be nuanced and provide the opportunity for a more contoured analysis. For example, if a high-status group member makes a statement that contradicts information in the group's knowledge base, lower status group members may not question or disagree with the statement even if they know that it is false. Furthermore, high-status members have greater range in the kinds of information they can offer without being challenged by the group. For example, a higher-status member might make a knowledge claim—a performance output that requires synthesis of information and an opinion—which thus carries greater social risk. A low-status member, on the other hand, is more likely to make a statement of fact, something that is already known to all group members, is less likely to be challenged, and carries less social risk as a result.[61] Given this, other behaviors to include in a measurement framework for hierarchy might include coordinating statements, claims of knowledge, statements of fact, and reversals of previous statements. These are all methods that group members may use to contribute to the overall task, and each conveys a different level of social risk, and possibly important nuances, suggestive of the group hierarchy.[61,71,75,85]

Finally, when measuring hierarchy, the performance of the group or team in a given task must be considered. The team performance literature offers a number of tools to measure the quality of teamwork and team communication.[86] Available tools range from methods of self-report to tools for use by observers. These tools are not designed to measure hierarchy directly within the team, but they may provide insight into how team hierarchy may be influencing individual and team performance. For example, the Safety Attitudes Questionnaire (SAQ) includes questions about speaking up, and while it may be an *indicator* of how hierarchical the team or organizational culture may be,[87] it is not intended to measure team hierarchy directly.

Other tools, such as the Oxford Nontechnical Skills Scale (NOTECHS),[88] Nontechnical Skills for Surgeons (NOTSS),[89] Observational Teamwork Assessment for Surgery (OTAS),[90] and Communication and Teamwork Skills (CATS),[91] measure various categories of team skills, such as coordination, cooperation, collaboration, leadership, performance monitoring, backup behavior, adaptability, team or collective orientation, shared mental models, synergy, mutual trust, and closed-loop communication. These tools are designed to be used by independent raters (typically content experts) using behaviorally anchored rating scales for observation of team interactions, either directly or by observing video recordings.

Why Does Hierarchy Matter?

In any organization, group, or team, hierarchies exist. When considering how to modify behaviors, improve processes, and transform healthcare delivery, it is essential to keep this in mind. The influence of social hierarchy can affect cognitive decision-making in a similar way as the cognitive biases discussed earlier in this chapter, so the healthcare delivery practitioner should be vigilant in looking for the influence of hierarchy when researching, designing, and developing innovations for use in a healthcare organization, whether at the bedside or in the boardroom.

For example, when assessing the performance of a healthcare team using any of the instruments previously described, the researcher must

Key Point

All organizations, groups, and teams have hierarchies.

be aware that tools relying heavily on human observations of the system (whether self-reported or observer-based) are particularly vulnerable to contextual influences and cognitive biases. For example, surveys used to measure nurse-physician interactions in the ICU or the operating room have consistently found that nurses and physicians differ in how they evaluate the quality of teamwork, with physicians making higher evaluations.[92,93] When evaluating key concepts such as cooperation and collaboration, nurses and physicians may interpret what constitutes satisfactory involvement and collaboration in different ways.[94] These varying perceptions are likely rooted in status and hierarchy, as well as the culture of the work environment.[95] In addition, multiple nurse-physician relationships most likely exist in the same clinical unit, and there will definitely be differences between clinical units, which further emphasizes both the influence of hierarchy at an individual level within the system and the influence of context between systems. Lastly, while the aforementioned measurement tools are not designed to measure hierarchy within teams, it is ironic that many of the measured dimensions of teamwork and what defines good teamwork skills are the very dimensions that can make teams more hierarchical.

TOOLS FOR UNDERSTANDING COMPLEX SYSTEMS

> *I never knew anybody ... who found life simple. I think a life or a time looks simple when you leave out the details....*
> —Ursula K. Le Guin, from "Solitude", in
> *The Birthday of the World and Other Stories*

Cognitive systems engineers and human factors scientists do many things: conduct experiments to assess interventions to prevent cognitive errors,[9] design and implement cognitive aids[96] and adaptive training systems,[97] and theorize on new models for understanding safety systems.[98,99] To accomplish these endeavors, we must *revel in the details* because most work environments are complex, and we cannot ignore that complexity because it is an inherent property of those environments that we are trying to understand and affect through research, design, and development.

To begin to understand these complex systems, we enlist a variety of tools that enable us to collect data about the system, analyze the data, and represent the information gleaned from those analyses to design and develop tools that will positively affect the system. Given the emphasis in healthcare on case-based reasoning and decision-making, we will describe two incident- or case-based methods to accomplish these tasks: the critical incident technique (CIT) and the critical decision method (CDM).

Critical Incident Technique (CIT)

As described by John Flanagan,[100] the critical incident technique (CIT) is a method developed to define the functional descriptions and parameters of activities conducted within a complex work system. The method uses incidents (i.e., specific situations, events, or behaviors) to anchor data-collection activities (i.e., conducting interviews, administering questionnaires, and making observations) conducted with experts who perform the work functions. Prior to conducting data collection, the purpose (or general aim) of the study must be described in order to further define whom to interview or observe; what incidents are of interest (i.e., they must be relevant to the aim of the study); and what questions to ask or tasks to observe.

Often, the researchers themselves conduct preliminary observations of the work domain to gain a basic understanding of the work, the types of situations and behaviors that occur, and the people conducting the work. An incident or behavior is considered critical when it contributes substantially to the outcome of the aim in question. For example, if a research team is studying how surgical teams respond to an emergency in the operating room, the members might focus on activities and behaviors surrounding such an event (what critical behaviors occurred just prior to, during, and just after the emergency). Conversely, the research team might not need to understand how the nurse manager schedules add-on surgical cases (i.e., this question is not relevant to the topic of interest). This is the key to the CIT—how best to scope the incidents of interest on which the team will collect and analyze data. Once data are collected on the behaviors exhibited during the critical incidents, they are analyzed and reported for dissemination and use.

From an analysis standpoint, Flanagan[100] cautioned that analysis should "increase the usefulness of the data while sacrificing as little as possible of their comprehensiveness, specificity, and validity," which is a good general rubric for all data analyses, regardless of the analytic technique. He describes the need to determine a frame of reference that will best enable clear descriptions and classifications of the behaviors collected. This frame of reference will depend on the general aim and requirements of the study, how the data are to be used (e.g., personnel selection, scenario requirements, device specifications), how the data

> **Key Point**
> The critical incident technique (CIT) defines functional descriptions and parameters of activities conducted within a complex work system.

should be reported (i.e., there may be requirements on how information should be reported), and if there are existing classification schemes for the types of data collected. Next, the data are categorized based on the defined frame of reference, starting with sorting a small number of incidents and behaviors into bins, which helps the researchers determine a tentative set of categories. As additional behaviors are categorized, the definitions of the categories may need to be updated, new categories created, or larger categories subdivided. Once all the incidents are categorized, the categories should be reviewed in the context of the behaviors they contain in order to verify and refine the category definitions. Once the behaviors are categorized, the categories themselves should be examined to determine if there are more general categories into which they can be sorted. Again, the analyses should not take away from the specific nature of the underlying data, so the initial categories chosen might be somewhat specific and granular; this next step is meant to aid in understanding the overall nature and organization of the information, while keeping in mind the purpose of the study.

The CIT has been used in a variety of domains, such as military aviation, air traffic control, leadership, and primary education, among many others. In healthcare and medicine, two studies stand out as good examples of the use of the CIT. In a study of residents' clinical performance in five anesthesia departments, Rhoton and colleagues used CIT via reported observations of anesthesia residents by attending anesthesiologists to understand how residents' nontechnical skills (e.g., confidence, interpersonal skills, and conscientiousness) affected near-misses (their defined "critical incidents") and overall clinical performance.[101] In another study, Yule and his colleagues[102] used CIT to conduct interviews with consultant (attending) surgeons to develop a classification scheme of their nontechnical skills. This resulted in the identification of five categories of skills that were further subdivided into 14 skill elements, for which observable, behaviorally anchored rating scales were developed (indicative of poor and good performance); these scales were instantiated into a prototype assessment system called Nontechnical Skills for Surgeons (NOTSS).

Critical Decision Method (CDM)

Expanding on the CIT, Klein and his colleagues developed the critical decision method (CDM).[103] Like CIT, the purpose of the CDM is to understand how work is done in the context of the actual work environment. The method relies on interviewing experts and asking them to provide information from memory on actual nonroutine

> **Key Point**
>
> The critical decision method (CDM) aims to understand how work is done in the context of the actual work environment. It focuses on actual non-routine events that experts have experienced, asking these experts to reflect on how they made their decisions, and what strategies they used.

> **Key Point**
>
> Cognitive task analysis (CTA) is a suite of scientific methods that help describe people's reasoning and knowledge— and how they relate to the outcomes people are trying to achieve. The CDM is one technique of cognitive task analysis.

events that they have experienced; in this way, it is an incident- or case-based approach, like CIT. However, the questions (or *probes*) used during CDM interviews are meant to encourage interviewees to "reflect on their own strategies and bases for decisions,"[103] which is a major departure from the CIT and puts CDM into a family of methods known as *cognitive task analysis (CTA)*. Crandell and her colleagues define CTA as "a family of methods used for studying and describing reasoning and knowledge ... [related to] the outcomes people are trying to achieve [within a complex cognitive system] ... [by means of] procedures for systematic, scientific examination to support description and understanding."[104]

Using CDM, information is gathered about how an expert approaches decision-making for a given situation, which can be used to develop and improve simulation-based training,[105,106] incident response systems,[107] computational models of human decision strategies,[108] and other systems. The CDM interview is conducted in four steps (known as *sweeps*) that build on the preceding step: selecting an incident, developing a timeline of the incident and identifying decision points along the timeline, deepening understanding of the incident at those decision points, and exploring hypothetical ("what if") situations at the decision points or for the incident overall.[109] For detailed instructions on how to conduct CDM, Crandall and her colleagues provided a thorough overview.[104] Once the data are collected via the interviews, they need to be analyzed, which generally involves ensuring that the data set is complete, structuring the data into discrete elements, identifying meaningful insights, and communicating the findings.[104]

For the CDM, Wong[110] described two analysis methods: the *emergent themes approach* and the *structured approach*. The former is more exploratory and qualitative, in that the data themselves help define the analysis framework, and it may be best used when the domain parameters are not well defined.[110] Using this method, interview transcripts are combed through to find common patterns in the data; these patterns reveal broad categories of information for grouping the transcript data. Once grouped, the data within each broad category are organized into more specific concepts, or *themes*. These specific themes are explored and further structured into a framework that helps explain the key elements within each one. Finally, these structured data are used to create a representation (e.g., a story, graphic, or figure) that explains the thematic concepts in a meaningful manner.

On the other hand, the structured approach is better used when the domain is well-defined and the researcher has some notion of the concepts that will emerge from the data, which allow the use of an "*a priori* classification framework."[110] Wong[110] outlines five steps for analyzing the CDM data using the structured approach:

1. Create a decision chart that illustrates how decisions were made by combining the initial interview timeline with the information gleaned during the "deepening" step of the CDM interview.
2. Create a narrative that summarizes the key information for the incident.
3. Create decision analysis tables by using an analytic framework (such as the recognition-primed decision model[111]) to group transcript data that further deepen understanding of the key decision points, as exposed by the decision chart and incident summary.
4. Identify items of interest based on the study goals and the artifacts of the previous steps.
5. Find commonalities across all the incidents under investigation by comparing their items of interest, which enables the researcher to make better sense of the data and link data from across incidents to possible explanations of the experts' decision-making strategies.

For an example of using the structured approach, Harenčárová[112] provides a detailed description of using this method to study decision-making under uncertainty in emergency response.

Other Techniques

These techniques are just a sample of the methods that have been developed to understand complex systems from the human's perspective. In fact, Crandall and her colleagues[104] list over 100 techniques for knowledge elicitation. Some other CTA techniques include applied CTA (ACTA)[113] and function-based CTA.[114] ACTA actually includes a family of interview techniques—knowledge audits, simulation interviews, and task diagrams—and it was developed to streamline the CTA process for more practical use in developing fieldable applications. Function-based CTA was developed to understand nascent or novel domains and systems with which other expert-centered methods (such as CDM) would be difficult to use.

Finally, several researchers recommend not relying on any single method, given that each system is different and each method provides different efficiencies to the research team and different perspectives on the domain of interest.[104,115] So, when planning studies of complex human systems, be cognizant of the goals and objectives of the research and choose a combination of methods that will provide the most insightful results while conserving the resources available. As an example, Craig and his colleagues[116] used a blend of techniques, including CDM and knowledge audits, to conduct their study of key decision points in laparoscopic surgery.

CONCLUSIONS

We live in a world of complex systems, within which humans work and navigate on a daily basis. In healthcare, it especially is imperative to understand this complexity in order to support workers at the bedside and in the boardroom so they can provide seamless, safe, and effective patient care. Human factors is the scientific and engineering discipline that provides the theories and tools to understand this complexity so that systems can be designed and developed to support humans' efforts to be at their best and limit the failings that are part of being human. This chapter has provided a glimpse of these theories, focusing on biases in decision-making and social hierarchy, as well as on tools such as CTA. This peek "under the hood" of human factors has provided a grounding that will allow you to better consider the human element of a particular system when studying and designing interventions to improve healthcare delivery.

KEY POINTS

- Human factors is both a science (the study of how humans use their cognitive, physical, and social psychological capabilities to interact with the systems around them) and an engineering discipline (optimizing the fit between humans and other elements within these systems through design and development).
- Humans are not purely rational decision-makers; they often use more heuristic decision-making strategies when under the pressures of uncertainty and time. The biases that sometimes emerge through the use of these strategies may be mitigated through training, reflective thinking, the design of decision-support tools, and enlisting the help of others in the work environment.
- Hierarchies exist in every organization, group, or team, and they can provide efficiencies to organizations by establishing order and coordination. However, social hierarchy can negatively affect group decision-making similarly to cognitive biases, so be vigilant about the influence of hierarchy when researching, designing and developing innovations for use at the bedside or in the boardroom.
- Work environments are complex systems, and human factors practitioners use various techniques to understand, rather than ignore or minimize, this complexity to positively affect human work within these systems. There is a plethora of cognitive task analysis (CTA) and knowledge-elicitation techniques to achieve this understanding, and it is generally wise to have multiple techniques at your disposal, as each provides different perspectives, as well as strengths and weaknesses, depending on the domain, resources available, and the time allotted to conduct the study.

REFERENCES

1. Institute of Medicine (US) Committee on Quality of Health Care in America, Kohn LT, Corrigan JM, Donaldson MS, eds. *To Err Is Human: Building a Safer Health System*. Washington, DC: National Academies Press; 2000. Accessed April 15, 2019, from https://doi.org/10.17226/9728.
2. Nutting PA, Miller WL, Crabtree BF, Jaen CR, Stewart EE, Stange KC. Initial Lessons From the First National Demonstration Project on Practice Transformation to a Patient-Centered Medical Home. *Ann Fam Med*. 2009;7(3):254–260.
3. Vetter TR, Goeddel LA, Boudreaux AM, Hunt TR, Jones KA, Pittet J-F. The Perioperative Surgical Home: how can it make the case so everyone wins? *BMC Anesthesiology*. 2013;13(6).
4. Carayon P. Human factors and ergonomics in health care and patient safety. In: Carayon P, ed., *Handbook of Human Factors and Ergonomics in Heath Care and Patient Safety*. 2nd ed. New York: CRC Press; 2012:3–15.
5. International Ergonomics Association (IEA). *Definition and Domain of Ergonomics*. Accessed August 6, 2018, from https://www.iea.cc/whats/.
6. Gilbreth FB Jr, Carey EG. *Cheaper by the Dozen*. New York: T.Y. Crowell Co.; 1948.
7. Ricci T. Frank Bunker Gilbreth. *Biography. American Society of Mechanical Engineers (ASME)*; 2012. Accessed October 13, 2018, from https://www.asme.org/engineering-topics/articles/construction-and-building/frank-bunker-gilbreth.
8. Meister D. *The History of Human Factors and Ergonomics*. Mahwah, NJ: Lawrence Erlbaum Associates; 1999.
9. Estock JL, Murray AW, Mizah MT, Mangione MP, Goode JS, Eibling DE. Label design affects medication safety in an operating room crisis: A controlled simulation study. *J Patient Saf*. 2018;14(2):101–106.
10. Ratwani RM, Savage E, Will A, et al. A usability and safety analysis of electronic health records: a multi-center study. *J Am Med Inform Assoc*. 2018; 25(9):1197–1201.
11. Hu YY, Parker SH, Lipsitz SR, et al. Surgeons' leadership styles and team behavior in the operating room. *J Am Coll Surg*. 2016;222(1):41–51.
12. Hoonakker PLT, Pecanac KE, Brown RL, Carayon P. Virtual collaboration, satisfaction and trust between nurses in the tele-ICU and ICUs: Results of a multi-level analysis. *J Crit Care*. 2017;37:224–229.
13. Alvarado CJ. The physical environment in health care. In: Carayon P, ed. *Handbook of Human Factors and Ergonomics in Heath Care and Patient Safety*. 2nd ed. New York: CRC Press; 2012:215–234.
14. Palmer G, Abernathy JH, Swinton G, et al. Realizing improved patient care through human-centered operating room design: a human factors methodology for observing flow disruptions in the cardiothoracic operating room. *Anesthesiology*. 2013;119(5):1066–1077.
15. Catchpole KR, De Leval MR, McEwan A, et al. Patient handover from surgery to intensive care: Using Formula 1 pit-stop and aviation models to improve safety and quality. *Paediatr Anaesth*. 2007;17:470–478.

16. Graber ML, Sorensen AV, Biswas J, et al. Developing checklists to prevent diagnostic error in Emergency Room settings. *Diagnosis (Berl)*. 2014;1(3):223–231.
17. Yeung N, Summerfield C. Metacognition in human decision making: confidence and error monitoring. *Philos Trans R Soc Lond B Biol Sci*. 2012;367(1594):1310–1321.
18. Mann K, Gordon J, MacLeod A. Reflection and reflective practice in health professions education: a systemic review. *Adv in Health Sci Educ*. 2009;14:595–621.
19. Reason J. *Human Error*. Cambridge, UK: Cambridge University Press; 1990.
20. Peterson CR, Beach LR. Man as an intuitive statistician. *Psychol Bull*. 1967;68(1):29–46.
21. James W. *Talks to Teachers on Psychology: And to Students on Some of Life's Ideals*. New York: Henry Holt and Company; 1899.
22. Simon HA. Bounded Rationality. In: Eatwell J, Milgate M, Newman P. eds. *Utility and Probability*. London: Palgrave Macmillan; 1990:15–18.
23. Gigerenzer G, Goldstein DG. Reasoning the fast and frugal way: Models of bounded rationality. *Psychol Rev*. 1996;103(4):650–669.
24. Gigerenzer G. The bounded rationality of probabilistic mental models. In: Manktelow KI, Over DE, eds. *Rationality: Psychological and Philosophical Perspectives*. London: Routledge; 1993:284–313.
25. Tversky A, Kahneman D. Judgement under uncertainty: heuristics and biases. *Science*. 1974;185(4157):1124–1131.
26. Tversky A, Kahneman D. Belief in the law of small numbers. *Psychol Bull*. 1971;76(2):105–110.
27. Kahneman D, Tversky A. Subjective probability: A judgment of representativeness. *Cogn Psychol*. 1972;3:430–454.
28. Kahneman D, Tversky A. On the psychology of prediction. *Psychol Rev*. 1973;80(4):237–251.
29. Tversky A, Kahneman D. Availability: A heuristic for judging frequency and probability. *Cogn Psychol*. 1973;5:207–232.
30. Epley N, Gilovich T. The anchoring-and-adjustment heuristic: Why the adjustments are insufficient. *Psychol Sci*. 2006;17(4):311–318.
31. Hardt O, Pohl R. Hindsight bias as a function of anchor distance and anchor plausibility. *Memory*. 2003;11(4–5):379–394.
32. Pohl R, Eisenhauer M, Hardt O. SARA: a cognitive process model to simulate the anchoring effect and hindsight bias. *Memory*. 2003;11(4–5):337–356.
33. Fischhoff B. Hindsight ≠ foresight: The effect of outcome knowledge on judgment under uncertainty. *Qual Saf Health Care*. 2003;12:304–312.
34. Stanovich KE, West RF. Individual differences in reasoning: implications for the rationality debate? *Behav Brain Sci*. 2000;23:645–726.
35. Kahneman D. *Thinking, Fast and Slow*. New York: Farrar, Straus, and Giroux; 2011.
36. Frankish K. Dual-process and dual-system theories of reasoning. *Philos Compass*. 2010;5(10): 914–926.
37. Croskerry P. Clinical cognition and diagnostic error: Applications of a dual-process model of reasoning. *Adv in Health Sci Educ*. 2009;14:27–35.

38. Moskowitz AJ, Kuipers BJ, Kassirer JP. Dealing with uncertainty, risks, and tradeoffs in clinical decisions: A cognitive science approach. *Ann Intern Med.* 1988;108(3):435–449.
39. Elstein AS. Heuristics and biases: Selected errors in clinical reasoning. *Acad Med.* 1999;74(7):791–794.
40. Hall KH. Reviewing intuitive decision-making and uncertainty: the implications for medical education. *Med Educ.* 2002;36(3):216–224.
41. Bhise V, Rajan SS, Sittig DF, Morgan RO, Chaudhary P, Singh H. Defining and measuring diagnostic uncertainty in medicine: A systematic review. *J Gen Intern Med.* 2018;33(1):103–115.
42. Greenhalgh T. Chapter 2: Uncertainty and clinical method. In: Sommers LS. Launer J. eds. *Clinical Uncertainty in Primary Care: The Challenges of Collaborative Engagement.* New York: Springer; 2013:23–45.
43. Mamede S, van Gog T, van den Berge K, et al. Effect of availability bias and reflective reasoning on diagnostic accuracy among internal medicine residents. *JAMA.* 2010;304(11):1198–203.
44. Sibbald M, Cavalcanti RB. The biasing effect of clinical history on physical examination diagnostic accuracy. *Med Educ.* 2011;45(8):827–834.
45. Croskerry P. Achieving quality in clinical decision making: Cognitive strategies and detection of bias. *Acad Emerg Med.* 2002;9(11):1184–1204.
46. Stiegler MP, Neelankavil JP, Canales C, Dhillon A. Cognitive errors detected in anaesthesiology: a literature review and pilot study. *Br J Anaesth.* 2012;108(2):229–235.
47. Stiegler MP, Tung A. Cognitive processes in anesthesiology decision making. *Anesthesiology.* 2014;120(1):204–217.
48. Sarker SK, Vincent C. Errors in surgery. *Int J Surg.* 2005;3:75–81.
49. Flin R, Youngson G, Yule S. How do surgeons make intraoperative decisions? *Qual Saf Health Care.* 2007;16(3):235–239.
50. Hicks EP, Kluemper GT. Heuristic reasoning and cognitive biases: are they hindrances to judgments and decision making in orthodontics? *Am J Orthod Dentofacial Orthop.* 2011;139(3):297–304.
51. Buckingham CD, Adams A. Classifying clinical decision making: interpreting nursing intuition, heuristics, and medical diagnosis. *J Adv Nurs.* 2000;32(4):990–998.
52. Banning M. A review of clinical decision making: models and current research. *J Clin Nurs.* 2008;17(2):187–195.
53. Thompson C, Yang H. Nurses' decisions, irreducible uncertainty and maximizing nurses' contribution to patient safety. *Healthc Q.* 2009;12(Sp):e178–e185.
54. Croskerry P. From mindless to mindful practice—cognitive bias and clinical decision making. *N Engl J Med.* 2013;368(26):2445–2448.
55. Croskerry P, Singhal G, Mamede S. Cognitive debiasing 1: origins of bias and theory of debiasing. *BMJ Qual Saf.* 2013;22:ii58–ii64.
56. Croskerry P. The importance of cognitive errors in diagnosis and strategies to minimize them. *Acad Med.* 2003;78(8):775–780.
57. Croskerry P, Singhal G, Mamede S. Cognitive debiasing 2: impediments to and strategies for change. *BMJ Qual Saf.* 2013;22:ii65–ii72.

58. Bornstein G, Yaniv I. Individual and group behavior in the ultimatum game: Are groups more "rational" players? *Exp Econ*. 1998;1:101–108.
59. Woods DD, Dekker S, Cook R, Johannesen L, Sarter N. *Behind Human Error*. 2nd ed. Farnham, UK: Ashgate; 2010.
60. Silver SD, Cohen B, Rainwater J. Group structure and information exchange in innovative problem solving. *Adv Gr Process*. 1988;5:169–194.
61. Silver SD, Troyer L, Cohen BP. Effects of status on the exchange of information in team decision-making: when team building isn't enough. *Adv Interdiscip Stud Work Teams*. 2000;7:21–51.
62. Galinsky AD, Magee JC, Gruenfeld DH, Whitson JA, Liljenquist KA. Power reduces the press of the situation: implications for creativity, conformity, and dissonance. *J Pers Soc Psychol*. 2008;95(6):1450–1466.
63. Berger JM, Fisek MH, Norman RZ, Zelditch M. *Status Characteristics and Social Interaction: An Expectation States Approach*. New York: Elsevier Scientific Publishing Company; 1977.
64. Bales RF, Strodtbeck FL, Mills TM, Roseborough ME. Channels of communication in small groups. *Am Sociol Rev*. 1951;16(4):461.
65. Berger JM, Cohen BP, Zelditch M. Status characteristics and expectation states. In: Berger J, Zelditch M, Anderson B, eds. *Sociological Theories in Progress*. New York: Houghton Mifflin; 1966:29–46.
66. Edmondson AC, Bohmer RM, Pisano GP. Disrupted Routines: Team learning and new technology implementation in hospitals. *Adm Sci Q*. 2001; 46(4):685–716.
67. Lingard L, Reznick R, Espin S, Regehr G, DeVito I. Team communications in the operating room: talk patterns, sites of tension, and implications for novices. *Acad Med*. 2002;77(3):232–237.
68. Marquet LD. *Turn the Ship Around! A True Story of Turning Followers into Leaders*. New Yorkm NY: Portfolio/Penguin; 2012.
69. Hong L, Page SE. Groups of diverse problem solvers can outperform groups of high-ability problem solvers. *Proc Natl Acad Sci*. 2004;101(46):16385–16389.
70. Woolley AW, Gerbasi ME, Chabris CF, Kosslyn SM, Hackman JR. Bringing in the experts: how team composition and collaborative planning jointly shape analytic effectiveness. *Small Gr Res*. 2008;39(3):352–371.
71. Lucas JW. Status processes and the institutionalization of women as leaders. *Am Sociol Rev*. 2003;68(3):464–480.
72. Johnson C. Gender and formal authority. *Soc Psychol Q*. 1993;56:93–210.
73. Johnson C. Gender, legitimate authority, and conversation. *Am Sociol Rev*. 1994;59:122–135.
74. Johnson C. Gender, legitimate authority, and leader-subordinate conversations. *Am Sociol Rev*. 2014;59(1):122–135.
75. Goar C, Sell J. Using task definition to modify racial inequality within task groups. *Sociol Q*. 2005;46(3):525–543.
76. Cohen EE. From theory to practice: the development of an applied research program. In: Berger J, Zelditch M, eds. *Theoretical Research Programs: Studies in the Growth of Theory*. Palo Alto, CA: Stanford University Press; 1993:385–415.
77. Johansson AC, Sell J. Sources of legitimation and their effects on group routines: a theoretical analysis. *Res Sociol Organ*. 2004;22:89–116.

78. Webster M, Hysom SJ. Creating status characteristics. *Am Sociol Rev.* 1998;63(3):351–378.
79. Webster M, Foschi M, eds. *Status Generalization: New Theory and Research*. Stanford, CA: Stanford University Press; 1988.
80. Berger J, Cohen BP, Zelditch M. Status characteristics and social interaction. *Am Sociol Rev.* 1972;37(3):241–255.
81. Boksem MAS, Kostermans E, Milivojevic B, De Cremer D. Social status determines how we monitor and evaluate our performance. *Soc Cogn Affect Neurosci.* 2012;7:304–313.
82. Sell J, Knottnerus JD, Ellison C, Mundt H. Reproducing social structure in task groups: the role of structural ritualization. *Soc Forces.* 2000;79(2):453–475.
83. Zelditch MJ, Walker HA. Legitimacy and the stability of authority. *Adv Gr Process.* 1984;1:1–25.
84. Ridgeway C, Johnson C, Diekema D. External status, legitimacy, and compliance in male and female groups. *Soc Forces.* 1994;72(4):1051–1077.
85. Love TP, Davis J. The effect of status on role-taking accuracy. *Am Sociol Rev.* 2014;79(5):848–865.
86. Baker DP, Gustafson S, Beaubien J, Salas E, Barach P. *Medical Teamwork and Patient Safety: The Evidence-Based Relation*. Rockville, MD: Agency for Healthcare Research and Quality (AHRQ); 2003.
87. Sexton JB, Helmreich RL, Neilands TB, et al. The Safety Attitudes Questionnaire: psychometric properties, benchmarking data, and emerging research. *BMC Health Serv Res.* 2006;10:1–10.
88. Mishra A, Catchpole K, Mcculloch P, Radcliffe J. The Oxford NOTECHS System: reliability and validity of a tool for measuring teamwork behaviour in the operating theatre. *Qual Saf Health Care.* 2009;18:104–108.
89. Yule S, Flin R, Maran N, Rowley D, Youngson G, Paterson-Brown S. Surgeons' non-technical skills in the operating room: reliability testing of the NOTSS behavior rating system. *World J Surg.* 2008;32:548–556.
90. Healey AN, Undre S, Vincent CA. Developing observational measure of performance in surgical teams. *Qual Saf Health Care.* 2004;13(Suppl 1):i33–i40.
91. Frankel A, Gardner R, Maynard L, Kelly A. Using the Communication and Teamwork Skills (CATS) Assessment to measure health care. *Jt Comm J Qual Patient Saf.* 2007;33(9):549–558.
92. Weiss SJ, Davis HP. Validity and reliability of the collaborative practice scales. *Nurs Res.* 1985; 34(5): 299–305.
93. Thomas EJ, Sexton JB, Helmreich RL. Discrepant attitudes about teamwork among critical care nurses and physicians. *Crit Care Med.* 2003;31(3):956–959.
94. Ferrand E, Lemaire F, Regnier B, et al. Discrepancies between perceptions by physicians and nursing staff of intensive care unit end-of-life decisions. *Am J Respir Crit Care Med.* 2003;167(10):1310–1315.
95. Khowaja-Punjwani S, Smardo C, Hendricks MR, Lantos JD. Physician-nurse interactions in critical care. *Pediatrics.* 2017;140(3):e20170670.
96. Neily J, DeRosier JM, Mills PD, Bishop MJ, Weeks WB, Bagian JP. Awareness and use of a cognitive aid for anesthesiology. *Jt Comm J Qual Patient Saf.* 2007;33:502–511.

97. Siu K-C, Best BJ, Kim JW, Oleynikov D, Ritter FE. Adaptive virtual reality training to optimize military medical skills acquisition and retention. *Mil Med.* 2016;181(5):214–220.
98. Carayon P, Schoofs Hundt A, Karsh B-T, et al. Work system design for patient safety: the SEIPS model. *Qual Saf Health Care.* 2006;15(Suppl I):i50–i58.
99. Hollnagel E. Resilience: The challenge of the unstable. In: Hollnagel E, Woods DD, Leveson N, eds. *Resilience Engineering: Concepts and Precepts.* Boca Raton, FL: CRC Press; 2006:9–17.
100. Flanagan JC. The critical incident technique. *Psychol Bull.* 1954;51(4): 327–358.
101. Rhoton MF, Barnes A, Flashburg M, Ronai A, Springman S. Influence of anesthesiology residents' noncognitive skills on the occurrence of critical incidents and the residents' overall clinical performances. *Acad Med.* 1991;66(6):359–361.
102. Yule S, Flin R, Paterson-Brown S, Maran N, Rowley D. Development of a rating system for surgeons' non-technical skills. *Med Educ.* 2006;40:1098–1104.
103. Klein GA, Calderwood R, MacGregor D. Critical decision making for eliciting knowledge. *IEEE Trans Syst Man Cybern.* 1989;19(3):462–472.
104. Crandall B, Klein G, Hoffman RR. *Working Minds: A Practitioner's Guide to Cognitive Task Analysis.* Cambridge, MA: MIT Press; 2006.
105. Geis G, Wheeler D, Bunger A, Taylor R, Militello L, Patterson M. 137: Leveraging critical decision method and simulation-based training to accelerate sepsis recognition. *Crit Care Med.* 2013;41(12 Suppl.):A28.
106. Patterson MD, Militello LG, Bunger A, et al. Leveraging the critical decision method to develop simulation-based training for early recognition of sepsis. *J Cog Eng Decision Making.* 2016;10(1):36–56.
107. Cattermole V, Horberry T, Burgess-Limerick R, Wallis G, Cloete S. Using the critical decision method and decision ladders to analyse traffic incident management system issues. In: Grzebieta RH, Armstrong K, Lewis I, Tunks L, Murray C, eds. *Proceedings of the 2015 Australasian College of Road Safety Conference* (pp. 1–11); Mawson ACT Australia: Australasian College of Road Safety; 2015.
108. Hutchins SG, Pirolli PL, Card SK. A new perspective on the use of the critical decision method with intelligence analysts. In: *Proceedings of the 2004 Command and Control Research and Technology Symposium;* 2004. Accessed May 28, 2019, from https://apps.dtic.mil/dtic/tr/fulltext/u2/a466054.pdf.
109. Hoffman RR, Crandall B, Shadbolt N. Use of the critical decision method to elicit expert knowledge: A case study in the methodology of cognitive task analysis. *Human Factors.* 1998;40(2):254–276.
110. Wong BLW. Critical decision method data analysis. In: Diaper D, Stanton NA, eds. *The Handbook of Task Analysis for Human-Computer Interaction.* Mahwah, NJ: Lawrence Erlbaum Associates; 2004:327–346.
111. Klein G, Calderwood R, Clinton-Cirocco A. Rapid decision making on the fire ground: The original study plus a postscript. *J. Cog Eng Decision Making.* 2010;4(3):186–209.
112. Harenčárová H. Structured analysis of critical decision method data: emergency medicine case study. *Hum Affairs.* 2015;25:443–459.

113. Militello LG, Hutton RJB. Applied cognitive task analysis (ACTA): A practitioner's toolkit for understanding cognitive task demands. *Ergonomics*. 1998;41(11):1618–1641.
114. Roth EM, Mumaw RJ. Using cognitive task analysis to define human interface requirements for first-of-a-kind systems. In: *Proceedings of the Human Factors and Ergonomics Society, 39th Annual Meeting*. Santa Monica, CA: Human Factors and Ergonomics Society; 1995:520–524.
115. Cooke N. Varieties of knowledge elicitation techniques. *Int J Hum Comput Stud*. 1994;41:801–849.
116. Craig C, Klein MI, Griswold J, Gaitonde K, McGill T, Halldorsson A. Using cognitive task analysis to identify critical decisions in the laparoscopic environment. *Hum Factors*. 2012;54(6):1025–1039.

6 HOW TEAMS WORK

In April 2018, the engine on Southwest Airlines Flight 1380 exploded as the plane approached cruising altitude. The explosion ruptured a window midflight and killed a passenger, a 43-year-old mother of two, who was partially sucked from the plane. "'Southwest 1380 has an engine fire', Captain [Tammie Jo] Shults radioed to air traffic controllers, not a hint of alarm in her voice. 'Descending'."[1] Despite the chaos of the event, the captain performed an emergency landing in Philadelphia as the flight attendants circulated through the aisle to make sure that passengers were secure, performed cardiopulmonary resuscitation (CPR) on the woman who had been pulled from the plane, and instructed passengers to position themselves for a crash landing.[2] No one on that flight, including the pilot, had ever been through anything like that. How did that team of people—the pilot, the copilot, and the flight attendants—succeed in landing the plane safely, despite terror, unfamiliarity, and loss of life?

Teams in healthcare are everywhere, and like the crew on Southwest Airlines flight 1380, many must function in high-stress, unfamiliar situations. Nursing and physician trainees are routinely thrown into new and terrifying clinical circumstances and must rely on their healthcare teams to keep control of the situation and keep patients safe. When healthcare teams fail, patients are put at direct risk.

How do we think about teams in healthcare? This chapter will address various types of these teams and the features of those teams, what teams need in order to succeed, what other industries have done to look at how teams function, and where healthcare is in this process. The previous chapter already began to dissect the ways in which hierarchy can overtly and subtly influence how teams function, including the idea of expectation states theory. As this chapter launches into a discussion of healthcare teams, consider how the inherent hierarchies of healthcare (e.g., between providers, between trainees and senior physicians, and between healthcare management and physician organizations) intersect with the urgency of the work of teams in healthcare.

TYPES OF TEAMS

In the 1950s, the Tavistock Institute began studying British coal mines. Previously, British coal miners performed their work deep in the mine, in small social groups that functioned independently from one another. However, after World War II, mining technology changed with the introduction of new coal-cutters and machinery that conveyed coal out of the mine. Now the mining company required that miners work in shifts and focus their energy on specialized tasks like cutting or loading. This new system eliminated many existing social networks, and as miners became increasingly unhappy, the mine saw rising absenteeism. The Tavistock Institute, conducting research on the mines, put forward a solution to this problem. They proposed giving more responsibility back to the teams while still maintaining some degree of specialization, a compromise that recognized the intersection between the mining teams and their larger context.[3,4] In the process, the Tavistock Institute helped launch a new field, the study of how teams work within larger organizations; this led to work on team-member characteristics, the life cycle of teams, and the context in which teams function.[5,6]

Teams are defined as a group of more than two people who join together for a shared purpose. Morgan and colleagues define the concept as "distinguishable sets of more than two individuals who interact interdependently and adaptively to achieve specified, shared, and valued objectives."[7] Not all teams are the same. This chapter will discuss three types of teams, derived from the organization proposed by Kline: crews, task forces, and standing teams.[3] These types of teams vary in how defined their roles are, what sort of resources the teams need, how much the members share a common goal, and how information moves. Not every team is the same.

Crews

In *crews,* the roles are rigidly defined and the team is pointed toward achieving a common short-term goal. Crews have an established way that information is shared. In many cases, given the clearly defined roles, team members can join a crew and immediately understand what is expected of them and everyone around them.

In particular, crews have established and clearly defined hierarchies. The leader of the crew is ultimately responsible for the outcome of the team. The explicit hierarchy and well-defined roles mean that members of the crew have clear lines and styles of communication with one another.

Examples of crews include airline cockpit crews (i.e., captain, co-pilot, flight attendants), sports teams (i.e., coach, quarterback, center), and firefighters. In healthcare, crews come together in the operating room and during cardiac arrests. The anesthesiologist arrives at the bedside of a patient in the operating room and knows his or her responsibilities to that patient. He or she would not begin to perform the operation, nor hand instruments to the surgeon, because these tasks are clearly assigned to other members of the crew.

When crews break down, it is because one of these elements isn't there. For example, each member of the crew needs to have the skills to perform their role. A medical student rotating through his or her surgical clerkship would not be prepared to step into the attending surgeon's role in the operating room. Unless the task is clearly assigned, such as the resuscitation of a patient, a flight to Denver, or an appendectomy, a crew cannot function smoothly.

Task Forces

A *task force* is a team formed to address a specific, common goal; unlike a crew, however, task forces are temporary, the roles are not clearly defined, and the steps to achieve the task are not set. The resources and needs for a task force differ from those of a crew. Much of the time the task force spends together is focused on identifying the individual steps toward the goal and assigning temporary roles for each participant. The direction and style of communication between task force members are not previously established and must be created with the formation of the team.

Kline points out that participants in task forces are rarely included because of their specific skills, but rather because they represent different political constituencies in the larger organization or because they are responding to external contextual forces. Identifying both the skills of participants and the political requirements of each member of the task force is critical to moving the task force forward.[3] Unlike in other team structures, unskilled or more junior team members are motivated and permitted to make an outsized contribution, given the absence of explicit hierarchy.

Given the political nature of participation and the lack of a well-defined path, task forces work through consensus rather than through clear decision-making. Task forces need clear objectives, usually externally derived, to continue to move forward and maintain shared goals.

Healthcare has many task forces. Specialty societies frequently use task forces to establish a consensus about healthcare delivery, evidence, and areas of uncertainty (e.g., multiple critical care societies establishing a plan for necessary research[8]). Small groups of healthcare providers may be assigned to a task force to identify how to improve the care of patients in an outpatient practice or reduce the length of stay of hospitalized patients in oncology. Other task forces are created for political purposes, to give all members of a healthcare organization an opportunity to discuss an ongoing controversy in a clinic or the hospital. In all cases, the overall goal is delineated, but the incremental steps to achieve that goal must be determined by the members of the task force.

Standing Teams

With *standing teams,* tasks come and go, but the team remains the same. The goals of standing teams are more general than other teams, such as a standing committee to hire new staff. Communication is used only as needed and is frequently performed through established patterns, such as at regularly scheduled meetings. The members work together for long periods of time and are defined by their roles rather than their skills; in fact, many members will have similar or overlapping skills. There are many goals and individual tasks, and they vary over time. The absence of a specific common objective makes it hard for these teams to function well, with individual members frequently defaulting away from the overall team and back into their preexisting individualized roles in the larger organization. Standing teams differ from crews due to the long-term nature of the standing team versus the short-term goals of crews (e.g., flying a plane from New York to Boston).

Standing teams in healthcare are common. Most clinical groups have standing teams that meet for payment policy and for operations. Other standing teams, like steering committees for different parts of the clinic or hospital, may have different political objectives. In the absence of routine realignment of their goals with the larger organization, standing teams may become focused on objectives that are in the interest of individual members. Like task forces, standing teams are frequently places where hierarchy is implicit rather than explicit, and junior members of the team may assume outsized roles given the absence of required expertise.

Where do clinical teams fit into these models? We will first get at the tools for teams to succeed and return to teams that deliver healthcare later in the chapter.

WHAT DO TEAMS NEED TO SUCCEED?

Resources

Basic resources for teams often go overlooked. Resources can include physical supplies, like physical space or computer software to facilitate online meetings, and financial resources. Human resources are often the most important need for teams. They may need support to facilitate and coordinate the group, or to contribute actual members to the team itself. Despite the tendency of task forces and standing teams to lack specific roles for individual members, expertise and skills are still essential. For example, if the group will build measures to follow over time, does the group have the ability, skill, and permission to access necessary health data cleanly (but with all of the caveats discussed in Chapter 11)? Does the group need statistical expertise? Does the task force or standing team need someone skilled at presenting to healthcare leadership or at writing clear reports? And fundamentally, do the individual team members have time set apart from other responsibilities to achieve the overarching goal or objective? Does a task force in a hospital assigned to reduce surgical-site wound infections have hours set aside each week to meet and complete its objectives? Does a crew like the cardiac arrest team have time assigned to practicing with simulations?

Organizational Support

How does the larger organization interact with the team, and where does the team fit into the larger organizational context? Does the organization actively identify and promote high-functioning teams? For example, the leadership structure for a hospital could choose to promote high-functioning nurse leaders to a task force designed to reduce patient falls, and they could provide adequate leadership training to participants. Is the organization invested in and interested in the products of the team? Does the organization have any way of measuring how the team is performing and rewarding successful teams? Larger organizations who support teams also create environments in which they can work successfully. For example, a hospital could put members of a team together in a physical location so that both informal and formal interactions are possible.

Organizations can further support teams by recognizing the value to the individual team members of participating in teams. In particular, teams are useful for making individuals feel fulfilled at work because they advance the individual within the organization, they build new skills, and they identify meaning in work.[3,9] Using the opportunities of team participation to further advance the professional development of participants demonstrates organizational support for the results of the team, the process, and individuals.

POORLY FUNCTIONING TEAMS IN HEALTHCARE

If teams are so common in healthcare, why do healthcare providers have such trouble working well in them? To start with, teams in healthcare are often poorly defined. Operating rooms and cardiac arrest teams have clear boundaries. However, many parts of the hospital, such as the intensive care unit (ICU), emergency department (ED), or inpatient floors, shift back and forth between the three definitions of teams, sometimes functioning as task forces and other times as crews with blurry boundaries. Multiple standing teams exist as part of healthcare administration. Different types of teams have different rules, and a constantly shifting team environment makes effective participation in teams difficult.

Compounding this problem, hierarchy in healthcare often emerges from informal roles influenced by status, as outlined in expectation states theory (as described in Chapter 5). Power may come from the defined leader of the team, like an attending physician or a senior nurse. Alternatively, expectation states theory says that other signals may also produce informal hierarchies, such as assumptions about clinical knowledge or ability to function well under stress, or assumptions based on gender or race. Whether team members will speak up in the larger group is influenced by these unspoken dynamics.

Perhaps even more challenging is that sometimes there is explicitly intimidating, disrespectful, and inappropriate behavior among healthcare providers that is pervasive and often tolerated. Openly threatening behavior further stifles the ability of junior or less powerful members of teams to speak up and participate actively. Physicians, already powerful within the group, may be aggressive, demeaning nurses and students routinely and publicly in many healthcare settings. Insidious behavior also comes in the form of passive disrespect, sometimes manifesting itself as failure to return pages or calls in a timely manner, if at all.[10,11] A constant threat of public humiliation or retaliation can create passivity among less powerful members of the team.

What can breakdowns in a high-functioning team mean for a patient? Imagine a patient admitted to the ICU for severe pancreatitis in the middle of the night by a second-year medical trainee. The ICU attending physician is at home. Before she left that night, she told the resident, "Call me about anything," but the medical resident isn't certain what qualifies as "anything." Would she want to hear about this patient newly admitted to the ICU now, or only if he does worse? And how much worse? When the patient arrived to the ICU, he was already severely ill and requiring mechanical ventilation for his concomitant respiratory failure, so the medical resident holds off calling, assuming that the attending probably heard about the patient from the ED. As the hours pass, the patient's abdomen becomes increasingly tense and the medical trainee is having trouble ventilating the patient. The trainee, however, thinks that he should be able to solve this problem. He thinks that if he just understood ventilators better, he'd know what to do. So as to not appear foolish, he decides again not to call his attending. But to get another opinion, the medical trainee contacts a surgical trainee for a general surgical evaluation of the patient's belly.

On the phone with the surgery resident, the medical trainee underplays the severity of the patient's clinical decline, as he worries that the patient is doing worse because of his own knowledge gaps. The surgical resident arrives in the ICU and evaluates the patient. He finds the exam concerning for abdominal compartment syndrome. He is scared and a bit uncertain about what to do next, but worries that looking uncertain shows he's not much of a surgeon yet. To the medical resident, he puts on a confident face, telling him, "This is what severe pancreatitis looks like." For his part, the surgical resident wonders about calling his own attending, but he is nervous about waking the attending surgeon overnight. He has seen this doctor yell at a scrub nurse just the day before and doesn't want to be on the receiving end of that sort of abuse. He delays discussing the case with the attending surgeon until early the next morning. Meanwhile, the hours tick on and the patient gets worse and worse.

This crew of physicians—the medical trainee, the surgical trainee, and their attendings—is haphazard at best. There is no shared goal; while they all worry about the clinical well-being of their patient, they are acting as individuals. No one is willing to signal to higher members of the hierarchy that a problem is unfolding. And everyone is responding to the hierarchy based on the perceived status of different actors in the group. And for simplicity in this scenario, we have left out the extensive multidisciplinary team of nurses, respiratory therapists, and pharmacists, all of whom would be moving in and out of this crew of clinicians. This environment, across disciplines, professions, and departments, makes establishing reliable rules and clear communication in high-functioning teams difficult to achieve. And the patient is the one who carries the cost.

TEAMS IN AVIATION AND THE BIRTH OF CREW RESOURCE MANAGEMENT (CRM)

Other high-stakes industries, such as aviation, have tackled the challenge of creating high-functioning teams from strong personalities with implicit and explicit hierarchies. Crew resource management (CRM) training is the dominant method that aviation uses to train cockpit crews. CRM emerged following several high-profile airline crashes in the late 1970s, including the crash of United Airlines Flight 173, which crashed in suburban Portland in 1978 when the plane ran out of fuel while the members of the cockpit were otherwise focused on what they believed to be a landing-gear problem. Research driven by the National Aeronautics and Space Administration (NASA) focused the attention of aviation on the role of human errors in crashes and harms. CRM came from the idea that interpersonal interactions in the cockpit could be trained and improved to prevent human errors before they happen and to mitigate the effects of them when they do.[12] Using the work of Reason and others, CRM and another method termed *threat and error management (TEM)*[13] trained crews to create multiple lines of defense against error, due both to things that can be expected and can't be expected. The first line of defense is avoiding errors altogether via increased situational awareness. If that doesn't work, the crew tries to identify and manage errors before there are any consequences (so-called "trapping" errors). Finally, if an error does occur, TEM trains crews to mitigate it.

To keep as many candidate errors from occurring as possible, CRM formally teaches crews about human factors, how to improve situational awareness, and how to use varying levels of assertiveness to communicate about concerns. CRM doesn't try to break down the hierarchies of cockpit crews. The hierarchy is necessary. As in any crew, the pilot is ultimately responsible for achieving the goal: a safe flight. But CRM creates an expectation, in explicit language, that any member of the crew can raise an alert about troubling signals or findings. In these instances, the hierarchy is briefly flattened so that all members of the cockpit can have a shared understanding of any dangers or threats. For less urgent issues, CRM normalizes raising questions and proposing interventions that might or would be necessary for a safe flight. In more urgent settings, CRM instructs members of the crew to make "an assertive comment… [that is] de-personal, specific, and may contain brief information to update the others' situational awareness. It will often contain an instruction or solution."[14] CRM has become standard training for airline crews, with broad acceptance throughout aviation.[15,16]

CRM IN HEALTHCARE

Human factors and problems with communication play large roles in healthcare errors as well. Communication problems are at the root of many adverse events and surgical harms.[17,18] However, physicians still fail to exhibit the self-awareness about human factors that could lead to harms. In Sexton's work comparing physicians to cockpit crew members, physicians routinely overestimated their ability to perform when fatigued. Nearly one in three ICU physicians failed to acknowledge that they made mistakes.[16]

As a result, several healthcare organizations have required team training to improve safety and crew functioning. Dunn et al. described the experience at the Veterans Health Administration (VHA) implementing CRM over a four-year period in more than 40 medical centers.[19] A subsequent analysis by Neily and colleagues found nearly a 50% relative reduction in risk-adjusted surgical mortality for patients cared for at VA hospitals that had implemented team-training programs compared to hospitals that had not implemented such programs.[20] Multiple additional healthcare organizations have implemented team-training strategies, with improvement in operating room communication, turnover, and mortality.[21–23] However, several other institutions who implemented team training strategies, often in the setting of randomized controlled trials, found no change in patient outcomes.[24–27]

Team Strategies and Tools to Enhance Performance and Patient Safety (TeamSTEPPS)

In an effort to train teams in healthcare more uniformly, the U.S. Department of Defense, along with the Agency for Healthcare Research and Quality (AHRQ), developed a standardized approach to team training for healthcare called Team Strategies and Tools to Enhance Performance and Patient Safety (TeamSTEPPS). Figure 6-1 outlines the concepts that are addressed in the program, many of which were drawn directly from the aviation field.[28]

> **External Resource**
>
> The instructor guide and other information on TeamSTEPPS are available at www.ahrq.gov/teamstepps.

> **External Resource**
>
> The AHRQ patient safety culture survey is available to the public at https://ahrq.gov/sops/surveys/hospital.

The program begins with the identification of champions and an assessment of readiness for change. The publicly available AHRQ Hospital Survey on Patient Safety Culture provides one validated tool to identify current attitudes and culture about patient safety, establish candidate metrics, and build a sense of urgency. The program then trains the local leaders, who then implement the predefined workshops, featuring simulation, scenarios, and development of unit-specific action plans. The skills are then practiced and sustained in clinical environments and formally evaluated using the identified metrics. TeamSTEPPS and its component parts of team training have been used in multiple clinical settings, including the ICU,[29–31] obstetric care and neonatology,[32–34] and outpatient care.[35,36]

LEADING TEAMS THROUGH CHANGE

This chapter has focused entirely on the internal dynamics of groups of individuals working within healthcare, the intersection of these groups with the larger healthcare environment, and how crews can be trained to

Barriers	Tools and Strategies	Outcomes
• Inconsistency in team membership • Lack of time • Lack of information sharing • Hierarchy • Defensiveness • Conventional thinking • Complacency • Varying communication styles • Conflict • Lack of coordination and follow-up with co-workers • Distractions • Fatigue • Workload • Misinterpretation of cues • Lack of role clairty	• Brief • Huddle • Debrief • STEP • Cross monitoring • Feedback • Advocacy and assertion • Two-challenge rule • CUS • DESC script • Collaboration • SBAR • Call-out • Check-back • Handoff	• Shared mental model • Adaptability • Team orientation • Mutual trust • Team performance • *Patient safety!!*

Figure 6-1. A summary of the TeamSTEPPS curriculum. *(From Figure 6–2, King et al. (2008).)*

function more reliably to prevent or respond to threats to patient safety. The discussion moves to the area of implementation science in Chapter 7, a field that helps us plan for and understand how teams live within larger contexts as we seek to lead change in healthcare delivery.

KEY POINTS

- A number of types of teams work in healthcare, including crews, task forces, and standing teams. The resources and requirements to make each of these teams run well are different.
- Teams in healthcare often have fuzzy borders, which makes creating and running a well-functioning team difficult.
- Crew resource management (CRM) is a formal training program derived from aviation that acknowledges how human factors can lead to errors. One key CRM tool is the flat hierarchy—the expectation that all individuals on a team can call out dangerous or concerning situations up the hierarchy. For example, any member of the operating room team should be able to raise an alert if sterility is broken.
- Do not underestimate the power of unspoken hierarchies, often derived from expectations about power and status, to stifle participation by all members of a team.
- Healthcare team training has been established and refined by the AHRQ and is available for free at www.ahrq.gov/teamstepps.

REFERENCES

1. Haag M. Southwest pilot of Flight 1380 is Navy veteran hailed for her "nerves of steel." *The New York Times* 2018. Accessed May 31, 2019, from https://www.nytimes.com/2018/04/18/us/southwest-pilot-tammie-jo-shults.html.
2. Healy J, Hauser C. Inside Southwest Flight 1380, 20 minutes of chaos and terror. *The New York Times* 2018. Accessed May 31, 2019, from https://www.nytimes.com/2018/04/18/us/southwest-plane-engine-failure.html.
3. Kline T. *Remaking Teams: The Revolutionary Research-Based Guide That Puts Theory into Practice*. San Francisco: Jossey-Bass/Pfeiffer; 1999.
4. Trist EL. *The Evolution of Sociotechnical Systems: A Conceptual Framework and an Action Research Program*. Toronto, Ontario, Canada: Ontario Quality of Working Life Centre; 1981.
5. Steiner ID. *Group Processes and Productivity*. New York: Academic Press; 1972.
6. Tuckman BW. Developmental sequence in small groups. *Psychol Bull*. 1965;63:384–399.
7. Morgan BB Jr, Glicmak AS, Woodward EA, Blaiwes AS, Salas E. *Measurement of Teams Behaviors in a Navy Environment*. (NTSC Tech Report No TR-86-014), Orlando, FL, Naval Training Systems Center; 1986:3.
8. Deutschman CS, Ahrens T, Cairns CB, Sessler CN, Parsons PE, Critical Care Societies Collaborative USCITG Task Force on Critical Care Research. Multisociety task force for critical care research: key issues and recommendations. *Crit Care Nurse*. 2012;32(1):16–18.
9. Hackman JR. *The Design of Work Teams*. Englewood Cliffs, NJ: Prentice Hall; 1987.
10. Leape LL, Shore MF, Dienstag JL, et al. Perspective: a culture of respect, part 1: the nature and causes of disrespectful behavior by physicians. *Acad Med*. 2012;87(7):845–852.
11. Saxton R, Hines T, Enriquez M. The negative impact of nurse-physician disruptive behavior on patient safety: a review of the literature. *J Patient Saf*. 2009;5(3):180–183.
12. Helmreich RL, Merritt AC, Wilhelm JA. The evolution of Crew Resource Management training in commercial aviation. *Int J Aviat Psychol*. 1999;9(1):19–32.
13. Reason J. The contribution of latent human failures to the breakdown of complex systems. *Philos Trans R Soc Lond B Biol Sci*. 1990;327(1241):475–484.
14. Authority CA. *Flight-Crew Human Factors Handbook*. West Sussex, UK: Civil Aviation Authority; 2014:143.
15. Salas E, Burke CS, Bowers CA, Wilson KA. Team training in the skies: does crew resource management (CRM) training work? *Hum Factors*. 2001;43(4):641–674.
16. Sexton JB, Thomas EJ, Helmreich RL. Error, stress, and teamwork in medicine and aviation: cross-sectional surveys. *BMJ*. 2000;320(7237):745–749.
17. Gawande AA, Zinner MJ, Studdert DM, Brennan TA. Analysis of errors reported by surgeons at three teaching hospitals. *Surgery*. 2003;133(6):614–621.
18. Sutcliffe KM, Lewton E, Rosenthal MM. Communication failures: an insidious contributor to medical mishaps. *Acad Med*. 2004;79(2):186–194.

19. Dunn EJ, Mills PD, Neily J, Crittenden MD, Carmack AL, Bagian JP. Medical team training: applying crew resource management in the Veterans Health Administration. *Jt Comm J Qual Patient Saf*. 2007;33(6):317–325.
20. Neily J, Mills PD, Young-Xu Y, et al. Association between implementation of a medical team training program and surgical mortality. *JAMA*. 2010;304(15):1693–1700.
21. Wolf FA, Way LW, Stewart L. The efficacy of medical team training: improved team performance and decreased operating room delays: a detailed analysis of 4863 cases. *Ann Surg*. 2010;252(3):477–483; discussion 483–475.
22. Awad SS, Fagan SP, Bellows C, et al. Bridging the communication gap in the operating room with medical team training. *Am J Surg*. 2005;190(5):770–774.
23. Schmutz J, Manser T. Do team processes really have an effect on clinical performance? A systematic literature review. *Br J Anaesth*. 2013;110(4):529–544.
24. Nielsen PE, Goldman MB, Mann S, et al. Effects of teamwork training on adverse outcomes and process of care in labor and delivery: a randomized controlled trial. *Obstet Gynecol*. 2007;109(1):48–55.
25. Duclos A, Peix JL, Piriou V, et al. Cluster randomized trial to evaluate the impact of team training on surgical outcomes. *Br J Surg*. 2016;103(13):1804–1814.
26. Fransen AF, van de Ven J, Schuit E, et al. Simulation-based team training for multi-professional obstetric care teams to improve patient outcome: a multi-center, cluster randomized controlled trial. *BJOG*. 2017;124(4):641–650.
27. Van de Ven J, Fransen AF, Schuit E, et al. Does the effect of one-day simulation team training in obstetric emergencies decline within one year? A post-hoc analysis of a multicenter cluster randomized controlled trial. *Eur J Obstet Gynecol Reprod Biol*. 2017;216:79–84.
28. King HB, Battles J, Baker DP, et al. TeamSTEPPS: Team strategies and tools to enhance performance and patient safety. In: Henriksen K, Battles JB, Keyes MA, Grady ML, eds. *Advances in Patient Safety: New Directions and Alternative Approaches* (Vol. 3: Performance and Tools). Rockville. MD: Agency for Healthcare Research and Quality; 2008:5–20. Accessed April 14, 2019, from https://www.ncbi.nlm.nih.gov/books/NBK43686/pdf/Bookshelf_NBK43686.pdf.
29. Haig KM, Sutton S, Whittington J. SBAR: a shared mental model for improving communication between clinicians. *Jt Comm J Qual Patient Saf*. 2006;32(3):167–175.
30. Reader TW, Flin R, Mearns K, Cuthbertson BH. Developing a team performance framework for the intensive care unit. *Crit Care Med*. 2009;37(5):1787–1793.
31. Figueroa MI, Sepanski R, Goldberg SP, Shah S. Improving teamwork, confidence, and collaboration among members of a pediatric cardiovascular intensive care unit multidisciplinary team using simulation-based team training. *Pediatr Cardiol*. 2013;34(3):612–619.
32. Nielsen PE, Goldman MB, Mann S, et al. Effects of teamwork training on adverse outcomes and process of care in labor and delivery: a randomized controlled trial. *Obstet Gynecol*. 2007;109(1):48–55.

33. Riley W, Davis S, Miller K, Hansen H, Sainfort F, Sweet R. Didactic and simulation nontechnical skills team training to improve perinatal patient outcomes in a community hospital. *Jt Comm J Qual Patient Saf*. 2011;37(8):357–364.
34. Thomas EJ, Sexton JB, Helmreich RL. Translating teamwork behaviours from aviation to healthcare: development of behavioural markers for neonatal resuscitation. *Qual Saf Health Care*. 2004;13(Suppl 1):i57–i64.
35. Jesmin S, Thind A, Sarma S. Does team-based primary health care improve patients' perception of outcomes? Evidence from the 2007–08 Canadian Survey of Experiences with Primary Health. *Health Policy*. 2012;105(1):71–83.
36. Paul ME, Dodge LE, Intondi E, Ozcelik G, Plitt K, Hacker MR. Integrating TeamSTEPPS((R)) into ambulatory reproductive health care: Early successes and lessons learned. *J Healthc Risk Manag*. 2017;36(4):25–36.

LEADERSHIP AND CULTURE CHANGE

Implementation Science Frameworks

7

Healthcare has a really hard time changing. Time and time again, we see delays in putting evidence into practice. In outpatient medicine, we frequently miss quality targets for care with high-quality evidence rankings.[1–3] In hospital medicine, we routinely discharge patients without needed secondary prevention.[3,4] In intensive care medicine, we continue to fail to provide lifesaving, lung-protective ventilation.[5] Why is this? Healthcare providers are not actively trying to deliver bad care. Doctors and nurses are not actively choosing to fail their patients. Frequently, what may be missing is an implementation path forward.[6,7]

This chapter will focus on two major topics: how to effectively function as a healthcare leader, and how to incorporate the insights of implementation science. These two areas are fundamentally tied together, although they often are taught separately. As healthcare delivery scientists, we are called both to identify the tools of change and, in some cases, the path forward to lead that change. Encouraging change, creating urgency, and inspiring colleagues all will require the building blocks of teams from Chapter 6 to lead a group of people. Implementation science provides us the tools to see a path forward. In this chapter, we add three well-established theories of implementation science to your growing toolkit and consider how to use these methods to lead change.

LEADING CHANGE IS DIFFICULT

Leading change in healthcare can be exhausting and frustrating. We believe that there are three major ways that we stumble, which we will discuss here, although we would caution the reader that this is not a comprehensive list.

Culture Change Is Usually the Outcome of Successful Change, Not the Intervention

When the culture of a health system is problematic, patients, families, and clinicians all suffer. Outcomes are worse, care is less safe, and staff are less engaged.[8,9] This leads many to believe that the best way to improve the quality of care is to try to intervene to improve the culture. While that makes intuitive sense, empirically it turns out that attempts to improve safety culture have been a less-effective-than-hoped-for intervention.[10,11] In our experience, intervening to change clinicians' behavior (e.g., standardizing practice with evidence-based pathways) often *results* in culture change. The culture that surrounds us is not fixed. It changes when forces act on it and reframe the experience of the actors contained within it; by definition, change in an existing culture is an outcome.[12] Culture change, itself, is almost never the intervention–it is the outcome of successful quality and patient safety improvement.

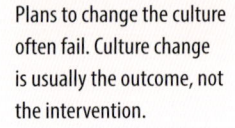

> **Caution**
>
> Plans to change the culture often fail. Culture change is usually the outcome, not the intervention.

Consider the following example. Over ten years ago, a culture existed at a Boston teaching hospital that discouraged junior trainees from seeking help from their more senior residents or from the attending physician of record. The sense from the doctors in training was that they should be able to take care of sick patients, and if they called for more support from senior physicians, they were bothering them or advertising their own lack of expertise. The term applied to this, "being weak," illustrated the decrease in self-worth that junior clinicians incorporated into the decision to seek help.

Junior clinicians not calling for help is clearly a problem. Newly minted doctors, just starting in their careers, are not yet capable of knowing what they know and don't know. These doctors, in an effort to appear that they had knowledge that they didn't have, were potentially risking the lives of their patients. But no intervention to change the culture of how junior doctors confront uncertainty was going to correct this pervasive problem in a durable, meaningful way. Imagine what such an intervention might look like. Maybe the training program would add education sessions or discussions about dangerous trainee behavior. If anything, though, telling harrowing tales of training might make the residents involved seem more heroic. When individual faculty members tried to confront this culture, their efforts did little to change it.

Instead, they went with a completely different intervention. The hospital implemented a new rapid response system, which put in place mandatory actions to take care of patients getting sicker. When a patient had an unexpected, seriously abnormal vital sign, or the nurse or family was concerned about the well-being of the patient, the senior physician (attending) and senior nurse had to be contacted, no matter the time of day or night. This activation of the senior clinicians was formally documented and electronically recorded. No longer were junior physicians deciding if they should notify their senior colleagues; they had to do so and then document what they did. Senior physicians would be upset if they weren't contacted because they too knew what was expected of everyone involved. Following the implementation of the program, and after several years when the entire training staff of physicians had turned over, residents went from saying they would call the attending 40% of the time to 65% ($p < 0.001$), and they felt more comfortable calling their attending.[13] Fundamentally, this external intervention changed the perceptions associated with calling a senior physician for guidance. A rapid response system changed the culture of the training program and removed the negative pressures that acted against calling for help.

We Take On Too Many Interventions at Once

Healthcare providers are fixers. We look for problems and try to solve them. We create series of lists and check boxes and take pleasure in checking them off. As a result, many quality and safety programs become plagued by multiple simultaneous projects. An informal snapshot of a single inpatient medical floor at a hospital in Boston yielded the following simultaneous efforts to improve care:

- New efforts to change how we get patients out of bed and provide physical therapy
- New plans to make sure that discharge medications are communicated to outpatient providers
- Efforts to make sure that families are included in discharge planning
- New data to be documented on discharge from the hospital about outpatient opioid use and risk of opioid-use disorder
- A new patient assignment strategy to minimize the number of patients who are cared for by a floor that does not specialize in that field (e.g., a cardiac patient on a surgical floor)

Each of these points is important. Each of these has champions. Each of these has solid face validity that the intervention should improve care, and most of them have measurement strategies to make sure that there is improvement. Many of these projects have urgency to them. But there is real risk to trying to accomplish all of them at once.

Innovation burnout can be fatal to successful implementation of evidence-based interventions.[14,15] Consider the daily work of a bedside inpatient floor nurse in the United States, caring for six patients. Each patient requires six medications, all administered twice a day in a timely way; each patient should be safely toileted several times a day; and half the patients need to travel to a study off the inpatient floor for 30 minutes each. We have already used up half of a bedside nurse's day, and we have yet to include the time that he or she spends on multidisciplinary rounds

Caution

We often take on too many changes at once. If everything is important, nothing is.

with the physicians, rounds with case management to evaluate for safe discharge, collaborative work with physical therapy, or taking care of his or her own personal care needs like lunch or bathroom breaks. All this can be calculated as follows:

> Medication administration = 6 pts × 6 meds × twice a day × 2 min per administration = 144 min
> Toileting = 6 pts × twice a day × 10 min = 120 min
> Travel to studies = 3 pts × 30 min = 90 min
> Total = 354 minutes (49% of the total of 720 minutes in a 12-hour shift or 74% of an 8-hour shift)

Any change or improvement layered onto the daily workload already has only half of the bedside nurse's day to work with, and that's assuming his or her day is reduced only to these three tasks. (We recognize that the example above is over-simplified, since nurses will often work with other team members such as patient care assistants—but it indicates the challenges of simply adding new requirements to clinicians' daily work.) For nurses and physicians, there is a constant need to increase throughput, reconcile conflicting financial and patient-focused demands, and deliver high-quality patient care. But this also represents the tension of continuing to add interventions and innovations to the bedside provider's work. The result is providers who are deeply burned out at their jobs. Burnout has become an increasingly candid and frequent topic in the medical and nursing literature.[14–17] When everything is deemed important, then nothing is important.

We Overweight the Value of Evidence Rather Than Spend Time Understanding the Context

Caution

A fantastic healthcare delivery intervention is not enough. We have to understand context—the complex adaptive system that we are going to try to change.

How we deliver care can vary dramatically from provider to provider, from day to day, from clinic to clinic. Each of these systems is among the complex adaptive systems described in Chapter 2. Introducing a new healthcare delivery intervention will shift and pull on each of these complex adaptive systems differently; healthcare delivery interventions are rarely like a dose of a medication. When we oversimplify the process of introducing a new healthcare delivery intervention and rely on the power of prior evidence, our interventions often fail spectacularly.

Mary Dixon-Woods and her coauthors describe an example of the power of the larger healthcare context in their paper, "Explaining Matching Michigan: An Ethnographic Study of a Patient Safety Program," which looked at what happened when clinicians in the United Kingdom attempted to replicate the success of a landmark study on central-line infections in Michigan.[18] In the initial Michigan project, called the Keystone Initiative, over 100 intensive care units (ICUs) in Michigan lowered their rates of central venous catheter bloodstream infections with a cohort study design, and decreased the in-hospital mortality in most of the intervention ICUs.[19,20] After 22 months, mortality among participating ICUs was nearly 25% lower for patients in the participating hospitals compared to the surrounding hospitals.[20]

Based on this compelling success, multiple hospitals in the United Kingdom undertook the same project to replicate the Keystone Initiative, but they failed to achieve the same results. Dr. Dixon-Woods' investigation used implementation science to understand why. She found that ICUs with prior experience with top-down infection control policies, individual healthcare providers who had previous negative experiences with quality improvement initiatives, and the role of leaders in the various sites all modified the institutions' ability to see any benefit from the Matching Michigan work.[18] It wasn't enough that the project in Michigan worked. Healthcare providers and infection control specialists had to understand the *how* and *why* of implementation, not just the *what*.

Key Point

Healthcare delivery scientists need to understand the *how* and *why* of implementation, not just the *what*.

WHERE TO START

Healthcare providers (researchers, nurses, physicians, pharmacists, and others) must lead clinical teams every day. But education for many healthcare providers creates solo actors, such as the clinician taught to solve all problems on his or her own. Many people in leadership roles within healthcare, such as department chairs and clinical directors, earned those roles through scholarship and research, their work as educators, or their service to the local microcosm within the healthcare organization, like the division or department. But despite the enormous size of the healthcare industry and the leadership roles assigned to many individuals, we routinely fail to provide the skills necessary to lead.[21] To that end, we propose three critical behaviors for any healthcare leader, from Peter Drucker's paper "What Makes an Effective Executive?"[22]: identify the true needs of an organization; take responsibility; and think in terms of "we," not "I." We introduce these concepts to help build a foundation of leadership skills for the reader, but we also add two more for healthcare: Be clear about your vision, and keep patients at the center of your work.

"What Needs to Be Done Now?"

Leaders in healthcare need to target their efforts. You should work toward one change (or at most two) at any given time. The scope of this change will be related to your role: a medical director of a clinic has a different scope than a hospital's CEO. But regardless, focus leads to better execution. Tied to the question of what needs to be done now is how the task relates to the larger vision and mission of the organization. Are you identifying a goal that is entirely consistent with them? In the setting of healthcare, what is the most urgent threat to the safety of your patients? To the success of your healthcare organization? To your values as a clinical team?

Take Responsibility

As a leader trying to influence change, you need to have a sense of responsibility for the action of the group, the communication that the group receives, and the sustainability of the project. This means seeing new opportunities available to the group, connections to be made with other parts of the organization, keeping the conversations meaningful within the group, and building the necessary infrastructure to keep the change moving, all before leaving the project and moving on to the next cycle.

Own the Idea of "We"

Drucker advises leaders to unfailingly practice saying "we," not "I," to your team. Fundamentally, for some in the leadership role, using the power of "we" runs counter to the clinical structure in which healthcare providers function, which has providers delivering care autonomously. Instead, what are the opportunities to extend the boundaries of leadership, ownership, and management, formally and informally? With whom can you share the success of your work?

Be Clear About the Vision

Making a change, putting in place a new strategy, and leading a healthcare organization in a new direction necessitate clarity in why and where everyone is headed. Tom Lee, MD, the former network president for Partners Healthcare in Boston, writes that "the vision expressed by leaders in health care must convey both understanding and resolve."[21] *Understanding*, in this case, has two meanings. First, we must understand that the providers and participants in this change may have difficulty with a new process or plan. But second, we must also understand that these same providers come to healthcare with altruism and a need to improve the care of their patients. A leader must lay down a vision that integrates both types of understanding with a larger determination about the direction of the organization.

Keep Patients as the Center of What We Do

As discussed in Chapter 4, patients are routinely *not* at the center of healthcare. Reimbursement systems cause hospitals, interested in maximizing reimbursement in a fixed-payment system (i.e., treating more patients for shorter periods of time), to compete against physicians who are paid based on billing for more complex care (i.e., treating more complex patients for longer periods of time). Both of these financial objectives center around individual care encounters rather than a patient's trajectory of health and need for care. Outcomes measured and reported to payers are certainly important (e.g., mortality), but they often fail to incorporate what patients truly value (e.g., returning home, as opposed to spending several days in a rehabilitation hospital).[23] As we lead change in healthcare, we have an ethical obligation to return to the true customers (i.e., the patients), which both increases the legitimacy and transparency of any change that we are hoping to lead.

WHAT IS IMPLEMENTATION SCIENCE?

We turn next to a series of tools in the field of implementation science in order to consider how to move our change efforts forward. All models are flawed, but some are useful. Implementation science is no exception. The term *implementation science* refers to the scientific study of methods and strategies to promote the translation of evidence into clinical practice by examining how and why adoption occurs or fails. Implementation science often uses theories and frameworks to guide implementation design—how can you understand what barriers there are to your intervention? How will you evaluate your implementation process to know whether it was successful or not? But before selecting a framework, you must first identify that you have an evidence-based intervention, ready for implementation. Fundamentally, the frameworks that we will discuss in this chapter provide a common language to communicate these results to other scientists in the field.

IMPLEMENTATION SCIENCE FRAMEWORKS

More than 100 models, theories, and concepts have been proposed, but the implementation science frameworks presented in this chapter are among the most commonly used and found by many to be the most effective.

Many funding agencies are also using implementation science frameworks to evaluate and organize the review of candidate proposals.[24–26] We will discuss three frameworks next. Each has its shortcomings. However, consider each one for the healthcare delivery science intervention that you are undertaking as a potential tool and select the right tool for the job. To determine which framework is appropriate to your healthcare delivery intervention, consider the following diagnostic questions:

- Are you trying to select one of several projects to implement? Frameworks may be helpful to identify which one has the greatest chance of success. An evaluation of success may include which project has the strongest evidence, the strongest advocates, or the most receptive context.
- Are you interested in identifying what obstacles lie in your way?
- Are you interested in knowing whether your project is succeeding?
- Are you looking to communicate larger challenges to other healthcare delivery scientists?

Case

How can Arbitrary Regional General Hospital open its ICU rounds to families?

To examine each of these frameworks, we will use a similar candidate healthcare delivery intervention: the inclusion of a patient's family in multidisciplinary rounds in the ICU. We will consider how each of these frameworks could be used to address this idea in a hypothetical hospital following the description of each one.

Healthcare Delivery Science Intervention: Including Families in ICU Rounds

Let's say that you are the nurse director of an adult ICU at Arbitrary Regional General Hospital. The intervention that you want to introduce is the inclusion of a patient's family when you conduct multidisciplinary rounds in the morning. You work in an eight-bed ICU where the physicians' rounds start at 8 a.m. and are finished by 10 a.m. Rounds include the bedside nurse and the respiratory therapist, when available. Currently, the family is not included. Instead, members of the team may meet with the family later to discuss the patient's current clinical status and goals for the day. However, the family's only current interaction with rounds is to encounter the physician when he or she examines the patient.

Your institution wants to try something different. It wants to implement inviting the family to hear all of rounds, joining rounds as one of the members of the team taking care of the patient. You will ask the family member if he or she has anything to add at the conclusion of the daily plan.

What is the existing evidence for this intervention? Evaluating the level of evidence is an important step in implementing any healthcare delivery intervention. In the pediatric community, parents and family members have been routinely incorporated into rounds in both ICUs[27] and wards,[28] with families more likely to receive consistent information and report positive satisfaction scores, without differences in length of stay (although some senior trainees report reduced autonomy).[29-31] Bringing this idea to adult ICUs is more limited.[32,33] In the current state of care of adult patients in the ICU, there is a substantial need to improve care for patients' families. Many families report inadequate communication with providers, have multiple unmet needs, and have persistent symptoms of anxiety and depression following the experience of having a family member admitted to the ICU.[34-36] However, it's not clear that including families on rounds will solve all these problems. Only one-third of family members in one survey wanted to participate in rounds, although over 80% of caregivers felt this should be offered to families as an option.[29]

Based on these data, you elect to implement including interested families in ICU rounds. You imagine the intervention will look like the following: The patient's nurse will ask any available family member to join rounds when they start. The family will join the team as a part of rounds, and family members will be invited to participate at a given point in rounds, after the plan is presented, to offer any clarifications or concerns.

Some members of your nursing staff are concerned that this new routine will make rounds last longer. Others are worried that listening to clinical information will be confusing and cause anxiety in patients. Still others feel it shouldn't be their responsibility to get the family at the start of rounds, and that they prefer not to attend rounds anyway, as it interrupts their morning workflow. Several champions for this idea step forward in the nurse and physician group and are excited at the prospect of including families, having heard about the practice at national and regional critical care meetings. One nurse experienced family inclusion on rounds when her son was admitted to a neighboring children's hospital.

As you pause to consider these reactions from others on the team, you ask: Is this a good idea? How do we think about leading change among our teams and using this intervention?

Frameworks

In the next several sections, we will outline three frameworks from implementation science: the Consolidated Framework for Implementation Research (CFIR), the Promoting Action on Research Implementation in Health Services (PARiHS) model, and RE-AIM. We will return to the family-on-rounds intervention following the discussion of the individual frameworks and see how they can be helpful.

Consolidated Framework for Implementation Research (CFIR)

CFIR is a consolidation of a number of different implementation frameworks that was developed through a systematic review process. It can be viewed as a summary of many different frameworks. CFIR is often very applicable to organizational interventions compared to other frameworks that may focus on individual behavioral interventions. CFIR has five domains, described next. In general, this framework is most useful when seeking to identify the obstacles and advantages of implementing your proposed intervention.[37]

Intervention

The *intervention* encompasses the core details and elements of the evidence-based practice to be implemented. Included as part of the assessment of the intervention are the following:

- Where the intervention comes from (e.g., is it derived from a colleague in the organization, or imported from an external source, or from somewhere else?)
- How likely stakeholders are to anticipate the success of the intervention
- Whether the intervention has an advantage over other possible interventions
- If the intervention can be piloted on a smaller scale
- How difficult the intervention appears
- The perceived costs, including opportunity costs, of the intervention

Outer Setting

The *outer setting* is the larger context in which the project will take place. This includes elements like the political, economic, and financing environments for a healthcare delivery intervention. The outer setting also includes how engaged stakeholders are with other external organizations and, similarly, how many other similar organizations may be competing in the clinical area of the intervention.

Inner Setting

The *inner setting* represents the local, specific context for the intervention, such as a hospital or a clinic; it can encompass a wide range of themes and concepts. This might include the culture of an organization, its willingness to change and readiness to do so, the informal and formal networks contained within it, and the characteristics of the organization itself, like its maturity.

Individuals

The *individuals* are the stakeholders themselves, particularly those involved in the project, as well as their characteristics. Examples include the individuals' understanding of the intervention itself, including their beliefs and knowledge; their perception of the larger organization; and their willingness and readiness for change.

Implementation Process

The final element is the *implementation process* itself, by which the intervention will be carried out. This concept becomes more of a planning tool for the on-the-ground performance of the intervention itself. Regular steps of the implementation process include planning, engaging the stakeholders, carrying out the plan, and evaluation.

CFIR is particularly useful in organizing the range of potential obstacles standing in the way of a new intervention. Its shortcomings include relegating the evaluation of the implementation to a subtheme without substantial weight, failing to incorporate a method of adapting to unexpected forces inside or outside the organization, a recognition that there may be a gap between the expected results and the true results, and a plan for sustainability if the intervention is a success.

PARiHS (Promoting Action on Research Implementation in Health Services)

PARiHS[38-42] relies on three dominant drivers to understand successful implementation of evidence-based strategies: evidence, context, and facilitation. Taken together, these are the three elements of successful implementation, described in equation format as follows:

$$SI = f(E,C,F)$$

where SI = successful implementation, E = evidence, C = context, and F = facilitation, and f() is read "is a function of."

Evidence is described as knowledge that is agreed upon by multiple stakeholders. In PARiHS, it can include local knowledge or scientifically derived knowledge, and guidance is not provided on ranking or priorities of these two types of evidence. *Context* is the setting in which the intervention will be implemented. Here, this concept incorporates broad understanding of the culture, the capacity of providers, the larger organization, and any environment for the intervention. *Facilitation* is the method by which the team will be supported to carry out the work. This includes how to identify the key stakeholders, clarity of the question to be

> **Key Point**
>
> The PARiHS framework asserts that successful implementation is a function of only three things: strength of evidence, the context in which the implementation is carried out, and facilitation strategies.

answered, any understanding of the process and how it will change, measurement to identifying a meaningful change, and integration of success in existing processes.

The PARiHS model incorporates the diagnostic part of implementation (evidence and context) and the therapeutic part (facilitation) into a single model and knits together enormous concepts under broad labels (e.g., including the physical, social, cultural, structural, systematic, and professional contexts under one general heading). The model itself has several limitations, and although it has been used in different clinical settings and across different countries, it still has the following disadvantages[43–46]:

- There is no definition of *successful implementation.*
- The quality of evidence is neither defined nor required.
- Facilitation remains largely underdefined, lacking more clearly developed candidate strategies for success.

RE-AIM

RE-AIM is particularly useful as a tool to understand if we've been successful in our efforts at implementing change. Its name stands for *Reach, Effectiveness, Adoption, Implementation,* and *Maintenance.* Each of these elements can be transformed into candidate outcomes, as explored next.[47]

Reach

Reach describes both the number of participants in any given intervention and how well the participants represent who they are meant to represent. You can use Reach to consider whether the implementation of your project affected the people of interest. Examples might include:

- What proportion of diabetics in your city received an invitation to participate in a new public health intervention designed to improve diet in diabetics?
- What proportion of patients responded to your office-based health questionnaire?
- How many nurses, out of all emergency department (ED) nurses, attended the simulation-based training session you conducted?
- How many patients and families agreed to be part of your new patient-and-family advisory council, out of the total who were asked?

Critical to Reach is also understanding how the patients, providers, families, and other respondents represent the larger population from which they are drawn. In the examples given here, did only female patients respond? Did ED nurses come to the training only if they were scheduled for the day shift? Did the patients and families who agreed to participate in the advisory council also include members of underrepresented or disenfranchised groups that your hospital serves? Critical to getting Reach right is checking whether there is a difference between those you reach and those you typically serve.

Effectiveness or Efficacy

Critical to determining the success of any intervention, the *efficacy* (the performance of your intervention in the idealized state) and *effectiveness* (the performance of your intervention in real-world conditions) are reported at the level of the individual (the patient, the family, the provider, etc.). To examine the efficacy or effectiveness, the healthcare delivery scientist needs to establish a meaningful effect size and identify outcomes of interest, as you would with any of the methods described in Part III of this book. Of note, the evaluation should also include balancing outcomes that highlight possible negative consequences or unintended outcomes that might result from your intervention.

Adoption

Adoption describes how many locations, sites, or individuals have implemented your program. Similar to Reach, this can be reported as proportions or numbers, but should extend beyond the individuals involved. As an example, if an office's scheduling tool is introduced to multiple primary-care offices to establish same-day office visits for patients, which practices choose to adopt this intervention? Also similar to Reach is the importance of studying the differences between the adopting and non-adopting groups in order to fully understand the representativeness and explanations behind any variation of adoption.

Implementation

Recognizing that any protocol or plan may not be implemented in the exact way you intend, *implementation* is useful for understanding the difference between the intended plan and the real-world implementation of it. This concept also includes the costs and time that implementation requires. Continuing from the previous example, where you are thinking of creating a patient and family advisory council for your hospital, what would that council actually look like? How much staff time would it require to put in place? What were the key elements you would use, as compared with other models in the literature?

Maintenance

Maintenance is critical to understanding the longevity of your change in healthcare delivery. You can measure this at a system level or at an individual level. Maintenance is a vastly underreported feature of most protocols and interventions. Maintenance of interventions is rarely described; it may include how to sustain quality improvement interventions, changes in processes of care, or alterations in systems of care delivery.

We would recommend considering RE-AIM as a helpful model to understand how well your intervention is succeeding or failing, guiding the development of a range of outcomes rather than assisting with the identification of barriers or accelerators of success. Additionally, RE-AIM may help you decide where to focus your resources. For example, if your intervention reaches 90% of potential patients and has 90% efficacy, but only has 5% adoption, you are likely to have more impact by working to improve adoption than by trying to achieve perfect reach or efficacy.

A Working Example: Returning to Family-on-Rounds

Let us return to our intervention, to include patients' families on rounds in our ICU. In Figure 7-1, we have used CFIR and RE-AIM to clarify our implementation challenges.

CFIR brings to the foreground the issues and obstacles around getting families on ICU work rounds implemented. You will notice that the CFIR illuminates challenges around the willingness of our providers to try something new and acknowledges that this may be influenced both by the institution's willingness to change and its larger knowledge base about other ICUs in the region, including families on ICU work rounds. But where does it fall short? CFIR does include the implementation process, but little involves the measurement of success or the maintenance of work. It does not help us to identify any expected gap between ideal and real-world implementation. It fails to acknowledge that not all the new ideas implemented in healthcare delivery will be successful or helpful, and CFIR fails to give us any tools to know when our project isn't actually helping patients and families.

What about RE-AIM? This model picks up where CFIR leaves off, offering several guiding areas for outcome development and allowing us to have ways to find out if poor participation represents poor representation. If we have only a few families participating in rounds, is this because not all types of nurses are inviting them at the start of rounds, or maybe because younger nurses don't feel comfortable doing so? Is low participation because of nursing concerns, or because only families with adult children feel comfortable participating? Or are families not available at the time of work rounds, so there is no one to invite? RE-AIM gets to the

CHAPTER 7 | LEADERSHIP AND CULTURE CHANGE

CFIR

Inner Setting: Are there particular groups of clinicians or ICUs that are more receptive to including families on rounds?

Outer Setting: Have providers heard about families on rounds at national meetings?

Current Care: Families isolated from rounds

Improved Care: Families included on rounds

Implementation Process: What change is needed to involve families reliably on rounds?

Individuals: What are clinicians' attitudes about including families?

Intervention: How are families included on rounds?

Re-AIM

Reach: What proportion of ICU nurses participated in education about families on rounds?

Effectiveness: By how much does including families on rounds reduce family stress in the ICU?

Adoption: What proportion of nurses/physicians invited available families to rounds?

Implementation: How much time was spent training clinicians on including families in rounds?

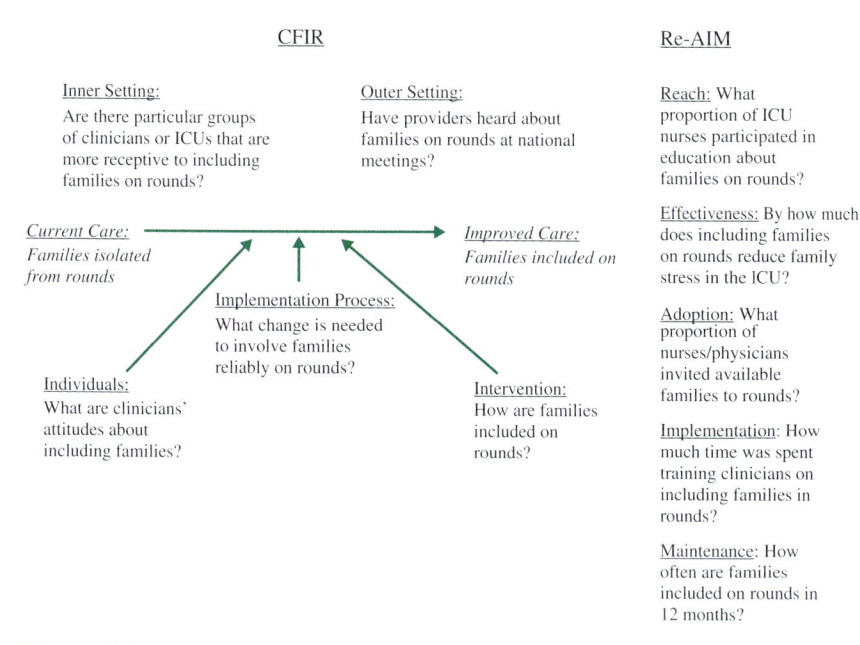

Maintenance: How often are families included on rounds in 12 months?

Figure 7-1 • An illustration of two implementation science frameworks: CFIR and RE-AIM, as applied to a hypothetical project to integrate families into rounds in the ICU. CFIR is useful for understanding the barriers and facilitators for a new project, while RE-AIM is useful to identify outcomes of interest.

bottom of this. But to design these measures and outcomes in advance, we need to have some understanding of the individuals, their characteristics, their culture and motivation, and their concerns and understanding of the literature—something absent in RE-AIM by itself.

However, we can knit together our findings from CFIR and RE-AIM to see how PARiHS can be helpful to us. We've already identified key external *evidence* about the usefulness and value of our intervention,[48–50] but we would now want to focus on how our stakeholders view and interpret that evidence. Do they find the pediatric literature useful, or is it too different from their work environment to be helpful? Does the narrative of your ICU nurse with personal experience of families on rounds in a pediatric environment change how the evidence is evaluated locally?

Our investigation into CFIR has helped us clarify the *context* in which we will be working. What are the cultural, local, institutional, and community constraints to our context? Is our ICU part of a close-knit community, where families are generally known to the providers and live locally? Or are we at a tertiary care center, where the families must travel and are unlikely to visit in the morning during business hours? Do we work in an ICU that has tried new, quality-focused interventions in the past? Do we view families as part of the team?

Finally, *facilitation* of our intervention gives us some time and space to reflect on the details of the intervention process, albeit an exceedingly large topic to tackle. Have we identified key stakeholders who want to lead local change? Do we know who the opinion leaders are? Do we plan to pilot this intervention or just start? What is our process?

Wrap-up: Implementation Science Frameworks

While we have described their shortcomings, consider each of these frameworks to be new tools in your healthcare delivery science toolkit. To identify the right tool, ask these questions:

- Do I need to understand the facilitators and barriers to implementation? → Consider CFIR
- How will I know if I succeed, fail, and reach the right people? → Consider RE-AIM
- How will I know if my intervention lasts? → Consider RE-AIM
- How can I think about the implementation of the process itself? → Consider PARiHS

Key Point

Use implementation science frameworks as they are useful to your intervention.

Further, despite the various theorists and extensive literature that underpin the implementation science models, knit together models to solve different problems—a technique accepted by many implementation science authors.

INTEGRATING IMPLEMENTATION SCIENCE FRAMEWORKS FOR THE PURPOSE OF CHANGE MANAGEMENT

Change management represents the process of moving from the current state to the necessary future state. Outside healthcare, the literature incorporates planned change management—moving between two fixed states—and emergent change management, which focuses on the dynamic interactions between context and processes within organizations. Implementation science frameworks give us the architecture and language to discuss both states.

Central to planned change management is the work of Kurt Lewin, which frames change management in three parts: unfreezing the current system, moving toward the future state, and then refreezing the system in the new state.[51] Integrating the implementation science work we've already done, we can use CFIR to understand the current healthcare organization, care unit, or healthcare practice, and then to recognize the organizational, cultural, and individual barriers to change. To move toward change, we can engage the PARHiS structure to build out the details of the implementation strategy, and RE-AIM to measure our success or failure. Finally, when we arrive at refreezing in the new state, we can engage RE-AIM to ensure that we maintain the ground we've made.

Fundamentally, however, these and other approaches to change management within healthcare necessitate studying, accommodating, and influencing all levels of the system. Perhaps most important, there are no reliable formulas for initiating, leading, and sustaining all change. This returns us to where we started in this chapter: In healthcare, change is hard, but necessary.

The next chapter will delve deeply into the implementation strategy of any framework, describing in detail some methods and tools for improvement. Consider, as you acquire this next set of tools, how each of these elements is layered with each other, from the overall planning process and vision to the detailed, daily strategies for change.

KEY POINTS

- Leading change in healthcare is a hard task.
- Healthcare delivery interventions are the equivalent of giving a new medication to a healthcare system. Context is important.
- Elements essential to effective leadership include: establish urgency and focus; take and demonstrate responsibility; live with "we," not "I"; establish and promote vision; and keep patients at the center of all healthcare work.
- Integrate implementation science frameworks to understand how to put new healthcare delivery interventions in place and communicate that process to other scientists.
- The three major implementation science frameworks can be used for different needs. Refer to our diagnostic questions to determine which one makes sense for the challenge ahead.

REFERENCES

1. Boyd CM, Darer J, Boult C, Fried LP, Boult L, Wu AW. Clinical practice guidelines and quality of care for older patients with multiple comorbid diseases: implications for pay for performance. *JAMA*. 2005;294(6):716–724.
2. Fonarow GC, Yancy CW, Heywood JT; ADHERE Scientific Advisory Committee; Study Group, and Investigators. Adherence to heart failure quality-of-care

indicators in US hospitals: analysis of the ADHERE Registry. *Arch Intern Med.* 2005;165(13):1469–1477.
3. Jencks SF, Cuerdon T, Burwen DR, et al. Quality of medical care delivered to Medicare beneficiaries: A profile at state and national levels. *JAMA.* 2000;284(13):1670–1676.
4. McGlynn EA, Asch SM, Adams J, et al. The quality of health care delivered to adults in the United States. *N Engl J Med.* 2003;348(26):2635–2645.
5. Bellani G, Laffey JG, Pham T, et al. Epidemiology, patterns of care, and mortality for patients with acute respiratory distress syndrome in intensive care units in 50 countries. *JAMA.* 2016;315(8):788–800.
6. Shekelle PG, Pronovost PJ, Wachter RM, et al. Advancing the science of patient safety. *Ann Intern Med.* 2011;154(10):693–696.
7. Auerbach AD, Landefeld CS, Shojania KG. The tension between needing to improve care and knowing how to do it. *N Engl J Med.* 2007;357(6):608–613.
8. DiCuccio MH. The relationship between patient safety culture and patient outcomes: a systematic review. *J Patient Saf.* 2015;11(3):135–142.
9. Daugherty Biddison EL, Paine L, Murakami P, Herzke C, Weaver SJ. Associations between safety culture and employee engagement over time: a retrospective analysis. *BMJ Qual Saf.* 2016;25(1):31–37.
10. Weaver SJ, Lubomksi LH, Wilson RF, Pfoh ER, Martinez KA, Dy SM. Promoting a culture of safety as a patient safety strategy: a systematic review. *Ann Intern Med.* 2013;158(5 Pt 2):369–374.
11. Morello RT, Lowthian JA, Barker AL, McGinnes R, Dunt D, Brand C. Strategies for improving patient safety culture in hospitals: a systematic review. *BMJ Qual Saf.* 2013;22(1):11–18.
12. Pager D, Quillan L. Walking the talk? What employers say versus what they do. *American Sociology Review.* 2005;70:355–380.
13. Stevens J, Johansson A, Lennes I, Hsu D, Tess A, Howell M. Long-term culture change related to rapid response system implementation. *Med Educ.* 2014;48(12):1211–1219.
14. Okie S. Innovation in primary care—staying one step ahead of burnout. *N Engl J Med.* 2008;359(22):2305–2309.
15. Vahey DC, Aiken LH, Sloane DM, Clarke SP, Vargas D. Nurse burnout and patient satisfaction. *Med Care.* 2004;42(2 Suppl):II57–II66.
16. McHugh MD, Kutney-Lee A, Cimiotti JP, Sloane DM, Aiken LH. Nurses' widespread job dissatisfaction, burnout, and frustration with health benefits signal problems for patient care. *Health Aff (Millwood).* 2011;30(2):202–210.
17. Shanafelt TD, Boone S, Tan L, et al. Burnout and satisfaction with work-life balance among US physicians relative to the general US population. *Arch Intern Med.* 2012;172(18):1377–1385.
18. Dixon-Woods M, Leslie M, Tarrant C, Bion J. Explaining Matching Michigan: an ethnographic study of a patient safety program. *Implement Sci.* 2013;8:70.
19. Pronovost P, Needham D, Berenholtz S, et al. An intervention to decrease catheter-related bloodstream infections in the ICU. *N Engl J Med.* 2006;355(26):2725–2732.

20. Lipitz-Snyderman A, Steinwachs D, Needham DM, Colantuoni E, Morlock LL, Pronovost PJ. Impact of a statewide intensive care unit quality improvement initiative on hospital mortality and length of stay: retrospective comparative analysis. *BMJ*. 2011;342:d219.
21. Lee TH. Turning doctors into leaders. *Harv Bus Rev*. 2010;88(4):50–58.
22. Drucker PF. *What Makes an Effective Executive*. Boston: Harvard Business Review Press; 2017.
23. Porter ME. What is value in health care? *N Engl J Med*. 2010;363(26):2477–2481.
24. Weiss CH, Krishnan JA, Au DH, et al. An official American Thoracic Society research statement: implementation science in pulmonary, critical care, and sleep medicine. *Am J Respir Crit Care Med*. 2016;194(8):1015–1025.
25. Gross PA, Greenfield S, Cretin S, et al. Optimal methods for guideline implementation: conclusions from Leeds Castle meeting. *Med Care*. 2001;39(8 Suppl 2):II85–II92.
26. Perkins MB, Jensen PS, Jaccard J, et al. Applying theory-driven approaches to understanding and modifying clinicians' behavior: what do we know? *Psychiatr Serv*. 2007;58(3):342–348.
27. Aronson PL, Yau J, Helfaer MA, Morrison W. Impact of family presence during pediatric intensive care unit rounds on the family and medical team. *Pediatrics*. 2009;124(4):1119–1125.
28. Mittal VS, Sigrest T, Ottolini MC, et al. Family-centered rounds on pediatric wards: a PRIS network survey of US and Canadian hospitalists. *Pediatrics*. 2010;126(1):37–43.
29. Latta LC, Dick R, Parry C, Tamura GS. Parental responses to involvement in rounds on a pediatric inpatient unit at a teaching hospital: a qualitative study. *Acad Med*. 2008;83(3):292–297.
30. Rappaport DI, Cellucci MF, Leffler MG. Implementing family-centered rounds: pediatric residents' perceptions. *Clin Pediatr (Phila)*. 2010;49(3):228–234.
31. Kuo DZ, Sisterhen LL, Sigrest TE, Biazo JM, Aitken ME, Smith CE. Family experiences and pediatric health services use associated with family-centered rounds. *Pediatrics*. 2012;130(2):299–305.
32. Cypress BS. Family presence on rounds: a systematic review of literature. *Dimens Crit Care Nurs*. 2012;31(1):53–64.
33. Azoulay E, Pochard F, Chevret S, et al. Family participation in care to the critically ill: opinions of families and staff. *Intensive Care Med*. 2003;29(9):1498–1504.
34. Pochard F, Azoulay E, Chevret S, et al. Symptoms of anxiety and depression in family members of intensive care unit patients: ethical hypothesis regarding decision-making capacity. *Crit Care Med*. 2001;29(10):1893–1897.
35. Azoulay E, Chevret S, Leleu G, et al. Half the families of intensive care unit patients experience inadequate communication with physicians. *Crit Care Med*. 2000;28(8):3044–3049.
36. Azoulay E, Pochard F, Chevret S, et al. Meeting the needs of intensive care unit patient families: a multicenter study. *Am J Respir Crit Care Med*. 2001;163(1):135–139.

37. Damschroder LJ, Aron DC, Keith RE, Kirsh SR, Alexander JA, Lowery JC. Fostering implementation of health services research findings into practice: a consolidated framework for advancing implementation science. *Implement Sci.* 2009;4:50.
38. Helfrich CD, Damschroder LJ, Hagedorn HJ, et al. A critical synthesis of literature on the Promoting Action on Research Implementation in Health Services (PARIHS) framework. *Implement Sci.* 2010;5:82.
39. Kitson A, Harvey G, McCormack B. Enabling the implementation of evidence-based practice: a conceptual framework. *Qual Health Care.* 1998;7(3):149–158.
40. Rycroft-Malone J, Harvey G, Seers K, Kitson A, McCormack B, Titchen A. An exploration of the factors that influence the implementation of evidence into practice. *J Clin Nurs.* 2004;13(8):913–924.
41. Rycroft-Malone J, Kitson A, Harvey G, et al. Ingredients for change: revisiting a conceptual framework. *Qual Saf Health Care.* 2002;11(2):174–180.
42. Kitson AL, Rycroft-Malone J, Harvey G, McCormack B, Seers K, Titchen A. Evaluating the successful implementation of evidence into practice using the PARiHS framework: theoretical and practical challenges. *Implement Sci.* 2008;3:1.
43. Hunt JB, Curran G, Kramer T, et al. Partnership for implementation of evidence-based mental health practices in rural federally qualified health centers: theory and methods. *Prog Community Health Partnersh.* 2012;6(3):389–398.
44. Hill JN, Guihan M, Hogan TP, et al. Use of the PARIHS framework for retrospective and prospective implementation evaluations. *Worldviews Evid Based Nurs.* 2017;14(2):99–107.
45. Stevens B, Riahi S, Cardoso R, et al. The influence of context on pain practices in the NICU: perceptions of health care professionals. *Qual Health Res.* 2011;21(6):757–770.
46. Bergstrom A, Peterson S, Namusoko S, Waiswa P, Wallin L. Knowledge translation in Uganda: a qualitative study of Ugandan midwives' and managers' perceived relevance of the sub-elements of the context cornerstone in the PARIHS framework. *Implement Sci.* 2012;7:117.
47. Glasgow RE, Vogt TM, Boles SM. Evaluating the public health impact of health promotion interventions: the RE-AIM framework. *Am J Public Health.* 1999;89(9):1322–1327.
48. Davidson JE. Family presence on rounds in neonatal, pediatric, and adult intensive care units. *Ann Am Thorac Soc.* 2013;10(2):152–156.
49. Au SS, Roze des Ordons A, Soo A, Guienguere S, Stelfox HT. Family participation in intensive care unit rounds: Comparing family and provider perspectives. *J Crit Care.* 2017;38:132–136.
50. Ingram TC, Kamat P, Coopersmith CM, Vats A. Intensivist perceptions of family-centered rounds and its impact on physician comfort, staff involvement, teaching, and efficiency. *J Crit Care.* 2014;29(6):915–918.
51. Lewin K. *Field Theory in Social Science: Selected Theoretical Papers.* New York: Harper; 1951.

STANDARD QUALITY IMPROVEMENT TOOLS AND TECHNIQUES 8

INTRODUCTION

Chapter 3 reviewed the overwhelming evidence that healthcare today is neither safe nor high quality. We learned that the best available data indicate that in any given healthcare encounter we receive only about half of the right care,[1] and that patients are also injured by care at an alarming frequency, resulting in tens or hundreds of thousands of preventable deaths per year.[2,3] Fortunately, significant practical and scholarly work has created a set of tools that can help you improve both the safety and quality of care. In this chapter, we focus on standard healthcare improvement tools. Then, Chapter 9 will cover tools derived from Lean production.

PREVENTING ADVERSE EVENTS AND IMPROVING PATIENT SAFETY

Sometimes things do not go as expected, and patients are harmed by the process of care. These adverse events are *patient safety events*. They happen because of the care process, not because of the underlying disease (Table 8-1). Many tools for the healthcare improvement practitioner revolve around responding to and preventing these kinds of events.

Some Definitions

Some terms are commonly used by patient safety practitioners, and healthcare delivery scientists should be familiar with them.[4]

- **Adverse event:** Often defined as an injury caused by care, not by the underlying disease. This injury results either in increased care (e.g., more monitoring) or a worse outcome (including death) for the patient. By definition, an adverse event results in harm to a patient.

Key Point

An adverse event is one that results in patient harm. A near miss does not reach a patient, but it still represents an error that we can learn from.

Table 8-1 QUALITY AND PATIENT SAFETY

	Questions to Ask	Examples of Problems in Each Domain
Patient Safety	Did something bad happen to a patient that is *not* caused by the disease?	A patient admitted for a knee replacement gets pneumonia. A patient admitted for pneumonia gets deep venous thrombosis (DVT). A patient in clinic is prescribed a medication to which she is allergic, resulting in anaphylaxis.
Quality	Did we do everything that we should have to give this patient the best chance of the best outcome?	A patient's hypertension is poorly controlled, increasing her risk of stroke. A patient is not offered age-appropriate colon cancer screening. A patient hospitalized with sepsis from pneumonia does not receive the right antibiotics.

Note: Whether distinguishing quality from safety is useful is debatable (and debated). Many authors subsume safety as an element of quality. In fact, the Institute of Medicine defined the Six Aims of healthcare quality as being safe, effective, efficient, timely, patient-centered, and equitable.

- **Preventable adverse event**: *Preventability* is difficult to define. The core idea is that an error in care occurred, and if that error hadn't happened, the patient wouldn't have been harmed.[5] While that approach has great face validity, it has numerous practical challenges. A common approach is to define a *preventable adverse event* as one that could have been stopped by any means currently considered as a reasonable standard of care.[4]
- **Unpreventable adverse event**: Some harms to patients are not preventable with science's current level of understanding. Some patients will have anaphylaxis after their first dose of an antibiotic. Some patients will have serious complications of surgery even when the surgery is technically executed well.
- **Near-miss**: A near-miss occurs when there is an error in care, but this error does not result in harm to a patient. For example, a physician might order a drug that a patient is allergic to, but this order might be intercepted by an electronic system, a nurse, or a pharmacist. A patient might even take a drug to which he has a known allergy, but this time he suffers no ill effects from it. Alternatively, a technical error might occur during a procedure, but without any harm to a patient.
- **Medical error**. Medical error represents the combination of preventable adverse events and near-misses.

- **Serious safety event (SSE), serious reportable event (SRE), sentinel events, and never events.** Some states and other agencies require the reporting of certain categories of events. In general, these are events that result in serious harm to patients or ones that should not occur at all during usual care processes. Because simple analytic methods make it hard to understand how or why these events could occur, they are sometimes called *never events,* though we do not prefer that term. Examples of these kinds of events include wrong-side or wrong-patient surgery, unintentional retained foreign objects after surgery, and deaths from medication errors. These events often have significant reporting requirements; the National Quality Forum maintains a list of SREs (http://www.qualityforum.org/Topics/SREs/List_of_SREs.aspx), and the Joint Commission has a significant program focused on sentinel events (https://www.jointcommission.org/sentinel_event.aspx). Individual states often have regulations or laws that apply to these types of events as well.

External Resource

The National Quality Forum maintains a list of Serious Reportable Events (SREs) (http://www.qualityforum.org/Topics/SREs/List_of_SREs.aspx).

IDENTIFYING PATIENT SAFETY EVENTS

It is hard to improve patient safety if you don't know when problems occur. Health systems with good safety cultures (discussed in Chapter 7) actively work to identify patient safety events. In fact, hospitals that have a better safety culture also have higher rates of reported safety events[6] because providers feel more comfortable reporting events. There are several approaches to identifying patient safety events, each with its strengths and weaknesses.

Voluntary Reporting

Voluntary reporting systems allow physicians, nurses, and other providers to identify safety events and near-misses. These reporting systems take different forms, ranging from a phone line with verbal reporting to sophisticated electronic systems.

All health systems should have a voluntary reporting mechanism for patient safety events. Electronic systems allow aggregation and analysis of data, but an important caution is to make the entering of information as frictionless as possible to encourage reporting. Ideally, these systems are integrated directly into clinicians' workflow to reduce barriers to reporting. What happens after a report is filed is extremely important in terms of encouraging (or suppressing) future reporting. Experience has shown that feedback about what happens with the report helps encourage future reporting. Letting frontline staff know about the analysis and—even better—improvement in patient safety that results from their reporting creates positive incentives for future reporting. Blame, or even just adding lots of additional paperwork, discourages future reporting.

Billing-Based Patient Safety Indicators

Numerous approaches for identifying adverse events from billing records exist. The most common of these are the Agency for Healthcare Research and Quality (AHRQ) Patient Safety Indicators. The major advantage of this approach to identifying safety events is that nearly every patient has a bill that is generated, and that these are usually available in an accessible electronic format. For example, the AHRQ Patient Safety Indicators require only standard discharge billing information (such as Diagnosis-Related Group (DRG), and International Classification of Diseases (ICD9 or ICD10) procedure and diagnosis codes). The ubiquity of the ability to calculate these indicators means that they are often used for pay-for-performance programs. For example, they are incorporated into Medicare's Value-Based Purchasing program for hospitals.

However, the downsides of billing-based patient safety indicators are numerous. First, they are *gameable*—meaning that discretionary billing practices can markedly influence observed event rates. Second, systematic reviews have found that the majority of these indicators do not meet criteria for validity.[7] Third, and perhaps most concerning, hospitals with quality accreditations, teaching hospitals, and safety net hospitals are all penalized more often by programs that use billing-based patient safety indicators, suggesting that these approaches may not measure the underlying constructs of patient safety and quality.[8]

Manual, Sampled Chart Review (Trigger Tools)

Voluntary reporting systems significantly under-identify patient safety events. For example, in one study, the voluntary reporting system identified only 5% of patient safety incidents that resulted in harm.[9] A different approach is to randomly sample patient charts and review them for evidence of patient harm. The best-known of these approaches was developed by the Institute of Healthcare Improvement (IHI) and is called the Global Trigger Tool.[10] This tool was initially developed in 2003 and has since been used in numerous studies and improvement programs. In this approach, a random selection of hospital discharges is chosen (e.g., 10 discharges every 2 weeks). Charts are reviewed for a maximum of 20 minutes each, and reviewers search for the presence of triggers that may indicate an adverse event. Examples of triggers include transfusion, cardiac arrest, transfer to an intensive care unit (ICU), glucose <50 mg/dL, and receipt of antidote agents like vitamin K, naloxone, and flumazenil. The presence of a trigger does not define an adverse event, but it does flag a record for attention about whether an adverse event occurred. A study of three hospitals found that the Global Trigger Tool identified a startling 10-fold more serious adverse events than either voluntary reporting or the AHRQ Patient Safety Indicators.[11]

Although trigger tools began in the inpatient setting, they have since been extended to the outpatient setting, nursing facilities, medication-event-specific trigger tools, and other areas.

Key Point

Voluntary reporting identifies only about 10% of serious adverse events.

External Resource

The Institute of Healthcare Improvement (IHI) provides numerous tools to help providers and health systems implement trigger tools (http://www.ihi.org/resources/Pages/Tools/IntrotoTriggerToolsforIdentifyingAEs.aspx).

Healthcare-Associated Infections

The Centers for Disease Control and Prevention (CDC) maintains standards and guidelines for reporting healthcare-associated infections through the National Healthcare Safety Network (NHSN). The vast majority of U.S. hospitals now report healthcare-associated infections through NSHN, and some of these patient safety events are reported publicly by Medicare's Hospital Compare. Although there can be substantial interfacility variation in how these infections are reported,[12] NHSN-driven healthcare-associated infection surveillance remains an important tool for detecting patient safety events.

Electronic Patient-Safety Trigger Tools

Today, more than 90% of U.S. hospitals have an electronic health record (EHR) and have attested to using the EHR for meaningful parts of ongoing patient care,[13] and more than 80% U.S. office-based physicians also have an EHR.[14] This creates the opportunity to use more sophisticated electronic approaches to detect patient safety events. More transformationally, this digitization of healthcare makes real-time intervention possible to prevent or ameliorate the consequences of adverse events.

However, the performance of electronic trigger tools has been mixed and generally limited by poor positive predictive values, with high false positive rates for actual adverse events. For example, a 2012 systematic review of electronic tools to identify adverse drug events found extremely variable, and generally inaccurate, performance.[15] A more recent tool designed to detect adverse drug events only had a positive predictive value of 31%.[16] Electronic "sniffers" to detect serious events have also had mixed performance. For example, algorithms to detect acute respiratory distress syndrome in the ICU only had positive predictive values in the 40%–45% range.[17]

ROOT CAUSE ANALYSIS (RCA)

When an adverse event or a near-miss occurs, understanding what happened is important because it helps us design systems to prevent similar events in the future. A common approach to this is root cause analysis (RCA). It is important to note that an RCA is always retrospective: it happens in response to an adverse event or near-miss, trying to prevent future events.

Why *Root Cause Analysis (RCA)* May not Be the Right Term

A problem with the term *root cause analysis (RCA)* is that it implies that an event has a single, primordial cause. This is almost never the case. Rather, adverse events in healthcare almost always stem from multiple factors that combine in sometimes unpredictable ways. This has led some to prefer the term *contributing factors analysis*.

Latent (and Active) Failure Model: The Swiss Cheese Model of Patient Safety

Although healthcare systems are complex adaptive systems (see Chapter 2), a simpler model is often helpful for improvement. The most common is a model that recognizes both latent and active failures. This model originated with James Reason's seminal 1990 paper[18] and is called the *Swiss cheese model* of accidents (Figure 8-1) because it recognizes that most accidents arise when failures in multiple layers of defense line up in exactly the

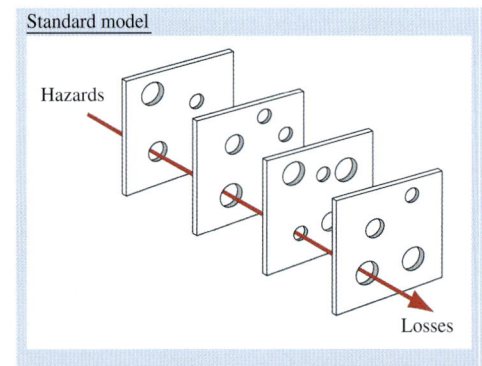

Standard model	Healthcare example
Hazards → [Swiss cheese layers] → Losses	An example hazard might be a physician entering an order for an antibiotic to which a patient has a serious allergy. For this error to reach the patient: • The computerized provider order entry system fails to allergy check (or doesn't have access to the allergy). • The pharmacist misses the allergy and provides the drug. • The nurse misses the allergy and administers the drug. • The bar-code-medication-administration software misses the allergy. The "loss" is the harm to the patient – in this case, a serious allergic reaction.

Figure 8-1 • Latent failure (Swiss cheese) model of accidents. *(Image source: By David Mack - Own work, CC BY-SA 3.0, https://commons.wikimedia.org/w/index.php?curid=31679759.)*

CHAPTER 8 | STANDARD QUALITY IMPROVEMENT TOOLS AND TECHNIQUES

right way to allow harm to reach a patient. RCA techniques attempt to elucidate all the layers of Swiss cheese—and how they failed—in order to create a picture of how the adverse event actually occurred.

Goals and Tools of RCA

The fundamental goals of RCA are to understand what actually happened and what actions might prevent similar adverse events in the future. RCA should focus on the systems of care, not on the individuals. It is not appropriate for cases when harm is intentionally caused or when there is flagrant negligence (e.g., criminal acts, or if a provider is intoxicated). Those events, which are rare, are referred to as *blameworthy*.

Who Should be on the RCA Team?

Although there is agreement that an RCA team should have real knowledge of both the event and the organizational processes around the event, there is disagreement about whether individuals involved in the event should be part of the team, or whether they should be interviewed separately from the process. Some health systems include patients and families on the team, and it is clear that having team members with more experience with RCA helps improve the process.

The Simplest RCA: The *5 Whys*

The true etiology of an adverse event is often not apparent. A general rule of thumb is that if you haven't asked "Why?" four or five times, you probably haven't reached the actual root cause. This technique is called the *5 Whys*. It is important to keep going because otherwise, you end up solving the wrong problem. Table 8-2 shows a hypothetical example of the technique for a woman whose treatment for sepsis was delayed, further described in Case 8-1.

Cause and Effect: *Ishikawa Diagrams*

Many RCA teams use an *Ishikawa diagram*, also called a *fishbone diagram* because of its visual appearance. The adverse event is placed on the right side of the diagram, and definite and potential causes are filled into the diagram's branches by the RCA team. This tool has the advantage of making it clear that there are many potential contributing factors, and it may also help to identify related areas for improvement that could have caused the same adverse event (even if they did not do so in the current case). Although the authors find this particular tool less helpful than others, many RCA teams find it very useful.

Case 8-1

A 38-year-old woman with a history of a splenectomy as a child comes to the Arbitrary General Regional Hospital's emergency department. She initially has a delayed diagnosis of sepsis (Figure 8-2). When she develops shock, antibiotics are ordered, but their administration is also delayed (Table 8-2).

Table 8-2 HYPOTHETICAL EXAMPLE OF THE 5 WHYS

Question	Analysis	Corrective Action
What happened?	Antibiotics were delayed for a septic shock patient, markedly increasing her risk of death.	None
Why? (1)	The nurse did not administer the antibiotics until 3.5 hours after they were ordered.	Discipline the nurse. (Wrong!)
Why? (2)	The antibiotics were not delivered to the ICU for 3 hours.	Discipline the transporter. (Wrong!)
Why? (3)	The pharmacy technician in the clean room did not prepare the antibiotics until 2 hours after they were ordered.	Discipline the pharmacy technician. (Wrong!)
Why? (4)	The pharmacy technician did not know the antibiotics had been ordered.	Discipline the pharmacy technician. (Wrong!)
Why? (5)	Signaling of the technician to prepare the antibiotics depends on a label printer—and the printer is (a) in a corner of the clean room with poor visibility, and (b) was out of labels.	Engineer a better signaling approach (move the printer, create an electronic queue, etc.). (Right!)

A common approach is to include the categories of People, Materials, Methods, Environment, and Equipment as branches on the diagram, although the categories commonly vary. Figure 8-2 illustrates an Ishikawa diagram for an imaginary RCA of the patient with delayed diagnosis of sepsis in the emergency department (ED), described in Case 8-1. In this hypothetical case, there were staffing issues (a sick attending physician, a new resident, and an agency nurse). Many RCAs would stop at this point, but the Ishikawa diagram helps enforce the rigor to think about other causes. In this case, multiple other causes were identified that are also important to address (each of which could be subjected to its own 5 Whys).

When using this tool, you should be particularly attentive to being adequately specific when identifying potential contributing factors for the adverse event. A common pitfall is to simply list items (or people) who were involved in the patient's care without drawing out the causal relationship to the adverse event. This can lead to very elaborate Ishikawa diagrams that give reassurance that the team has been systematic in their thinking, without actually being systematic or helping understanding the event. For example, listing "Phlebotomist," "Nurse," and "Physician" as branches in the People category would not contribute to understanding

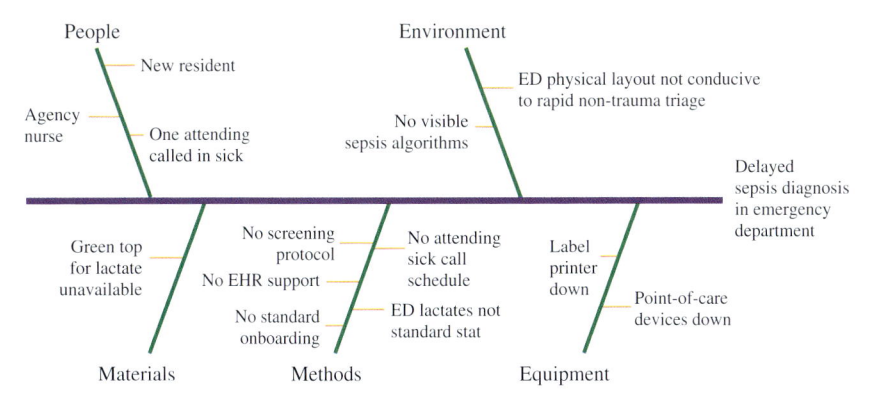

CHAPTER 8 | STANDARD QUALITY IMPROVEMENT TOOLS AND TECHNIQUES

Figure 8-2 • Example of an Ishikawa diagram.

what happened, whereas "Phlebotomist called to rapid response event," "Nurse off floor for CT scan," and "Physician intubating another patient" are helpful.

Process Mapping

Process mapping is commonly thought of as a tool for process improvement rather than for RCA, but in our experience, it is quite helpful for both. Process mapping is covered in detail in the section "Process Mapping," below, and also in Chapter 9.

Causal Mapping and the Cause Mapping® Method

An extension of an RCA is a tool that integrates mapping with beliefs and evidence about the actual cause of an event is a cause-and-effect diagram, sometimes called *rationale mapping*.[19] A commonly used technique for this approach to an RCA is called Cause Mapping®, which is implemented by and trademarked by ThinkReliability (https://www.thinkreliability.com/). This provides a visual approach that shows causal reasoning, handles multiple causes of single events well, and integrates evidence and remediation strategies into a single representation. In our experience, this approach has been quite intuitive to clinicians. An example is shown in Figure 8-3.

Pitfalls of RCA: Moving Beyond RCA to RCA²

Limitations and mixed effectiveness of RCA have caused national leaders to move toward an evolving framework of Root Cause Analyses and Actions, or RCA² ("RCA squared").[20] This approach focuses on the actions that create systematic, sustainable improvements.

External Resource

The IHI Open School has online courses with more detail about root causes analyses (RCA) http://www.ihi.org/education/IHIOpenSchool/resources/Pages/CourseRelatedResources.aspx#PS104.

External Resource

The National Patient Safety Foundation and IHI's RCA² provides detailed information about how to improve RCAs—and should be required reading for RCA practitioners (http://www.ihi.org/resources/Pages/Tools/RCA2-Improving-Root-Cause-Analyses-and-Actions-to-Prevent-Harm.aspx).

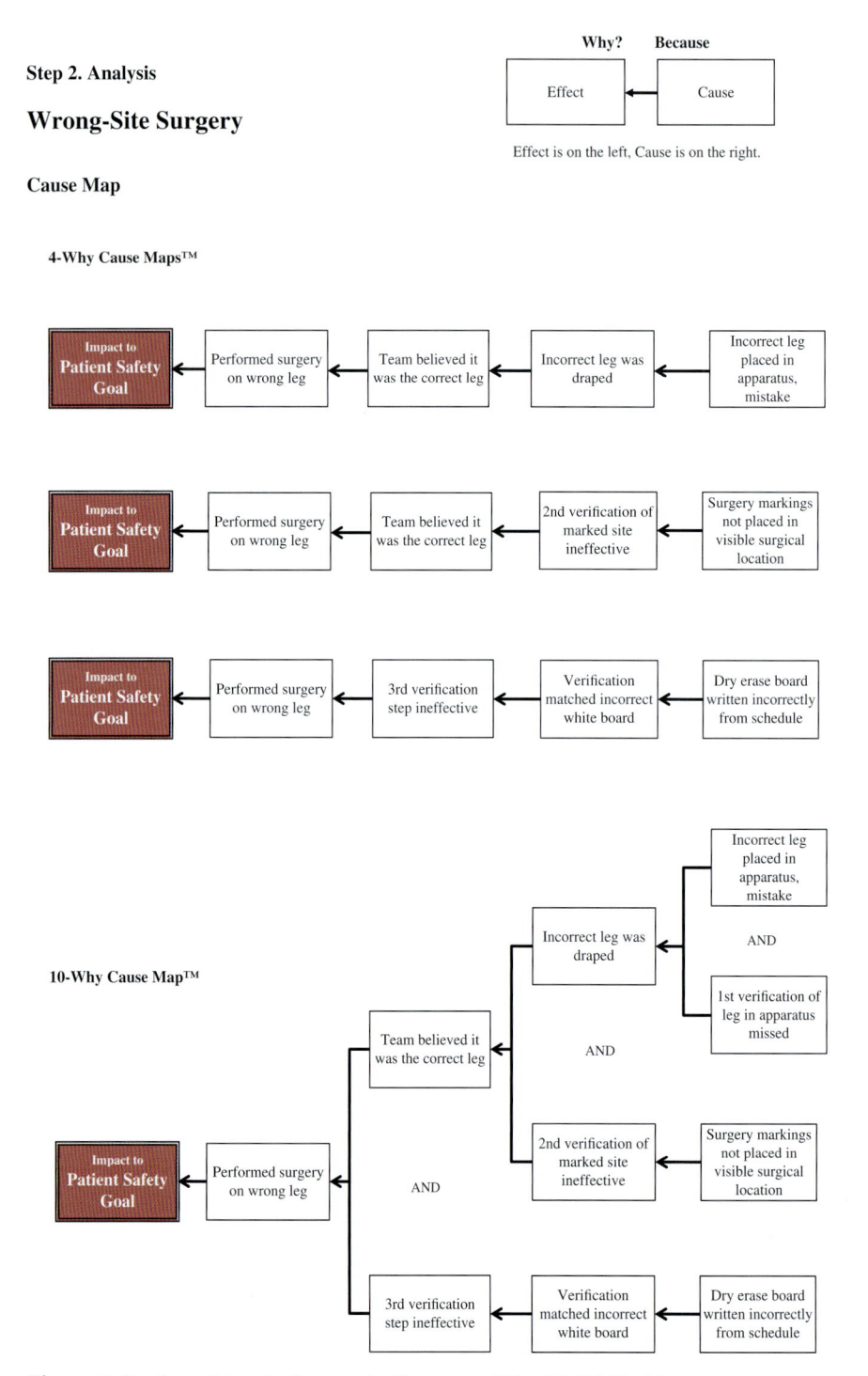

II | UNDERSTANDING HEALTHCARE DELIVERY SCIENCE

Step 2. Analysis

Wrong-Site Surgery

Cause Map

Why? Because
Effect ← Cause

Effect is on the left, Cause is on the right.

4-Why Cause Maps™

Impact to Patient Safety Goal ← Performed surgery on wrong leg ← Team believed it was the correct leg ← Incorrect leg was draped ← Incorrect leg placed in apparatus, mistake

Impact to Patient Safety Goal ← Performed surgery on wrong leg ← Team believed it was the correct leg ← 2nd verification of marked site ineffective ← Surgery markings not placed in visible surgical location

Impact to Patient Safety Goal ← Performed surgery on wrong leg ← 3rd verification step ineffective ← Verification matched incorrect white board ← Dry erase board written incorrectly from schedule

10-Why Cause Map™

Impact to Patient Safety Goal ← Performed surgery on wrong leg ← [Team believed it was the correct leg AND 3rd verification step ineffective]

Team believed it was the correct leg ← [Incorrect leg was draped AND 2nd verification of marked site ineffective]

Incorrect leg was draped ← [Incorrect leg placed in apparatus, mistake AND 1st verification of leg in apparatus missed]

2nd verification of marked site ineffective ← Surgery markings not placed in visible surgical location

3rd verification step ineffective ← Verification matched incorrect white board ← Dry erase board written incorrectly from schedule

Figure 8-3 • Cause Mapping® example. (Courtesy of ThinkReliability®.)

Blameworthy Events

Effective RCAs do not focus on individual error. In fact, "human error" is an inadequate finding as a root cause. However, a very, very small fraction of events are caused by individual actions that should be considered "blameworthy." These include harm caused by criminal acts, intentional harm of patients, or adverse events caused by a provider's alcohol or substance use. Organizations may also define specific types of actions that are deliberately unsafe and considered blameworthy. Although they are extremely rare, understanding that some events are caused by individual, intentional actions is an important part of the development of the Just Culture approach to handling adverse events.[21,22]

Prioritization

Medium-size and large healthcare organizations may receive thousands (or tens of thousands) of potential safety reports each year. Because resources are finite, some kind of prioritization must happen. Although the most common approach is to prioritize by the level of harm that occurs after an individual event, a better approach is one that looks toward future risk and that takes account of both the severity of an event and the probability/frequency with which it occurs.[20] The National Patient Safety Foundation uses the categories described in Table 8-3. It is important to note that, for near-misses, the worst-case outcome should be assigned for severity. These criteria are then used to prioritize available resources for analysis, action, and improvement, as described in Table 8-4.

The Five Rules of Causation

It is remarkably easy to be imprecise about causes in an RCA. The RCA^2 approach encourages us to be precise and clear when developing causal statements by applying the Five Rules of Causation. These rules originate from David Marx's work on aircraft maintenance safety,[23] and they were adapted from work by the U.S. Department of Veterans Affairs on RCA tools and incorporated into the National Patient Safety Foundation's RCA^2 approach. Table 8-5 lists the rules, along with correct and incorrect examples of them. In particular, it is important to note that human error and policy violations are not acceptable root causes: the fact that they occurred when well-intentioned providers were working in their normal environments implies (1) that they can happen again, and (2) that there are systemic causes that let the error occur.

> **Key Point**
>
> Human error and policy violations are not acceptable root causes: the fact that they occurred when well-intentioned providers were working in their normal environments implies (1) that they can happen again, and (2) that there are systemic causes that let the error occur.

Table 8-3 RCA² SEVERITY AND PROBABILITY CRITERIA

Severity	Probability
Catastrophic: Actual or potential death or major permanent loss of function	**Frequent:** Likely to occur again soon; may happen several times per year
Major: Permanent worsening of bodily function; or an event that requires surgery or results in disfigurement for any patient. Events that result in increased lengths of stay or higher levels of care for 3 or more patients are also considered major.	**Occasional:** Probable to occur; may happen several times in a 1–2-year period
Moderate: Increased length of stay or level of care for 1 or 2 patients	**Uncommon:** May happen in the next 2–5 years
Minor: Events without harm, or those not requiring increased length of stay or level of treatment	**Remote:** Unlikely to occur; may happen in a 5–30-year range

Near-misses, and actual events, can be assessed based on both their severity and the probability that they will recur. For near-misses, you should choose a severity based on a reasonable "worst case." For example, if a bar-code-medication administration system intercepted the administration of a potentially lethal dose of medication (e.g., a medication to which a patient has known anaphylaxis), but all preceding safety steps failed, it would be reasonable to classify that event as catastrophic even though no harm occurred.

Adapted from National Patient Safety Foundation (2016). Based on Department of Veterans Affairs, Veterans Health Administration, *VHA Patient Safety Improvement Handbook1050.01,* May 23, 2008. Available at http://cheps.engin.umich.edu/wp-content/uploads/sites/118/2015/04/Triaging-Adverse-Events-and-Close-Calls-SAC.pdf.

Table 8-4 RCA² MATRIX FOR SAFETY ASSESSMENT CODES

Probability	Severity			
	Catastrophic	**Major**	**Moderate**	**Minor**
Frequent	3	3	2	1
Occasional	3	2	1	1
Uncommon	3	2	1	1
Remote	3	2	1	1

Near-misses and actual events are assessed for probability and severity, and then plotted in the Safety Assessment Code Matrix. 3 = highest risk; 2 = intermediate risk; and 1 = lowest risk. These risk assessments can then be used to prioritize when analysis and improvement resources are limited.

Adapted from National Patient Safety Foundation (2016). Based on Department of Veterans Affairs, Veterans Health Administration, *VHA Patient Safety Improvement Handbook1050.01,* May 23, 2008. Available at http://cheps.engin.umich.edu/wp-content/uploads/sites/118/2015/04/Triaging-Adverse-Events-and-Close-Calls-SAC.pdf.

CHAPTER 8 | STANDARD QUALITY IMPROVEMENT TOOLS AND TECHNIQUES

Table 8-5 FIVE RULES OF CAUSATION FOR USE IN RCAs

	Rule	Incorrect	Correct
①	Clearly shows the cause-and-effect relationship.	The nurse was distracted.	The nurse was interrupted five times during preparation of a patient's medications, leading to confusion of two medications, resulting in a medication error.
②	Use specific and accurate descriptors for what occurred, rather than negative and vague words.	The medication label was poorly designed.	The medication label was written in 6-point type, with no distinction between the patient's name and the medication name and no signaling of high-risk medications.
③	Human errors must have a preceding cause.	The physician ordered the wrong medication dose.	The EHR defaulted to an incorrect dose for this patient, increasing the risk that a medication error would occur.
④	Violations of procedure are not root causes; they must have a preceding cause.	The nurse did not follow the sepsis screening protocol.	The hospital's sepsis screening criteria are time consuming and have a positive predictive value of <20%, causing many nurses to defer implementing screening during busy shifts.
⑤	Failure to act is only causal when there is a preexisting duty to act.	The hospitalist did not review the sodium lab result, resulting in a delay in therapy that was potentially life-threatening.	The renal consultant ordered labs on a hospital medicine patient. Because there is no mechanism by which the primary team is notified when orders are placed by a consulting service, the probability of delay in recognition of serious abnormalities is increased, resulting in a delay in therapy.

Adapted from National Patient Safety Foundation (2016). Based on The Five Rules of Causation developed by the Department of Veterans Affairs, Veterans Health Administration, and appearing in their *NCPS Triage Cards™ for Root Cause Analysis*.

Some Things Don't Work

An all-too-frequent outcome of RCAs is that they result in new policies, education, or training. Unfortunately, the empirical evidence shows that these interventions simply don't work to improve patient outcomes.[24] This leads to the idea that some interventions to improve patient safety are stronger than others, which is consistent with what we understand from human factors engineering. The RCA[2] process structures this as stronger, intermediate, and weaker actions (Table 8-6). When you reach the stage of

Table 8-6 ACTION HIERARCHIES

	Action Category	Example
Stronger Actions (these tasks require less reliance on humans to remember to perform the task correctly)	Architectural/physical plant changes	Replace revolving doors at the main patient entrance into the building with powered sliding or swinging doors to reduce patient falls.
	New devices with usability testing	Perform heuristic tests of outpatient blood glucose meters and test strips and select the most appropriate for the patient population being served.
	Engineering control (forcing function)	Eliminate the use of universal adaptors and peripheral devices for medical equipment and use tubing/fittings that can only be connected the correct way (e.g., IV tubing and connectors that cannot physically be connected to sequential compression devices or SCDs).
	Simplify process	Remove unnecessary steps in a process.
	Standardize on equipment or process	Standardize on the make and model of medication pumps used throughout the institution. Use bar coding for medication administration.
	Tangible involvement by leadership	Participate in unit patient safety evaluations and interact with staff; support the RCA^2 process; purchase needed equipment; ensure staffing and workload are balanced.
Intermediate Actions	Redundancy	Use two RNs to independently calculate high-risk medication dosages.
	Increase in staffing/decease in workload	Make float staff available to assist when workloads peak during the day.
	Software enhancements, modifications	Use computer alerts for drug–drug interactions.
	Eliminate/reduce distractions	Provide quiet rooms for programming PCA pumps; remove distractions for nurses when programming medication pumps.
	Education using simulation based training, with periodic refresher sessions and observations	Conduct patient handoffs in a simulation lab/environment, with after action critiques and debriefing.

Table 8-6 ACTION HIERARCHIES

	Action Category	Example
	Checklist/cognitive aids	Use pre-induction and pre-incision checklists in operating rooms Use a checklist when reprocessing flexible fiber optic endoscopes.
	Eliminate look- and sound-alikes	Do not store look-alikes next to one another in the unit medication room.
	Standardized communication tools	Use read-back for all critical lab values. Use read-back or repeat-back for all verbal medication orders. Use a standardized patient handoff format.
	Enhanced documentation, communication	Highlight medication name and dose on IV bags.
Weaker Actions (these tasks require more reliance on humans to remember to perform the task correctly)	Double checks	One person calculates dosage, another person reviews their calculation.
	Warnings	Add audible alarms or caution labels.
	New procedure/memorandum/policy	Remember to check IV sites every 2 hours.
	Training	Demonstrate correct usage of hard-to-use medical equipment.

From National Patient Safety Foundation. RCA[2] (2016).[20] Action Hierarchy levels and categories are based on *Root Cause Analysis Tools*, VA National Center for Patient Safety, http://www.patientsafety.va.gov/docs/joe/rca_tools_2_15.pdf.

defining your actions in response to a near-miss or an adverse event, you should focus on stronger and intermediate actions.

FAILURE MODE EFFECTS (AND CRITICALITY) ANALYSIS (FMEA AND FMECA)

RCA and RCA[2] evaluate processes after a failure has happened. Failure mode effects analysis (FMEA) and its cousin, failure mode effects and criticality analysis (FMECA) can be used to evaluate processes before a patient is harmed. FMECA was developed by the U.S. military in the 1940s[25] and extended for use in the Apollo space program, which released its FMECA procedure in 1966.[26] The Apollo program's definition of FMECA points out the key features relevant to healthcare today:

Failure Mode, Effects, and Criticality Analysis is a reliability procedure which documents all possible failures in a system design within specified ground rules, determines by failure mode analysis the effect of each failure on system operation, identifies single failure points, i.e., those failures critical to mission success or crew safety, and ranks each failure according to criticality category of failure effect and probability of occurrence.[26]

FMECA differs from RCA, in that it can be deployed when a new process is being designed, not just with existing processes. The second point to make about FMECA is that it helps prioritize among the potentially large number of targets for improvement in any healthcare process. It is designed to provide a rank order of process steps for improvement based on their risk of causing harm via failure. FMECA, therefore, can be particularly useful in identifying high-leverage points for improvement in complex processes—those that have a disproportionate impact on reducing risk to patients.

The core steps of a FMECA are as follows:

- **Crisply identify the process you want to evaluate.** This step can be trickier to execute than it sounds at first. It is important, but difficult, to understand the starting and stopping boundaries of the process on which your FMECA is focused. The difficulty comes because healthcare processes are so interconnected—and the decisions about boundaries will be somewhat arbitrary, but they should make clinical sense.
- **Assemble the team.** The team should include subject matter experts on the process you're addressing, plus a facilitator who focuses on the FMECA process.
- **Map the process.** In this step, create a process diagram, or process map (see "Process Mapping," below, and also Chapter 9). It is important to note that this is a map of the process itself, not necessarily a temporal map of an event. In this stage, you may find out that you've picked too large a scope and need to narrow the focus of the FMECA. In addition to the process map, you'll now have a list of all of the process steps, linked to the process map.
- **Consider how each step go wrong.** For each step in the process, brainstorm about ways the process could go awry. For example, when prescribing a medication, a physician might order the wrong

medication, order the wrong dose, or assign the order to the wrong patient. Each of these ways that something could go wrong is called a *failure mode.*

- **Determine how risky each of these failure modes might be, in three dimensions (probability, detectability, and severity).** For each failure mode, use your best judgment to rate the following items on a 1–10 scale:
  - *Probability:* Likelihood of happening (10 = most likely, 1 = least likely)
  - *Detectability:* Likelihood of the failure being detected before a patient is harmed (10 = least likely to be detected; 1 = most likely to be detected)
  - *Severity:* (10 = most severe outcome for the patient, 1 = least severe outcome for the patient)

Many clinicians feel uncomfortable at this stage because there are no strict guidelines, for example, on what a score of '8' means. The important aspect of this method is that you get the *relative* order right between failure modes. It matters less whether something is an 8 or a 9 and more whether the risks are out of order.

- **Calculate the risk of each failure mode.** Now, for each failure mode, calculate the risk priority number (RPN). There are different ways to do this, but in the schema given here, you just multiply Probability x Detectability × Severity. The maximum number you can get is 1,000 (10 × 10 × 10) and the smallest is 1 (1 × 1 × 1). (It is important to note that the scale for detectability is reversed: 10 is least likely to be detected.)
- **Use the RPN to prioritize among potential actions.** In a given FMECA, you might easily have 100 or more potential failure modes that your team identifies. Obviously, you can't work on all of them at the same time. Sorting by RPN will help you identify high-leverage failure modes—ones that are more likely to have a catastrophic outcome. Not all the high-RPN failure modes will be addressable or preventable, but this tool will help you focus your efforts on failure modes that are likely to have significant impacts.

Many clinicians find that the FMECA approach helps identify risky points in a process whose importance might not be immediately obvious. For example, when performing an FMECA on the medication administration process, you might find that "Putting medication into the wrong IV bag" is particularly highly ranked because—once the medication is in the bag—the error cannot be detected by any other prevention methods

> **External Resource**
>
> Additional tools for FMECA are available at
>
> - IHI: http://www.ihi.org/resources/Pages/Tools/FailureModesandEffectsAnalysisTool.aspx
> - CMS: https://www.cms.gov/Medicare/Provider-Enrollment-and-Certification/QAPI/downloads/GuidanceForFMEA.pdf
> - VA National Center for Patient Safety: https://www.patientsafety.va.gov/docs/hfmea/FMEA2.pdf

such as pharmacist review, nurse double-checks, or even barcode medication administration.

FMECAs are sometimes required by state and national regulatory agencies as part of a healthcare provider's accreditation process. Additional resources for this tool are available at the Institute for Healthcare Improvement (IHI), the Centers for Medicare and Medicaid Services (CMS), and the Department of Veterans Affairs National Center for Patient Safety.

SAFETY I AND SAFETY II

This chapter has primarily focused on identifying failures of safety—adverse events, patient harms, and near-misses. This is the dominant view of and approach to patient safety and is sometimes called *Safety I*. While it has undoubtedly led to significant improvements, recent scholarship has focused on a different conceptual approach, called *Safety II*. Proponents of this approach argue that safety should move from "preventing things from going wrong" to "ensuring that as many things as possible go right."

At first glance, these sound like the same thing, but they turn out to have important conceptual differences. For example, in Safety I, we generally assume that humans are the most variable component in a system, so they introduce hazards into a system. But a corresponding question might be, "If this is the case, why do things almost always go right?" Safety II takes a different view: namely, that systems are complex and interdependent, that conditions on the ground are variable, and that safety requires frequent, minute adaptions to real-world conditions in the moment. Safety II points out important differences between work-as-imagined (and encoded into policies and guidelines) and work-as-done, and the fact that advances in healthcare have led to healthcare itself being intractably complex (see also Chapter 2). This complexity means that cause and effect in healthcare may not be cleanly observable, particularly in retrospect, and when looking only at things that failed. Some key messages of Safety II include:

- Focus on processes that go right, not only those that go wrong.
- Pay attention to common processes and frequent events, not just those with patient harm.
- Remain vigilant for the possibility of failure.
- Recognize that there is almost always a tradeoff between efficiency and thoroughness.[27]

For more details about this approach, see Erik Hollnagel's excellent white paper[28] and book[29] on Safety II.

PROCESS IMPROVEMENT AND QUALITY IMPROVEMENT

Improving the reliability of care can improve both quality and safety (Table 8-1). Several tools are commonly used in healthcare quality improvement to help improve process reliability. In this chapter, we cover process mapping, PDSA/PDCA, and choice architecture interventions. Chapter 9 focuses on methods associated with the Toyota Production System/Lean.

Process Mapping

Process mapping is a lightweight tool that can be used to help you better understand a process before trying to improve it. (It also forms the foundation for Value Stream Mapping, an important Lean tool.) Process mapping can be used from the clinician's viewpoint and focus on technical aspects of care, but it can also start with the patient's viewpoint and focus on experience.[28] Even if it is a process that you personally perform every day, you often learn a lot about assumptions, options, and decisions inherent in the work via this method. There are many formalisms and techniques to process mapping, but our advice is to start simply— with paper and pencil, a whiteboard, or sticky notes and a wall. To begin, make sure to have people who know the process in the room, and to observe the process in the real world after you're done planning.

The first step is to define the start and end of the process you want to map. This is important so that you know what's in bounds and out of bounds. Then, map each activity and each decision in the process. For example, "Choose which antibiotics to give" might be a decision in a pneumonia pathway process, while "Infuse antibiotic over 1 hour" would be an activity. Although flowcharting formalisms use many more symbols, we recommend just starting with these four:

- ○ A circle indicates the first or last step in the process.
- □ A square indicates an activity.
- ◇ A diamond indicates a decision.
- → Draw arrows between circles, squares, and diamonds to indicate the process flow.

There are some common problems that people encounter when they use process mapping in healthcare. Picking the level of detail that you want to use can be quite daunting. Healthcare work is essentially fractal: you can keep getting more and more granular with every process. We recommend that you use your intuition and common sense about how

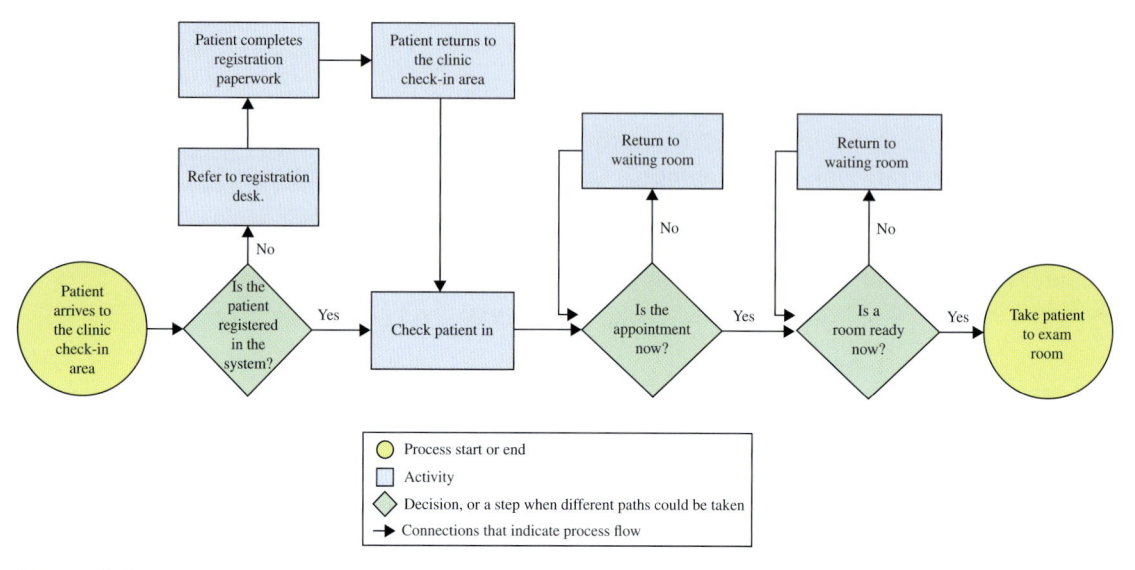

Figure 8-4 • A (very) simplified process map.
This figure shows a very simplified process map for a patient's journey between arriving to clinic and being taken back to the exam room. A real process map might have more details (for example, checking vital signs before going to the exam room).

granular to be, and that you be flexible to adapting as you do the work. For example, if you're working on ICU improvement, you probably don't want a box that just says "Manage sepsis," but neither do you want a process map with thousands of boxes that include details like "Pick up IV bag."

Additionally, there are some common problems with decision nodes (◇). First, each node should represent only a single decision, not multiple decisions. Multiple decisions should be represented in multiple nodes that follow each other. Second, the choices that come out of a decision node must be both mutually exclusive (i.e., they can't overlap each other) and exhaustive (i.e., there can't be other choices that are not represented). For example, a decision node that says, "Choose site to which discharge patient from ICU" should not just have "Hospital Ward" and "Home" as options because patients can go to numerous other locations Figure 8-4 shows an example of a simplified process map..

The Model for Improvement

Perhaps the most commonly taught method for improving processes in healthcare is the Model for Improvement Figure 8-5. Developed by Associates in Process Improvement, it draws on a long history of

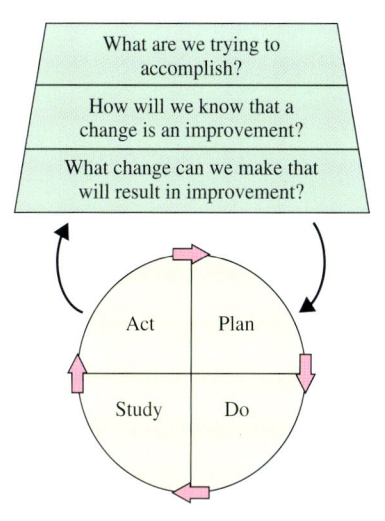

CHAPTER 8 | STANDARD QUALITY IMPROVEMENT TOOLS AND TECHNIQUES

Figure 8-5 • The Model for Improvement. *(Source: Langley et al. (2009))*

improvement techniques and is a method often taught by the Institute for Healthcare Improvement (IHI).

The technique involves setting aims, measures, and ideas, and then using a structured method for testing iterations of improvement. It is common for improvement teams to move quickly into testing iterations during the earlier component of the process, and we would emphasize the importance of following the model in order.

First, ask and answer three questions: (1) What are we trying to improve? (2) How will we know if a change is an improvement? (3) What is a change we can make that (we think) will result in an improvement? The first question sets aims, the second defines how we will evaluate changes, and the third develops a catalog of ideas for improvement.

Then, move to a structured approach to testing your ideas. In the Model for Improvement, this is referred to as *PDSA* (which stands for "Plan, Do, Study, Act"), but it is analogous to *PDCA* ("Plan, Do, Check, Act"; or "Plan, Do, Check, Adjust") which is also called the Deming Cycle or the Shewart Cycle in other methods. The steps for PDSA are as follows:

- **Plan:** Design your test of change (include measures, and your hypothesis about what the measures will show).
- **Do:** Implement the change, usually on a small scale. Collect enough data to understand whether things are working as you expected, or not.

External Resource

The IHI's guide on *How to Improve* focuses on the Model for Improvement and is available at http://www.ihi.org/resources/Pages/HowtoImprove/default.aspx.

- **Study:** Analyze the results. Did things go as expected?
- **Act:** Decide whether you've achieved your goal. If not, plan another PDSA cycle.

An absolutely critical component of this is that the PDSA cycles are meant to be iterations—and good improvement efforts usually have many sequential PDSA cycles before they achieve their goals.

For more details about the Model for Improvement, see the IHI's numerous resources on the subject, as well as Nolan et al.'s *Improvement Guide*.[31]

Choice Architecture: The Soft Tyranny of the Default Option

The field of behavioral economics has proved that how choices are structured strongly influences which choices people make. This is the case in diverse settings, ranging from schools to grocery stores to retirement planning. It turns out that this approach also helps improve quality in healthcare.[32,33] How can this work? Often, you may have a choice that you want a clinician to make (e.g., picking a particular guideline-based anticoagulant), but you know that there are numerous exceptions that occasionally influence the best medication choice. Instead of forcing a choice on a physician, or requiring approval by a third party (e.g., a clinical pharmacist), you can design choices to nudge the physician to the guideline-based anticoagulant. For example, the order in which medications are presented can change which medications physicians order. You can let the default order be the guideline-based medication. Or you can require a brief free-text explanation of why a physician is choosing a different medication. These often influence significant percentages of medication choices.

Choice architecture interventions can influence surprisingly personal types of healthcare behavior. For example, one study looked at how patients choose end-of-life advance directives. In this study, seriously ill patients with life-limiting illness were randomized to an advance directive with a default choice: comfort-oriented care, life-extending care, or a standard advance directive with no options checked. Patients who were randomized to the default option of comfort-oriented care were 34% more likely to choose comfort-oriented care in the end, compared to those who were defaulted to life-extending care.[34] The fact that even this most personal of decisions is influenced by default options shows the power of choice architecture. This has led some health systems to deploy *nudge units,* which focus on using behavioral economics techniques to improve care.[35]

KEY POINTS

- Adverse events are those that result in harm to patients; near-misses are errors in care that are intercepted or do not harm patients.
- Voluntary patient safety reporting systems are important, but they miss up to 90% of important patient safety events.
- RCAs focus on using tools like the 5 Whys to understand systematic causes of adverse events.
- Safety science shows us that some interventions (e.g., training, new policies, double-checks) do not work as well as others (e.g., engineering controls, removing unneeded steps in a process) to improve patient safety.
- Choice architecture (such as guideline-compliant default options) are often an effective approach to changing clinicians' behavior.

REFERENCES

1. McGlynn EA, Asch SM, Adams J, et al. The quality of health care delivered to adults in the United States. *N Engl J Med*. 2003;348(26):2635–2645.
2. Brennan TA, Leape LL, Laird NM, et al. Incidence of adverse events and negligence in hospitalized patients. Results of the Harvard Medical Practice Study I. *N Engl J Med*. 1991;324(6):370–376.
3. James JT. A new, evidence-based estimate of patient harms associated with hospital care. *J Patient Saf*. 2013;9(3):122–128.
4. Agency for Healthcare Research and Quality. Patient Safety Primer: Adverse Events, Near Misses, and Errors. 2017; Accessed April 16, 2018, from https://psnet.ahrq.gov/primers/primer/34/adverse-events-near-misses-and-errors.
5. Pronovost PJ, Colantuoni E. Measuring preventable harm: helping science keep pace with policy. *JAMA*. 2009;301(12):1273–1275.
6. Hutchinson A, Young TA, Cooper KL, et al. Trends in healthcare incident reporting and relationship to safety and quality data in acute hospitals: results from the National Reporting and Learning System. *Qual Saf Health Care*. 2009;18(1):5–10.
7. Winters BD, Bharmal A, Wilson RF, et al. Validity of the Agency for Health Care Research and Quality patient safety indicators and the Centers for Medicare and Medicaid hospital-acquired conditions: a systematic review and meta-analysis. *Med Care*. 2016;54(12):1105–1111.
8. Rajaram R, Chung JW, Kinnier CV, et al. Hospital characteristics associated with penalties in the Centers for Medicare and Medicaid Services Hospital-Acquired Condition Reduction Program. *JAMA*. 2015;314(4):375–383.

9. Sari AB, Sheldon TA, Cracknell A, Turnbull A. Sensitivity of routine system for reporting patient safety incidents in an NHS hospital: retrospective patient case note review. *BMJ*. 2007;334(7584):79.

10. Institute for Healthcare Improvement (IHI). *IHI Global Trigger Tool for Measuring Adverse Events.* Accessed April 16, 2018, from http://www.ihi.org/resources/Pages/Tools/IHIGlobalTriggerToolforMeasuringAEs.aspx.

11. Classen DC, Resar R, Griffin F, et al. "Global Trigger Tool" shows that adverse events in hospitals may be ten times greater than previously measured. *Health Aff (Millwood)*. 2011;30(4):581–589.

12. Lin MY, Hota B, Khan YM, et al. Quality of traditional surveillance for public reporting of nosocomial bloodstream infection rates. *JAMA*. 2010;304 (18):2035–2041.

13. Office of the National Coordinator for Health Information Technology. *Hospital Selection of Public Health Measures in Medicare EHR Incentive Program, Health IT Quick-Stat #16.* 2016. Accessed April 18, 2019, from http:///quickstats/pages/FIG-MU-Hospitals-Public-Health-Measure-Attestations.php.

14. Office of the National Coordinator for Health Information Technology. *Office-Based Physician Electronic Health Record Adoption, Health IT Quick-Stat #50.* 2016. Accessed February 22, 2017, from http:///quickstats/pages/physician-ehr-adoption-trends.php.

15. Forster AJ, Jennings A, Chow C, Leeder C, van Walraven C. A systematic review to evaluate the accuracy of electronic adverse drug event detection. *J Am Med Inform Assoc*. 2012;19(1):31–38.

16. Lim D, Melucci J, Rizer MK, Prier BE, Weber RJ. Detection of adverse drug events using an electronic trigger tool. *Am J Health Syst Pharm*. 2016;73(17 Suppl 4):S112–S120.

17. McKown AC, Brown RM, Ware LB, Wanderer JP. External validity of electronic sniffers for automated recognition of acute respiratory distress syndrome. *J Intensive Care Med*. 2017. doi:10.1177/0885066617720159.

18. Reason J. The contribution of latent human failures to the breakdown of complex systems. *Philos Trans R Soc Lond B Biol Sci*. 1990;327(1241):475–484.

19. Aurisicchio M, Bracewell R, Hooey BL. Rationale mapping and functional modelling enhanced root cause analysis. *Safety Science*. 2016;85:241–257.

20. National Patient Safety Foundation. *RCA2: Improving Root Cause Analyses and Actions to Prevent Harm.* 2016. Accessed April 8, 2018, from http://www.ihi.org/resources/Pages/Tools/RCA2-Improving-Root-Cause-Analyses-and-Actions-to-Prevent-Harm.aspx.

21. Wachter RM, Pronovost PJ. Balancing "no blame" with accountability in patient safety. *N Engl J Med*. 2009;361(14):1401–1406.

22. Petschonek S, Burlison J, Cross C, et al. Development of the just culture assessment tool: measuring the perceptions of health-care professionals in hospitals. *J Patient Saf*. 2013;9(4):190–197.

23. Marx DA, Watson J. *Maintenance error causation. Phase IX Progress Report on Human Factors in Aviation Maintenance and Inspection*. Washington, DC: Federal Aviation Authority Office of Aviation Medicine; 1999.

24. Shojania KG, Grimshaw JM. Evidence-based quality improvement: the state of the science. *Health Aff (Millwood)*. 2005;24(1):138–150.
25. Army U. *Procedure for Performing a Failure Mode Effect and Criticality Analysis. United States Military Procedure*. MIL-P-1629;1949. Accessed April 18, 2019, from http://www.fmea-fmeca.com/milstd1629.pdf.
26. National Aeronautics and Space Administration (NASA). *Procedure for Failure Mode Effects and Critical Analysis (FMECA)* [Apollo Program]. 1966. Accessed April 8, 2018, from https://ntrs.nasa.gov/archive/nasa/casi.ntrs.nasa.gov/19700076494.pdf.
27. Hollnagel E. *The ETTO Principle: Efficiency-Thoroughness Trade-Off: Why Things That Go Right Sometimes Go Wrong*. Burlington, VT: Ashgate; 2009.
28. Hollnagel E, Wears R, Braithwaite J. *From Safety-I to Safety-II: A White Paper 2015*. Accessed April 29, 2018, from https://www.england.nhs.uk/signuptosafety/wp-content/uploads/sites/16/2015/10/safety-1-safety-2-whte-papr.pdf.
29. Hollnagel E. *Safety-I and Safety-II: The Past and Future of Safety Management*. New York: CRC Press; 2014.
30. Trebble TM, Hansi N, Hydes T, Smith MA, Baker M. Process mapping the patient journey: an introduction. *BMJ*. 2010;341:c4078.
31. Langley GJ, Moen RD, Nolan KM, Nolan TW, Norman CL, Provost LP. *The Improvement Guide: A Practical Approach to Enhancing Organizational Performance*. San Francisco, CA: Jossey-Bass; 2009.
32. Nease RF, Glave Frazee S, Zarin L, Miller SB. Choice architecture is a better strategy than engaging patients to spur behavior change. *Health Aff (Millwood)*. 2013;32(2):242–249.
33. Halpern SD, Ubel PA, Asch DA. Harnessing the power of default options to improve health care. *N Engl J Med*. 2007;357(13):1340–1344.
34. Halpern SD, Loewenstein G, Volpp KG, et al. Default options in advance directives influence how patients set goals for end-of-life care. *Health Aff (Millwood)*. 2013;32(2):408–417.
35. Patel MS, Asch DA, Volpp KG. Nudge Units to Improve the Delivery of Health Care. *NEJM Catalyst (February 19, 2018)* 2018. Accessed April 30, 2018, from https://catalyst.nejm.org/nudge-unit-improve-health-care-delivery/.

9 LEAN IMPROVEMENT TECHNIQUES IN HEALTHCARE

> **Case**
>
> Throughout this chapter, we will return to Dr. Sanchez's experience of the process of central venous catheter placement in the ICU at Arbitrary Regional General Hospital. By way of quick explanation, the placement of a central venous catheter is necessary to give critically ill patients certain medications or fluids rapidly. The catheter, or central line, is often placed in the internal jugular, the subclavian, or the femoral vein, large veins that run near arteries; and is often placed with ultrasound guidance, as Dr. Sanchez intends to do. The process can be simplified to several critical steps, although substantial variation remains between providers and across hospitals.

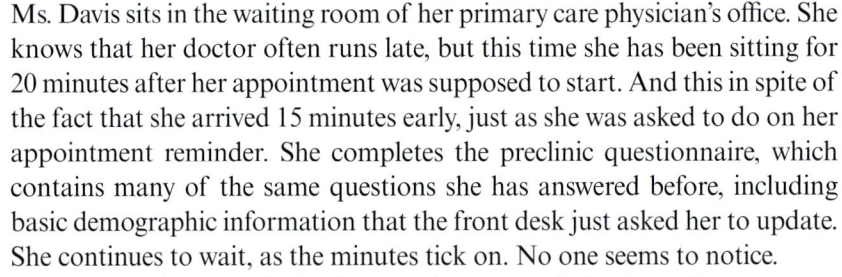

Ms. Davis sits in the waiting room of her primary care physician's office. She knows that her doctor often runs late, but this time she has been sitting for 20 minutes after her appointment was supposed to start. And this in spite of the fact that she arrived 15 minutes early, just as she was asked to do on her appointment reminder. She completes the preclinic questionnaire, which contains many of the same questions she has answered before, including basic demographic information that the front desk just asked her to update. She continues to wait, as the minutes tick on. No one seems to notice.

Dr. Sanchez stands in the supply room of the intensive care unit (ICU) at Arbitrary Regional General Hospital. She knows that the large-bore central venous catheter she is working with has to go in quickly. Her patient is rapidly losing blood but only has in place in her arms tiny intravenous (IV) catheters, so any blood that she wants to put back into her patient will go in very slowly. As she looks around, she finds that all the pieces she needs to put the central line in the patient safely are spread out on all of the towering shelves before her. Saline flushes… saline flushes… She finds the nonsterile flushes, but she needs the special sterile ones for the field. And she can locate sterile gloves and a gown (all in large sizes, not her size), but not the mask and hat she needs for the procedure. She feels her heart thumping in her chest as she knows the minutes spent in this room looking for supplies are minutes the patient cannot afford to lose.

Waste is everywhere in healthcare. We are constantly tolerating wasted time in ways that would never be acceptable in other industries. Imagine showing up for restaurant reservations but reliably sitting down to eat 30–45 minutes late–and without a word of apology. Waste can be disrespectful to patients, causing them to feel their time is considered less valuable than the providers' time. But in other cases, waste can actively be dangerous. What additional interventions will Dr. Sanchez's patient have to receive because her physician couldn't find the tools she needed, lost and pacing through a supply room stocked like a warehouse (but stocked with medical equipment designed for only one size of doctor)?

CHAPTER 9 | LEAN IMPROVEMENT TECHNIQUES IN HEALTHCARE

In this chapter, we will continue to add to the tools and techniques largely borrowed from other fields to unravel, understand, and improve healthcare. We will focus on specific tools taken from the *Toyota Production System (TPS)*, or *Lean production.* Initially, we will look at some specifics and further readings in this field, describing several of the tools available through this strategy, and then describe how Lean has been used (or failed to be used) in healthcare. We believe that many of these tools are useful on their own and can be married to other methods of improvement, although several Lean proponents in healthcare believe this method leads managers to "drown in techniques."[1,2]

A BRIEF HISTORY OF LEAN

Toyota changed manufacturing. And this car company pulled off this dramatic, unexpected business transformation in just a few decades. It changed from a small, struggling company in the stressed, post–World War II Japanese economy to a dominant international car manufacturer in the second half of the 20th century, in a story told by Womack and Jones in *The Machine that Changed the World*.[3]

Before Toyota, car manufacturing used assembly lines, a method that had previously revolutionized this industry in the 1910s and 1920s (and, later, other industries as well). Unfortunately for the individual worker, the job of working on the assembly line was repetitive and boring. The process of building a car required that any one step be completed before the next one could be started. If any one employee had to stop working, the entire line shut down for everyone. Supervisors were largely paid by the number of cars the line produced, making mistakes a common occurrence and largely not corrected until after the assembly was completed (if then). Given the lack of attention to errors, many mistakes weren't caught, and defective cars were sold to the public, with consumers having little alternative.

In the 1950s, devastated from World War II, Japan's Toyota car company transformed the manufacturing of cars to create products based on the demands of its customers and the desire to minimize waste. Originally based on observations (and the rejection) of the Ford Motor Company's production system, Eiji Toyoda and Taichii Ohno, two engineers, developed the TPS. TPS, or what has come to be called *Lean production,* is based on the value of *Kaizen,* or continuous improvement, and respect for both employees and customers. In contrast to the assembly model, any time an error is identified, the line is stopped and the system is examined to continuously improve and eliminate that and future similar errors.

The Lean production model values the worker as the person with the greatest expertise in any given specific manufacturing process. Workers have the freedom to experiment with new processes. Errors are investigated by repeatedly asking "why" to get to the root cause of a problem rather than individual blame.

The result was a production system that maximized flexibility and gave customers what they wanted, while minimizing inventory, waste, and anything the customer did not value. By the 1990s, Toyota had risen alongside the American automaking giants to capture a similar market share in the United States. The result was also the discovery of an appealing series of management and leadership strategies that help improve systems continuously, while giving power and leadership to the frontline worker.[2-4]

Those in healthcare saw the appeal and the easy crossover. Here was a field where the frontline provider felt largely unheard. But when those frontline providers made mistakes, those mistakes really mattered. Most important, here was an industry where healthcare providers came with an inherent sense of duty to the work that they do.

Lean began turning up in healthcare in the form of new organizations (e.g., www.lean.org), national meetings, and many individual tests of change. Several healthcare organizations embraced Lean throughout the management structure. Many healthcare organizations have embraced Lean or tools from Lean. Two that stand out are Virginia Mason and ThedaCare.

Virginia Mason Production System

In a collaboration with several purchasers of healthcare, Virginia Mason, a Seattle-area hospital, used Lean methods to focus on five specific domains of quality: patient satisfaction, use of evidence-based care, rapid access to care, rapid return to functioning, and cost.[5] The healthcare system used clinical value streams to identify care that did not add value, which resulted in decreased use of magnetic resonance imaging (MRI) for headaches (23%) and lumbar pain (23%) and computed tomography (CT) scans for sinus disease (27%).

ThedaCare Improvement System

Over a five-year period, the entire organization of ThedaCare Regional Medical Center in Wisconsin worked to continuously improve quality of the care they delivered, moving toward a goal of a 10% increase in productivity. The organization describes 18 units trialing over 3,600 improvements, including a 25% improvement in warfarin education for inpatient cardiology patients and a 70% reduction of inpatient falls in the oncology unit.[1]

Most organizations used the tools derived from Lean to perform individual tests of change. For example, consider the efforts to improve bloodstream infections from central-line catheters led by Peter Pronovost and others in a Michigan collaborative. Fundamentally, by generating a checklist for central line insertion, these investigators reduced the process to a series of predictable, measurable steps. This method borrows largely from Lean and has led to large national declines in central-line infections.[6,7] However, a comprehensive literature review of Lean in healthcare published in 2015 yielded 243 studies, with only 18 describing patient safety outcomes and 14 describing clinical quality.[8] Steven Spear notes that this may not run counter to the foundational work of Lean, that "people don't typically go in for big, dramatic cure-alls. Instead, they break big problems into smaller, tractable pieces and generate a steady rush of iterative changes that collectively deliver spectacular results."[9]

THE RULES OF LEAN

Despite the appeal of the Lean system, many industries have had difficulty replicating the approach. To attempt to understand the success of Lean, Spear traveled to Japan to interview and observe workers and managers at Toyota itself. He found that many Toyota workers couldn't articulate the rules they applied to their daily work. But Spear's observations brought four rules to light, which will be described next.[10]

Rule 1: Work is done is a highly repeatable, measurable way, with a clear process and order.

Spear observed that seats were installed in cars in U.S. manufacturing plants in an order determined by the worker: walk and get the bolts, wait for the car frame to arrive, install the seat, and tighten the bolts, one after another. Meanwhile, in a Toyota plant, a worker would have a series of prespecified steps and an expected amount of time to complete them. If the process took longer than expected or the steps were out of order, this would be quickly apparent to both the frontline worker and everyone else. This process would have all extra steps or waste removed.

Rule 2: All connections between people are simple and unambiguous.

Each interaction between people—suppliers and line workers, line workers and supervisors, etc.—was performed in a direct, clear, and prespecified way. And all communication had to fit into the expected time to complete a task described in Rule 1. In the Toyota plant itself, workers would use *Kanban,* or preprinted cards, to request what they needed to keep work moving forward. If the communication added time to the process, it would come to light as a problem. Note that Rule 2 means that all problems are out in the open. Workers are not to solve problems on their own because doing so means that workarounds are used and generalized knowledge is never gained or shared. Instead, problems are called out to supervisors because these are unlikely to be unique to the individual worker or worker/supervisor dyad.

Rule 3. The production path for every item (and person) is clear and prespecified.

Each item follows a clear, specified path, and each person has a specific person to look to for help. As Spear emphasizes, because each path is always the same, if there is a problem, delay, or ambiguous message, the path will release data that there may be an issue.

Rule 4. The workers closest to a particular task use the scientific method to improve their daily work.

Workers, in conjunction with their supervisor (who functions as their teacher), must make hypotheses, test them, and then share their successes with the larger factory. The frontline worker must be the one developing the hypotheses, however, because they are the ones with the most data.

A CONCRETE DEFINITION OF THE IDEAL

The final insight to be gained from Spear's work with TPS are the ideals all the workers strive for. The ideal in TPS is not a general mission statement, but an unambiguous, specific, and concrete goal for the entire organization. The team at Intermountain Healthcare, an organization that used Lean methods to improve care, translated the TPS ideal for healthcare as follows:[11]

> Exactly what the patient needs, defect free.
> One by one, customized to each individual patient.
> On demand, exactly as requested.
> Immediate response to problems or changes.
> No waste.
> Safe for patients, staff, and clinicians: Physically, emotionally, and professionally.

In Lean healthcare, the ideal becomes how to give patients only what they need and want, paring out all the additional waste, and keeping our focus solely on the patient's health.

Key Point

The ideal in Lean healthcare is to eliminate waste to give patients exactly what they need for health.

THE 8 WASTES

To begin to practice our Lean thinking, we start with learning to spot waste. Fundamental to the Lean ideal is to remove all waste from the process (hence the term *lean*) and distill each system down to only the most necessary elements. Ohno condensed all types of waste in any system into eight categories, which helps all members of the production team to spot and remove them:[12]

- **Idle time**—Time spent waiting is wasted. Waiting on the production line for the product to roll up in front of you means your skills are not being used. In healthcare, idle time in rampant. Ms. Davis waited for her physician in the waiting room at the start of this chapter. Physicians wait for other physicians to round on patients. Patients wait in waiting rooms to see providers. Providers sit on hold with insurance companies in search of coverage options for their patients. Everyone in healthcare waits all the time.
- **Inventory**—Inventory waiting to be used ties up resources in the form of sunk costs to purchase the materials and storage space and cost to keep it. If the end use for the inventory ends up evolving or improving (e.g., the office purchases a new printer), then all of the inventory that has been waiting to be used (e.g., unused printer cartridges for the prior printer) is completely wasted. An example from healthcare includes the huge, confusing supply closet in which Dr. Sanchez got lost.
- **Defects**—Defects or failures in the process require rework to fix them. Rework takes staff, resources, and time, all of which are not being used to make new products. In healthcare, a surgical error is a defect. A patient may have to return to the operating room because of that error, tying up all the capital costs associated with running the operating room, the surgeon's time, and, most important, the patient's health. Another example of a defect in healthcare is a central-line infection, which increases the patient's length of stay and/or his or her risk of death.[13]
- **Transportation**—The unnecessary movement of supplies or people adds to wasted time and possible defects due to not having the right equipment or right person in the right place at the right time. In healthcare, we can interpret this to mean the transportation of patients to multiple studies on different floors of a hospital, or asking outpatients to walk to one area to get their blood drawn, but other places to get a chest x-ray. Alternatively, *transportation* can

be the movement of a clinician trying to gather supplies for a procedure from multiple confusing places, increasing both time and the chance that a necessary item is missing.
- **Motion**—Unnecessary motion also increases wasted time and possible harm. In healthcare, many novice residents in the ICU will set up for a procedure with the patient in an uncomfortable position for both patient and provider. More experienced clinicians, however, have a specific process by which they perform a procedure, which minimizes extra movements that do not add value for the patient, thereby reducing the risk that an essential piece of equipment is overlooked or out of reach.
- **Overproduction**—Making too many products at the same time, or at inappropriate times, floods the system with unnecessary items. Drawing unnecessary labs that are disregarded, such as checking basic laboratory studies on the day of discharge, "just to be sure," increases waste for the patient (blood loss, cost, time), the laboratory (cost, time), and eventually the hospital (prolonged length of stay).
- **Overprocessing**—Excess care that provides no additional benefit to the patient represents overprocessing in the system. Unfortunately, overprocessing in healthcare is rampant. For example, there is substantial variation in specialty referrals, ICU transfers, and palliative care use by region and by availability of resources.[14] At least some proportion of this variation must be due to excess care or overprocessing.
- **Human potential**—The sheer volume of time spent on all of these other points wastes the thoughts, creativity, and engagement of healthcare workers. Healthcare worker burnout is a growing topic in the healthcare literature, a reflection of the sheer magnitude of time spent by providers on all of other wastes we described, and the consequence to human potential when the health system actively obstructs providers from working at the "top of their licenses", as described in Chapter 4.[15,16]

We now return to Dr. Sanchez's frantic search for central-line equipment in the supply room of the ICU. To put the practice of waste-spotting into practice, we have outlined here several types of waste she encountered,

CHAPTER 9 | LEAN IMPROVEMENT TECHNIQUES IN HEALTHCARE

in the order that they occur in her process (Note: we've highlighted the examples of waste in italics as you go through each example.):

Waste	Central-Line-Specific Wastes
Transportation	Dr. Sanchez *walked back and forth seven times* in the supply room, looking for and gathering the necessary tools for the procedure, which were spread out around the room. Eventually she gathered all of the necessarily pieces of equipment, her arms full as she rushes out of the supply room.
Inventory	In the process of gathering her tools, she grabbed five sterile saline flushes, knowing she didn't want to be without a necessary flush while doing the line (sterile flushes help make sure the catheter is working smoothly). Over the course of the procedure, however, she used only three flushes. *The extra two had to be thrown out after the procedure.*
Motion	During her setup, in her haste, Dr. Sanchez placed a crucial piece of equipment, the flexible wire, out of easy reach. She began the procedure, located the internal jugular vein with the ultrasound, and then inserted the sharp introducer needle into the vein. But now she needed her wire. *She contorted herself to reach for the wire* while the introducer needle was inserted into the patient's vein, which risked inadvertently advancing the needle without her knowing it.
Defects	*Because her needle moved by accident, Dr. Sanchez inadvertently hit the carotid artery,* which sat directly beneath the internal jugular vein. This error required that she stop the procedure temporarily and hold pressure over the puncture site. She then had to start the process over to locate the vein again, which she eventually did.
Idle time	After inserting the central venous catheter into the internal jugular vein and securing it with stitches and a sterile dressing, Dr. Sanchez wants to further confirm the location using a portable chest x-ray. She orders the x-ray. Dr. Sanchez *waits for the x-ray technician to arrive—and waits, and waits…*
Human potential	The stress of putting a greatly needed central line in the patient Dr. Sanchez distracts her from thinking about her next patient, as she continues to review what went wrong in her head.

As this example shows, there is waste all around us. Now let's move on to several foundational tools from Lean. Each of these tools allow us to delve into the details of a process, unpack it, and begin to refine the true costs of waste to the patient.

TOOLS FROM LEAN

Process Mapping

To improve a process, we typically start by understanding the current state. An excellent starting point and overview is the process map, which allows the user to break any given process down into the individual component parts. We have covered the detailed tools of process mapping in Chapter 8. We will now fold in concepts inherent in Lean, and then apply an example from Dr. Sanchez's work.

The first major step in mapping the current state is observing the process, in detail. Understanding each detail requires that the practitioner walk through the process from beginning to end, a process called going to *gemba,* the "place where value-creating work happens,"[17] but it is frequently used to mean going to the front line, where actual work happens, to uncover the truth in the process. We recommend starting with a quick summative walk, followed by a more in-depth walk to time each step and sketch out the process.[18] The more detail, the better.

A gemba walk through of Dr. Sanchez's central-line-insertion process can be seen in Figure 9-1. There appear to be five major steps: (1) getting all the necessary equipment; (2) getting the ultrasound so the central line can be inserted under direct visual guidance; (3) taking all the equipment to the room, setting up the patient and the equipment, and creating a sterile field; (4) inserting the central line; and (5) confirming the location with chest x-ray visualization. The process map serves as a good start. There are clearly very different processes taking place—the process in the supply room is different from that at the patient's bedside. The introduction of a chest x-ray means that the process of another area, radiology, intersects with the ICU's processes as well.

Get sterile equipment → Get ultrasound → Set up patient and equipment → Place central line → Confirm location with chest x-ray

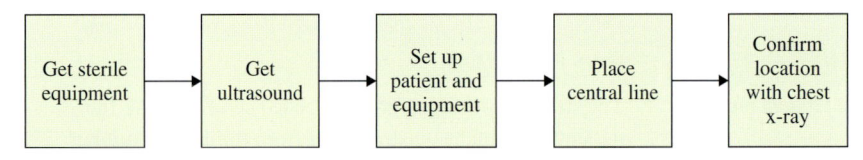

Figure 9-1 • Process map of the insertion of a central venous catheter. Depending on the improvement process being undertaken, each step could be broken down into its own multistep process map, as well.

Now we can start to see the shortcomings of process maps. While we can understand the process in broad strokes, we don't have any data or information about the details. Does getting the equipment take a lot of time? Why? How often are there problems getting the ultrasound, or finding that it wasn't plugged in the night before, so its battery is depleted? Which parts of the process actually matter to the patient? Put another way, do any of the parts of the process actually add to the patient's health? The next tool in our discussion, value stream mapping, helps us answer these questions.

Value Stream Mapping

Value stream mapping draws out all the value-added and nonvalue-added steps in any process, from start to finish. Under most circumstances where the user is trying to understand a process in detail, we recommend mapping the current state. When the user is looking to fundamentally transform a system or start from scratch, one can map a future state or process. Value stream maps have a substantial amount of data, usually taking the form of time. To gather time data, we recommend measuring each step and cycle by hand. Time counts collected for other purposes (e.g., admission, discharge and transfer tables that track patient movement) often lack the detail necessary for this tool.

The standard elements of a basic value-stream map are the following[18]:

Symbol	What It Means
Factory	**Factory**. This symbol describes the boundaries of the process.
Data Box	**Data Box**. These boxes contain the different types of data that make up the requirements for the customer.
Process Box	**Process Box**. These are the individual processes that make up the flow. Typically, these describe slightly larger processes, and a new box starts where there are breaks in the material or flow.

The material flow (or patient flow, in this case) goes from left to right on the bottom of the map. The information flow, designated by arrows, moves from right to left. At the bottom of the map, one draws a timeline, which documents the wait time between each step in the process and the cycle time for each step. The timeline can draw a distinction between time spent in the current state and the proportion that is time spent on value-added steps.

There are several elements of data that can be collected for each step of the process:

Data Element	Definition
Cycle time	The total time from one produced part to the next produced part.
Batch	The number of products you make at one time
Inventory (or Work in Progress)	The number of items waiting at any given stage (e.g., patients to be seen)
Changeover time	The time from making one part to making another part.
Number of people	The number of people required to operate the process.
Available working time	The total time, minus breaks, available for working (e.g., number of hours in a shift).
Value-added time	The total time spent creating a product that the customer is willing to pay for.
Lead time	The total time for a piece to move from start to finish in the value-stream process.

We have generated an oversimplified value stream map of Dr. Sanchez's problem of putting in a central line and gathering the necessary equipment to make that process happen (Figure 9-2). The total lead time, or the time spent on the entire process, is 56 minutes. This means that for Dr. Sanchez's patient to get the lifesaving intervention of rapidly infusing blood products, he or she needs to wait nearly an hour. And we have assumed no errors in placement (e.g., accidentally sticking the arterial vessel rather than the vein) and no rework.

By illustrating the process, even in general detail, we can see several glaring areas of waste, which we already suspected when we practiced

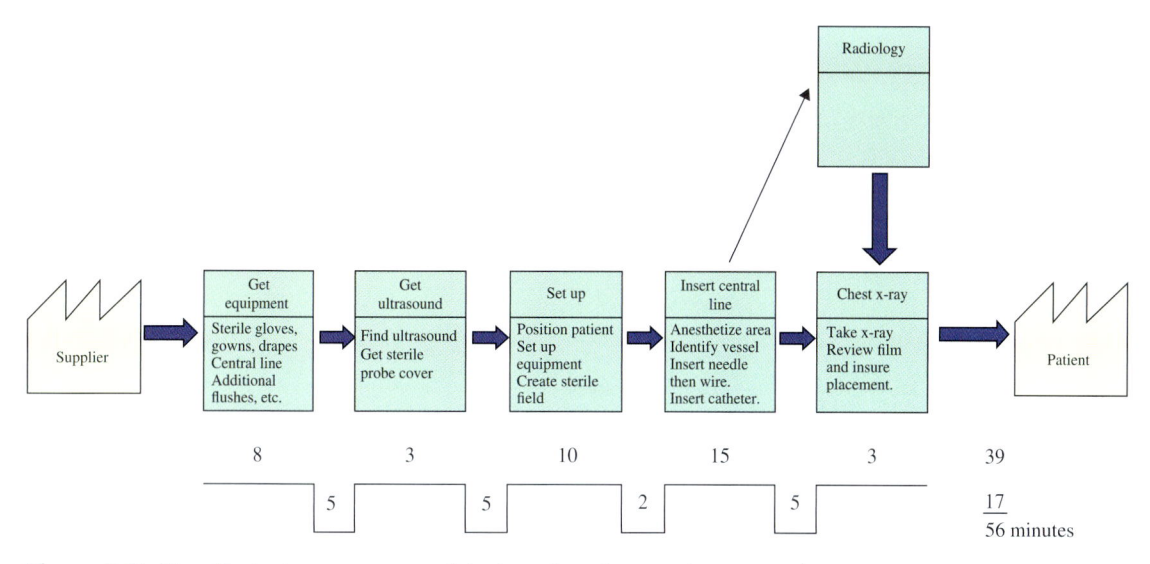

Figure 9-2 • Simplified value stream map of the insertion of a central venous catheter.

looking for waste earlier in the chapter. First, the process of acquiring the central-line equipment takes a long time (nearly 8 minutes). We would need to walk through that process carefully to understand, hypothesize, and test improvements to reduce that time.

Second, setting up the patient also seems to take a long time. This may be because this process is always done in a variable, haphazard way, with lots of opportunities to reduce variation. Perhaps using a stepwise, unambiguous checklist approach to central-line insertion would reduce time.

Third, Dr. Sanchez spent more time waiting for the radiology technician to arrive and take the x-ray (5 minutes) than she did using reviewing the x-ray (3 minutes), and the process involved substantial transportation as the x-ray technician pushed the machine to the ICU. What ways could we get the x-ray faster? Is it necessary at all?

Fourth, there does not appear to be much in the entire process that adds to patient health. The actual process of insertion appears to be the only true value-added part of the process (perhaps we could say 1 minute of additional value-added time earlier in order to ensure sterile equipment). The entire production yields only approximately 3 minutes of value-added time, but we kept the patient waiting nearly an hour. Our value stream map gives us plenty of targets for improvement. Now, how do we start identifying and testing hypotheses to make these improvements happen? More important, how do we gain consensus and build a team to make this happen? Our final tool, the A3, helps bring the task of improvement into focus.

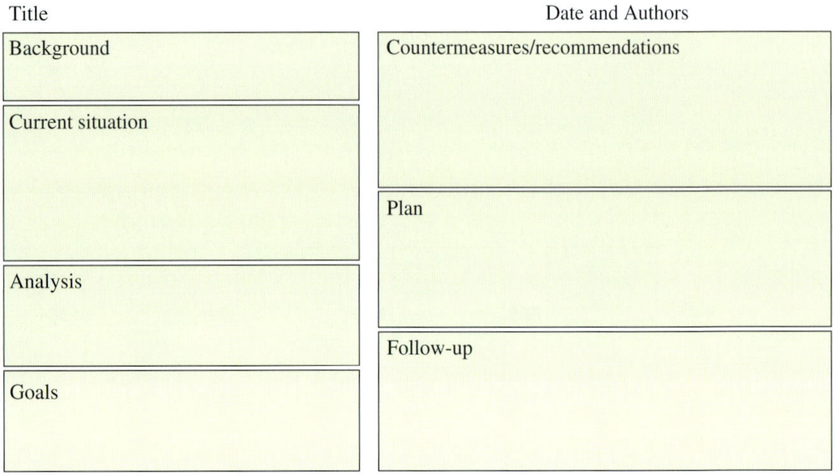

Title		Date and Authors
Background		Countermeasures/recommendations
Current situation		
		Plan
Analysis		
		Follow-up
Goals		

Figure 9-3 • A blank A3 template.

A3

The term *A3* refers to a specific size of paper, approximately 11 by 17 inches, designed to guide and focus a group of people collaborating on a process toward the "right thing to do."[17] To use the A3 process, one brings together a group to create a clear narrative of a specific challenge or problem, describe the current state, identify the goals and plan, and clarify all associated measures. The document contained in the A3 puts each of these elements in writing, a process that focuses all parties in the room on the process to change.

Figure 9-3 shows the basic framework of an A3. The sections should include the following: (1) a title and a place for the authors to sign; (2) the background; (3) the current condition or situation; (4) necessary goals and targets; (5) an analysis, which means a proposed root cause to the problem; (6) proposed countermeasures, or ways to tackle the current problems; (7) a plan for moving forward; and (8) the proposed follow-up. How different teams design their A3s and use them vary substantially. Note that the A3 process uses the concepts of analysis and countermeasures differently than other parts of quality improvement described in this text. *Countermeasures* here refers to the identification of the problems and a series of proposed solutions, rather than using the term to mean balancing measures ensuring that an improvement doesn't have unintended consequences. *Analysis* for an A3 is the proposed root cause, rather than a more detailed presentation of results.

The following prompting questions aid in the A3 development process (adapted from John Shook's *Managing to Learn: Using the A3 Management Process to Solve Problems, Gain Agreement, Mentor, and Lead*, which serves as a useful workbook and resource to delve into the A3 process in greater detail):[17]

- What is the problem?
- Who owns the problem?
- What are the root causes of the problem?
- What are our proposed countermeasures, "temporary responses to specific problems"?[19]
- How can we move toward agreement?
- How will we implement our plan?
- What's our follow-up plan?
- How will we share what we've learned?

External Resource

For other good examples of A3, please see Shook's *Managing to Learn* and Jimmerson et al's "Reducing waste and error: piloting lean principles at IHC."

The A3 tool is particularly useful in a couple of ways. For one thing, the development of a single, focused goal guides both the meeting where the A3 is derived and subsequent meetings, where the team can come together to evaluate and refine the work. For another, the A3 requires that all parties buy into the agreement and the goals in the document. In fact, A3s should be signed by the coauthors, further formalizing this agreement. Finally, the document itself becomes a way of communicating the process and telling its story. Shook recommends using a variety of tools beyond text alone, such as control charts, graphs, Gantt charts, process and future state maps, and sketches.[17]

Based on her experience in the supply room, Dr. Sanchez decides to lead an effort to remove waste from the process of inserting central lines in the hospital's ICU. She convenes a workgroup with members from materials and processing, nursing, and critical care at the hospital. She sets a goal to reduce the time of inserting central lines and proposes a plan to create premade central-line equipment bags, thereby reducing the random pacing and searching that stalled her in the supply room. Using an A3 as a tool for the various parts of the hospital to unify around, she could get the group to design and iterate on the goal of keeping all related supplies in one single place in the supply room. At the end of the A3 session, all members sign the document, thereby demonstrating their commitment to removing waste from the central-line insertion process.

SUMMARY

In this chapter, we have briefly reviewed the history of TPS (Lean) and its application to healthcare. The skills and tools that we covered are useful in examining any contained system or process and keeping our focus solely on what matters to patients. But consider those larger "factory" shapes in our value stream map, the symbols that mean entire industries, locations, teams, or places exist at the start and end of our processes. Any set of tools derived from industrial processes may have limits in the complex environment of healthcare. Lean tools may be best used in healthcare settings that best match industrial assembly lines or processes, such as central-line insertion, operating rooms, or emergency departments (EDs) that move patients in and out of a system.

Later in this book, we will return to several analytical methods that better accommodate the complexity of healthcare. In the next chapter, we will look beyond our individual, complicated tasks in healthcare and examine the larger, complex system of community-based organizations and policy organizations—the system that surrounds and makes up a larger health system.

KEY POINTS

- Lean healthcare, or the Toyota Production System (TPS), is based on respect for the frontline worker and the patient, removing waste, and focusing only on tasks that add value.
- Waste is rampant throughout healthcare.
- To understand a process, one must walk physically through the process in detail, collecting data in the form of time (known as **going to gemba**).
- Process and value stream maps clarify the current process in order to target improvements.
- A3s are useful for building consensus and sharing improvements.

REFERENCES

1. Barnas K. ThedaCare's business performance system: sustaining continuous daily improvement through hospital management in a lean environment. *Jt Comm J Qual Patient Saf*. 2011;37(9):387–399.
2. Womak J, Daniel J. *Lean Thinking: Banish Waste and Create Wealth in Your Corporation*. New York: Free Press; 2003.
3. Womack JP, Jones DT, Roos D, Massachusetts Institute of Technology. *The Machine That Changed the World: Based on the Massachusetts Institute of Technology 5-Million Dollar 5-Year Study on the Future of the Automobile*. New York: Rawson Associates; 1990.
4. Krafcik JF. Triumph of the Lean production system. *Sloan Management Review*. 1988;30(1):41–52.

5. Blackmore CC, Mecklenburg RS, Kaplan GS. At Virginia Mason, collaboration among providers, employers, and health plans to transform care cut costs and improved quality. *Health Aff (Millwood)*. 2011;30(9):1680–1687.
6. Pronovost P, Needham D, Berenholtz S, et al. An intervention to decrease catheter-related bloodstream infections in the ICU. *N Engl J Med*. 2006;355(26):2725–2732.
7. Centers for Disease Control and Prevention (CDC). Vital signs: central line-associated blood stream infections—United States, 2001, 2008, and 2009. *MMWR Morb Mortal Wkly Rep*. 2011;60(8):243–248.
8. D'Andreamatteo A, Ianni L, Lega F, Sargiacomo M. Lean in healthcare: A comprehensive review. *Health Policy*. 2015;119(9):1197–1209.
9. Spear SJ. Fixing health care from the inside, today. *Harv Bus Rev*. 2005;83(9):78–91, 158.
10. Spear S, Bowen HK. Decoding the DNA of the Toyota Production System. *Harv Bus Rev*. 1999 (September–October):97–106.
11. Jimmerson C, Weber D, Sobek DK2nd. Reducing waste and errors: piloting lean principles at Intermountain Healthcare. *Jt Comm J Qual Patient Saf*. 2005;31(5):249–257.
12. Catalyst N. What is Lean healthcare? 2018. Accessed December 30, 2018, from https://catalyst.nejm.org/what-is-lean-healthcare/.
13. Rosenthal VD, Guzman S, Migone O, Crnich CJ. The attributable cost, length of hospital stay, and mortality of central line-associated bloodstream infection in intensive care departments in Argentina: A prospective, matched analysis. *Am J Infect Control*. 2003;31(8):475–480.
14. Fisher ES, Bynum JP, Skinner JS. Slowing the growth of health care costs—lessons from regional variation. *N Engl J Med*. 2009;360(9):849–852.
15. Weeks WB. Physician burnout—overdiagnosis and unproven interventions. *JAMA Intern Med*. 2018;178(4):576–577.
16. Panagioti M, Geraghty K, Johnson J, et al. Association between physician burnout and patient safety, professionalism, and patient satisfaction: a systematic review and meta-analysis. *JAMA Intern Med*. 2018;178(10):1317–1330.
17. Shook J. *Managing to Learn: Using the A3 Management Process to Solve Problems, Gain Agreement, Mentor and Lead*. Cambridge, MA: Lean Enterprise Institute; 2008.
18. Rother M, Shook J, Lean Enterprise Institute. *Learning to See: Value Stream Mapping to Create Value and Eliminate Muda*. Brookline, MA: Lean Enterprise Institute; 2003.
19. Spear SJ. Learning to lead at Toyota. *Harv Bus Rev*. 2004;82(5):78–86, 151.

10 PARTNERING WITH COMMUNITY, PROFESSIONAL, AND POLICY ORGANIZATIONS

Sonia Y. Angell and Sarah Shih

INTRODUCTION

The healthcare delivery system is evolving. As described in Chapter 1, its historical simplification of being "a workshop for the physician" is no longer relevant; now it has "the complexity of a living organism." To take the analogy further, the healthcare delivery system, like most living organisms, is not the only creature in the community. Its borders can abut or meld with other evolving systems, and its intended outputs will be influenced by what's happening in the surrounding environment. Healthcare delivery systems research, therefore, cannot be conducted without an understanding of the influences outside its formal operations. Furthermore, that which is outside the formal healthcare delivery system can be a key asset to the study of healthcare delivery science itself. To tap into this added value and analytic insight most effectively, partnering with community, professional, and policy organizations becomes paramount.

This chapter will first set the stage for this discussion, describing what produces health and the context within which the healthcare delivery system itself resides. It will identify other institutions and organizations relevant to the goal of improved health and outline reasons why developing partnerships with relevant players outside of the healthcare delivery system should be of interest to healthcare delivery science through case examples. It will pay particular attention to public health departments because they are a common entity across all communities, and because they have unique standing with respect to mission, resources, and data. Finally, it will provide practical guidance for successful partnering with those outside the healthcare delivery system.

CHAPTER 10 | COMMUNITY, PROFESSIONAL, AND POLICY ORGANIZATIONS

HOW HEALTH IS CREATED

Health is the product of a lifelong interplay between individuals and their environments. Often underappreciated is that healthcare itself is a relatively small contributor to overall population health.[1,2] While individual-level conditions, such as genetic mutations, cardiovascular risk factors, or diseases, are often the target of medical interventions, a host of non-clinical, social, and economic factors are influencing health concurrently. These factors include those commonly referred to as the "social determinants of health," such as housing, education, income, discrimination, and safety.[3] They shape the conditions of places where we live, learn, work, play, and worship, molding the health of individuals, communities, and populations across the life course.[4] (See Figure 10-1.[5])

These factors, their quality, and their distribution across populations may enhance or impede health and contribute to inequities in health outcomes commonly documented today. For example, parks that are perceived to be unsafe are less likely to be used for physical activity by those who live in the community[6]; poorly maintained housing affected by mold, dust mites, or cockroaches can exacerbate asthma[7]; low family income can result in food insecurity, poor nutrition, and obesity[8,9]; and stress and discrimination are associated with increased blood pressure.[10] While our understanding of the causal pathways through which these factors influence health continues to evolve, appreciating that these external influences will affect the health outcomes measured in the study of healthcare delivery operations is key.

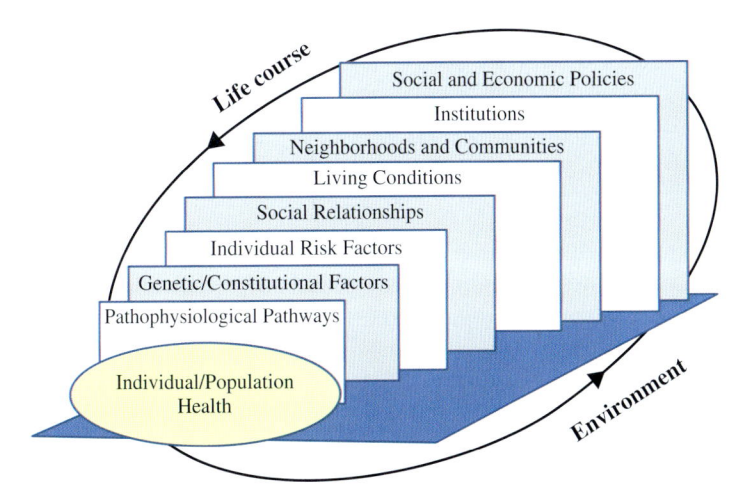

Figure 10-1 • Socioecological model, a multilevel approach to epidemiology described by Kaplan et al. (Used with permission from Kaplan GA, Everson SA, Lynch JW (2000).[5])

These place-shaping determinants historically have functioned untouched by the reach of clinical care delivery systems. Recently, however, changes in payment incentives and effects of healthcare reform have blurred those relationships and the boundaries of healthcare delivery systems themselves. Healthcare organizations are now partnering with community organizations, including those who have traditionally worked outside healthcare, and the reverse is true as well (see Boxes 10-1 and 10-2). These newly forged connections are essential to creating systems that link the clinical and nonclinical environments, with population health as the bridge between them. Although inclusion of community and social services as part of healthcare payment or operations may seem more recent, public health entities have long histories of looking across and involving multiple sectors to create health.

> **Key Point**
>
> Healthcare organizations are now partnering with community organizations, including those who have traditionally worked outside healthcare, and the reverse is true as well.

Box 10-1 CASE STUDY 1: PAYMENT REFORM

For decades, lawmakers, payers, and others have been attempting to address unsustainable growth in healthcare costs.[11] Policymakers are searching for ways to control costs while maintaining quality and improved health outcomes by testing new provider payment models.[12,13] Over time, various payment models have been tested for payments of discrete services (fee-for-service) as opposed to a payment for the total cost of care. One recent approach to reimbursing for the total cost of care is called *value-based payment*.[14] This arrangement aims to reimburse providers based on the value of care they provide to the patient—and, by extension, the payer—instead of reimbursing by volume and type of service provided.[15,16] Here is an example of one variant of value-based payment called shared savings:

- Dr. Gomez sees Mrs. Jones, who has diabetes.
- The insurance company has observed that, on average, care for patients like Mrs. Jones costs $5,000 per year in medical expenditures. Similar patients are hospitalized twice a year which costs an additional $10,000 per day of stay in the hospital.
- Dr. Gomez provides care to Mrs. Jones that costs the insurance company only $2,000 that year, and Mrs. Jones does not get hospitalized.
- Dr. Gomez and the insurance company split the savings between the expected cost and the actual cost—the patient, the doctor, and the insurance company are all "winners" in this system.

While this example is simplified, the concept remains the same—the amount that the provider gets paid is not linked to the services that they provide, but rather the health and savings that they create. This type of arrangement removes the need for discrete, billable services and instead

> **Box 10-2 CASE STUDY 2: COMMUNITY AND CLINICAL SYSTEM PARTNERSHIPS**
>
> As the healthcare delivery system seeks to influence the health of communities at large, it increasingly links to other health-related entities, both public and private, including those that address social determinants of health. In Summit County, Ohio, a multistakeholder coalition of over 70 partners across hospital systems, payers, community and faith-based organizations, and other groups have formed an accountable care community (ACC).[18] The ACC strives to meet the health needs of the local community, with a focus on chronic disease prevention and management, by strengthening connections between clinical and community resources, integrating clinical and public health approaches, and creating a robust health information technology (IT) infrastructure to support agency referrals and resource tracking.[19] The ACC in Summit County was one of the first of its kind, but the model is being adopted in other localities nationwide.[18]
>
> The Summit County ACC has adopted a "Health in All Policies" tactic to address its diabetes problem.[20] This approach considers the health impact of areas of policy that are not health-specific, such as transportation or housing. Through a multipronged approach that included activities like increasing access to healthy fruits and vegetables, and redesigning city streets in partnership with the local transportation authority, the partnership reported significant weight loss, diabetes control, and reductions in the cost of care for their participants with diabetes.[18]

brings resources to allow a provider to care for patients more holistically. This may include addressing social determinants by screening for social needs and connecting patients to resources. In other words, total-cost-of-care payment models create an opportunity to bring community and social services into the clinical setting.[17] Often, these arrangements are structured so that the provider is not judged by a payer based upon one patient, but rather on the outcomes of the *entire population* of patients that they see. Increasingly, a shift toward value-based payment forces the lines between healthcare delivery and public health to blur.

Key Point

Payment reform means providers' quality metrics and reimbursement structures may be judged on the *entire population* of patients that they see rather than any single patient.

KEY STAKEHOLDERS IN SHAPING HEALTH

Public health is a key system with the recognized responsibility for generating health. According to the U.S. Centers for Disease Control and Prevention (CDC), a common definition of public health systems is "all public, private, and voluntary entities that contribute to the delivery of

> **Box 10-3 TEN ESSENTIAL PUBLIC HEALTH SERVICES**
>
> In 1994, representatives of U.S. Public Health Service agencies and other major public health organizations convened the Core Public Health Functions Steering Committee, which developed the Ten Essential Public Health Services that public health systems should undertake.[21] (See Figure 10-2.) These services remain relevant today and act as a guiding framework for public health actions. The Ten Essential Public Health Services are:
>
> 1. Monitor health status to identify and solve community health problems.
> 2. Diagnose and investigate health problems and health hazards in the community.
> 3. Inform, educate, and empower people about health issues.
> 4. Mobilize community partnerships and action to identify and solve health problems.
> 5. Develop policies and plans that support individual and community health efforts.
> 6. Enforce laws and regulations that protect health and ensure safety.
> 7. Link people to needed personal health services and assure the provision of healthcare when otherwise unavailable.
> 8. Assure competent public and personal healthcare workforce.
> 9. Evaluate effectiveness, accessibility, and quality of personal and population-based health services.
> 10. Research for new insights and innovative solutions to health problems.

essential public health services within a jurisdiction"[21] (see Box 10-3). This includes a broad range of actors, from public health government agencies; to economic, environmental, recreational, educational, and human service agencies; to public, private, and philanthropic organizations. According to this definition, it also includes healthcare providers, illustrating the natural overlap between healthcare delivery and public health systems.

Within any community, there also resides a host of other actors who may not view themselves as providers of *essential public health services*; they may not even have "health" embedded in their defined responsibilities. Yet, their actions—and inactions—heavily influence health. An example may be a distributor of sugar-sweetened beverages in a community in which schools are considering removing sodas from their vending machines to decrease unhealthy beverage intake in youth. Alternatively, a developer may want to build a new building, and engage others to participate in design and construction—including city planning, developers,

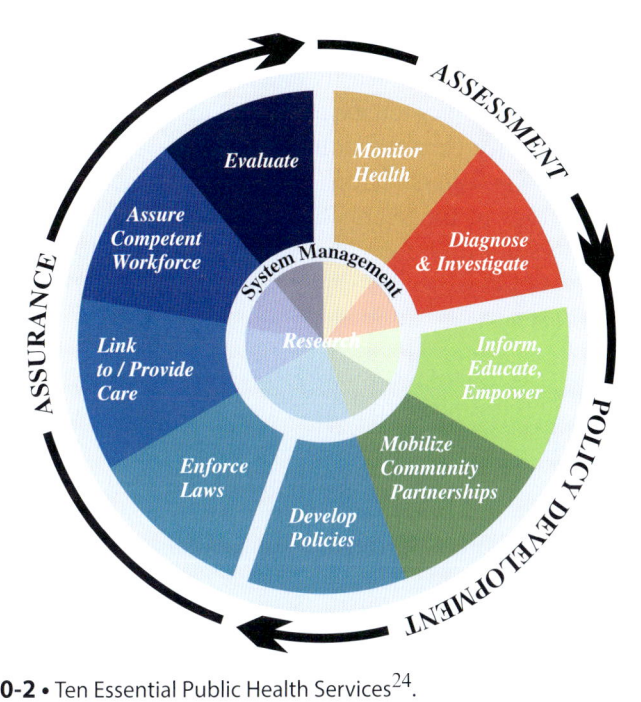

Figure 10-2 • Ten Essential Public Health Services[24].

architects, designers, etc.—all will make decisions that may or may not make the building space promote the health of residents. This includes planning for green spaces, access to light, and mixed-land use to increase access to grocery stores among residential units. As our understanding of the social determinants of health grows, so does the range of influential actors.

While it is beyond the scope of this chapter to describe the full universe of stakeholders shaping health, the following are examples of both nongovernmental and governmental actors.

Nongovernmental Organizations and Private Institutions and Businesses

Community-Based Organizations (CBOs)

Community-based organizations (CBOs) are groups of people, rooted in a particular community or small geographic area, that are committed to providing services that help meet the social needs of that community. The groups can align themselves along many different lines—some may define themselves by a neighborhood, a racial or ethnic group, religious grounds (what we refer to as *faith-based organizations,* or *FBOs*), or they may focus

Key Point

Within any community, there also resides a host of other actors who may not view themselves as providers of *essential public health services*; they may not even have "health" embedded in their defined responsibilities.

on specific medical conditions. The types of services CBOs may provide include providing for food insecurity (such as a food pantry), delivering education on various topics for social well-being, helping the community access legal assistance (immigration, housing, etc.), and others. CBOs tend to have a deep understanding of the specific needs of their community, connections to the people living there, and specific expertise in delivering services not traditionally provided by the healthcare system.

Advocacy Groups

Advocacy groups, as opposed to CBOs, tend to be less rooted in a particular community and less likely to deliver direct services. Instead, advocacy groups have a greater focus on a particular issue area and keep themselves apprised of policy and political issues to try to influence decision-making. The value in partnering with these organizations comes from their vast networks of connections to policymakers, including both legislative and nonlegislative bodies. Advocacy groups also drive communities to support various initiatives, raising awareness among elected officials in local communities. These groups can be organized professionals (like medical associations or labor unions), focused on a particular disease or class of diseases (such as the American Heart Association or American Diabetes Association); a specific population (such as a specific geography or special interest area); or other groups. Many CBOs and other organizations often have advocacy teams or dedicated staff in their organization, separate from stand-alone advocacy organizations.

Both CBOs and advocacy groups are often seen as representing the voices of their specific community or issues. When the healthcare sector begins considering interventions to make an impact on the social determinants of health, CBOs and advocacy groups can be vital partners in the planning, developing, and implementing the delivery of services, as well as evaluation of those programs. Likewise, they can be informants for identifying key issues or for advising on health systems research intended to address specific populations or issues.

Healthcare Payers

Organizations that purchase healthcare (e.g., government, insurance companies, unions, employers) can be public or private and have enormous influence over how healthcare is delivered. Payers have the final say over what and how healthcare treatments or services are reimbursed, and they generally have an ability to hold providers accountable for health outcomes and costs of care through reimbursement or incentive mechanisms. At the federal level, Medicare plays a unique role in setting minimum standards for various types of payments. Medicaid, at both the federal and state levels, also has a role in setting payment standards that other payers look to when establishing formularies and payment schemes. A common barrier to improving healthcare delivery is when services needed to improve health are identified but not currently covered.[22,23] Having a payer (or many of them) involved in the research and implementation of services can be a great asset to understanding how the needs of a population can be met and increase the likelihood of payer adoption following successful testing. Payers also are the gatekeepers to a treasure trove of medical claims data that, when used effectively, can be the basis for groundbreaking research on the effectiveness and economics of healthcare delivery.

Private Industry

Private industry—the producers and distributors of the goods and services that surround us—make decisions that have an impact on our health as a part of their businesses. Design, formulation, placement, price, and promotion all play a role in determining the choices we have as consumers, which in turn influences our behavior. From producers of the foods we eat, to the entertainment we engage in, to the types of work we pursue, these stakeholders are a diverse group. That said, companies or corporations are often well organized. When focusing on a sector, their business associations can serve as important connectors on specific issues.

Of interest in this category are community-based pharmacies, which assume a rapidly evolving intermediary role in community-clinical connections. The introduction of clinical care services in big-box stores with embedded pharmacies, like Walmart, Costco, and Target, along with limited-service or drop-in clinics in pharmacy chains like CVS, brings an additional dimension of healthcare access in new environments. Because these care delivery sites may or may not be linked to traditional healthcare delivery systems, they may warrant particular consideration in the design of healthcare delivery systems research.

Government Entities

Government has an important stake in health, along with the ability to influence health through a variety of levers. In the United States, there is hardly any government agency whose work does not touch health at some point. From the Department of Transportation (e.g., clean-energy vehicle requirements that decrease air pollution) to the National Park Service (e.g., investment in green spaces in urban areas that entices physical activity) to the Department of Justice (e.g., decisions to reduce the prison population by redirecting those with mental health issues into community-based treatment programs), they and other agencies influence the health of our communities and should be considered potentially relevant to the study of healthcare delivery systems.

Public Health Agencies

Public health agencies may provide the most direct and natural entry for healthcare delivery researchers into nonhealthcare delivery areas of government. Public health agencies vary in structure, responsibility, and scope of authority at the federal, state, and local levels across the country. They are generally responsible for ensuring that the public health system—the collection of public, private, and nonprofit actors defined earlier—performs its ten essential functions (see Box 10-3).[24]

Federal public health agencies are largely focused on broad policy changes and the provision of funding for research and implementation efforts nationwide. At the state and local levels, much more emphasis is placed on the direct planning and implementation of services and supports to serve constituencies. Public health agencies are typically active in policy development and assessment, and data collection and reporting are part of their core functions. Because they have the ability to be more flexible, both politically and financially, than federal agencies, and due to their concentrated knowledge about particular populations, state and local health departments have produced some significant innovations in health, including through engagement with networks of community partners that focus on different aspects of health and related fields.

ENGAGING WITH LOCAL PUBLIC HEALTH AGENCIES

Public health agencies are unique entities to engage with on healthcare delivery research because they provide broad insight into the community, access to population-level data, ability to convene stakeholders, and positioning to draft, develop, and influence policy.

Insight

Public health agency programming and policies will affect variables of interest to healthcare delivery science. Researcher awareness of when and how relevant actions will be implemented by health departments can provide insight into the planning and design of healthcare delivery research.

For example, New York City (NYC) passed a local regulation in 2006 that restricted the use of *trans fatty acids* (artificial trans fats) in all its restaurants—25,000 of them.[25] Artificial trans fats were targeted because they are associated with increased risk for coronary events, understood to be mediated by their unfavorable impact on lipid profiles. At the time of the policy's launch, trans fats were commonly used for cooking, frying, and baking. This policy was quickly adopted by other cities and states across the country. A study of changes in the purchases of chain restaurants in NYC showed a decline in the amount of trans fats in their meals after the implementation of the policy, and pre-post analysis of serum levels of trans fat in NYC showed a decline after policy implementation.[26,27]

Ecologic studies of the impact of local trans fats regulations associated them with reductions in myocardial infarction-related hospitalizations and cardiovascular disease mortality.[28,29] It is difficult to isolate the relative contribution of specific population-based policies on clinical outcomes. However, without awareness of these external policy assumptions, studies related to healthcare delivery operations, in particular emergency department (ED) use in NYC during this time, may have made incorrect assumptions about the impact of internal healthcare delivery operations.

This is just one example of the myriad ways in which local health department actions may affect healthcare delivery system uses and outcomes. From involvement in nicotine replacement distribution, to the promotion of postexposure human immunodeficiency virus (HIV) prophylaxis, to water tower disinfection following Legionnaires' disease outbreaks, health departments are actively engaged in areas that influence healthcare delivery systems and their patients' outcomes. Establishing relationships with health department leadership can provide deeper insight into potential areas to consider in research design.

Data Access and Analysis

Health is about context, and context is defined not only by variables that are measurable within the healthcare delivery system, but also within the community. In some cases, these data may provide the missing link allowing healthcare delivery research to consider their findings within the context of community trends overall. You may recall that in the Cleveland Health Quality Choice Program (as discussed in Chapter 1), researchers would have more immediately understood the relevance of their findings had the program's analysis been concurrently compared to mortality data in the area or region, avoiding misattribution of results to their quality-improvement efforts.

Government agencies, in particular public health departments, have access to a plethora of data that can be meaningful to healthcare delivery systems research. In fact, the majority of the Ten Essential Public Health Services (see Box 10-3) require the collection, analysis, and use of data.

Table 10-1 provides a categorical overview of various types of data available at specific organizations, largely (although not exclusively) held

Table 10-1 EXAMPLES OF DATA SETS FROM WHICH LOCAL HEALTH INFORMATION CAN BE DEVELOPED

Data type	Data set	Provider organization
Mortality by cause of death Natality (births)	Vital statistics	Local/state health departments
Health behavior and risk factors	Behavioral Risk Factor Surveillance System (BRFSS) and Youth BRFSS	Centers for Disease Control and Prevention; state health departments
Health status and disability	National Health Interview Survey (NHIS)	National Center for Health Statistics (NCHS)
Access to care	State and local health surveys	Examples: California, Hawaii, New York City
Disease prevalence	Cancer incidence and treatment	State or regional cancer registries; National Cancer Institute
	Communicable disease (reported by physicians or laboratories)	Local/state health departments
	Chronic disease (Self-reported)	State and local health surveys: NHIS
Health insurance coverage	Current Population Survey	Census Bureau
	State and local health surveys	Examples: California. Hawaii. New York City
Healthcare use	Hospital discharges, ER use	State health department or hospital association
	Variation in use of services	*Dartmouth Atlas*
	Medicare claims data	Centers for Medicare and Medicaid Services
	Medicaid claims data	State health departments or Medicaid agencies
	Childhood immunization rates; (National Immunization Survey)	NCHS
	Use of services and access barriers	State and local health surveys; NHIS
Healthcare spending	Medical Expenditure Panel Survey	Agency for Healthcare Research and Quality (AHRQ)
Healthcare quality	National Healthcare Quality Report	AHRQ
	Cardiac surgery outcomes	State health departments (New York)

Data type	Data set	Provider organization
Public program participation	Childhood health screening results	State health departments
	Child and maternal nutrition	State Women, Infants, and Children (WIC) agencies
Environmental health	Air quality	Environmental Protection Agency
	Water quality, aquifer patterns	Local/state health departments
Neighborhood and local environment	Mortgage lending patterns (Home Mortgage Disclosure Act data)	Fannie Mae
	School enrolment, quality, prevalence of reduced-price lunches	School districts: state education departments; National Center for Education Statistics
	Reported crimes	Local police departments, Department of justice
	Neighborhood quality-of-life indicators	Community Indicators Consortium members
	Social Capital Community Benchmark Survey	Roper Center/Institute for Social Inquiry
	Housing quality	Local tax accessors/housing inspectors
Bioterrorism-related data	Syndromic surveillance data (ER patient symptoms, OTC drug sales)	Local health departments or regional health information organizations
Local economic conditions	Employment and labor force	Bureau of Labor Statistics
	Income, economic activity	Bureau of Economic Analysis
Demographics (population, age, race/ethnicity, employment, poverty, education)	Decennial census and American Community Survey	Census Bureau
	Survey of Income and Program Participation and other surveys	Census Bureau or other federal agencies (many available online via DataFerrett)
	Earned Income Tax Credit patterns	Internal Revenue Service
	Business and marketing databases	Private date providers (payment required)

SOURCE: Examples provided by participants at a meeting on local health information convened by the Robert Wood Johnson Foundation, Princeton, New Jersey, April 2004.

NOTES: ER is emergency room. OTC is over the counter.

Used with permission from Luck et al. (2006).[31]

by government. Their availability will vary depending upon locality. For example, a city-wide diabetes registry in NYC was created through a change in local health code, resulting in a data source not available in most municipalities (see Box 10-4). There also may be limitations on the use of publicly held data sets, be they related to statistics (e.g., samples too small) or to privacy protection requirements, regulatory or otherwise. It is

> **Box 10-4   CASE STUDY 3: USING DATA COLLECTED THROUGH THE CLINICAL ENCOUNTER FOR PUBLIC HEALTH: NEW YORK CITY'S HEMOGLOBIN A1C (HBA1C) REGISTRY**
>
> New York City's registry for hemoglobin A1c (HbA1c) laboratory test results was established in 2005 through regulation that requires mandatory reporting of all HbA1c laboratory results ordered by providers in the city to the Health Department, thereby allowing them to monitor and develop programming to address diabetes.[34] Information reported to the registry includes the facility and care provider ordering the test; name, gender, age, and residence of patient; and date of the test. This limited information has been used by the Health Department to create point-density maps of populations with persistent poor HbA1c control (HbA1c level >9.0) and, combined with other data sources (e.g., poverty status, public housing, food access), to design programs or prioritize action.[35,36] Figure 10-3 shows the persistent high levels of poor HbA1c control, including one area that spans across several blocks of public housing in the city. Based upon this geographic understanding of need, the city developed a demonstration community health worker program that conducts outreach to the public housing residents, connects them to healthcare systems, and to other community-based resources in the neighborhood.

External Resource

National Information Center on Health Services Research and HealthCare Technology (NICHSR), https://hsric.nlm.nih.gov/hsric_public/display_links/722

External Resource

New York City's EpiQuery, available at https://a816-healthpsi.nyc.gov/epiquery/.

also important to consider that data types and sources are not static; for example, the use of syndromic surveillance data continues to evolve beyond bioterrorism and is often used to assess trends in ED visits. Online data repositories exist and will continue to emerge, as technology supports a rapid proliferation of databases. An example is the National Information Center on Health Services Research and HealthCare Technology (NICHSR) at the National Institutes of Health (NIH), which includes federal and state databases.[30] A general appreciation for the diversity of types of data available is useful as researchers consider connecting with health authorities.

Local health departments may maintain interfaces to make querying and mapping local health statistics broadly available. An example is New York City's EpiQuery, an online query system that provides data on the health of New Yorkers derived from a variety of sources, including surveys, surveillance data, and vital records (which includes birth and death records). As the goals of public health and clinical care delivery systems converge, health departments are also increasingly engaged in accessing and using data from clinical encounters, including electronic health records (EHRs).

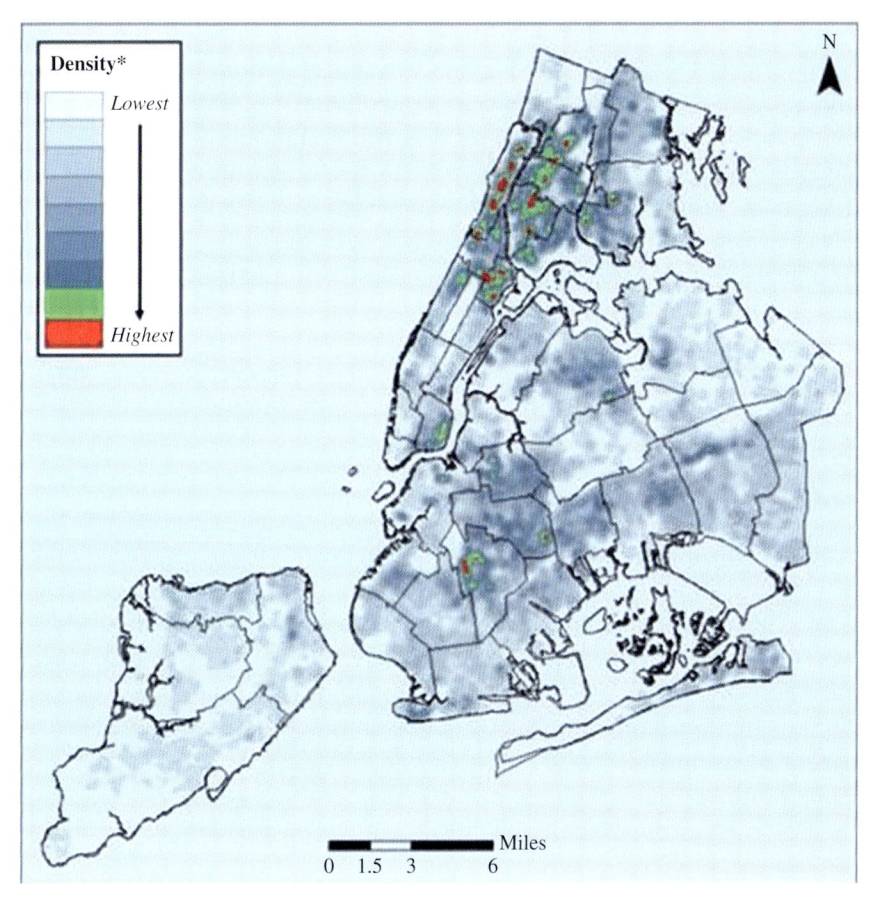

CHAPTER 10 | COMMUNITY, PROFESSIONAL, AND POLICY ORGANIZATIONS

Figure 10-3 • Point-density map of HbA1c. (Source: New York City Department of Health and Mental Hygiene.)

While all data sources may not be available for public use, collaboration with local health departments on specific queries may be possible. For example, many states and regions now have health information exchanges (HIEs) or regional health information organizations (RHIOs), which act as "hub-and-spoke" models for multiple settings (clinical or nonclinical organizations) to share a limited health data set (e.g., hospital discharge events, patient health status summaries, alerts for hospitalization, patients entering or leaving prison or jail systems).[32] Because of the potential broad reach of health information across a region, these more recent data sources derived from healthcare delivery are often shared with public health agencies for population health surveillance and disease outbreak investigation activities.[33]

Public health agencies and their partners have research and evaluation competencies and approaches to data collection that can complement and add value to healthcare delivery system research. Using principles of epidemiology, public health researchers are trained to look for information and data sources to address root causes or identify factors that are associated with population health issues, with the intent to take action, the development of guidance for prevention, or the revision or promotion of specific local, state, and federal policies.[37] In addition, public health researchers often combine existing data sources (e.g., structured surveys, vital statistics, medical records, and healthcare claims) with issue-specific information (e.g., key informant interviews, case studies, and storytelling) to better understand the effects or causes of a health gap.

Convening

Another role commonly assumed by public health agencies is the ability to convene multiple sectors or parties around a common goal or health issue. Public health agencies can act as a trusted third party (e.g., an entity who facilitates interactions between parties who trust the entity), where an organization is responsible for guiding a group's vision and strategy, supporting the alignment of activities, helping to establish shared indicators or measurement, building public will, advancing policies, and mobilizing funding.[38]

An example in which public health convened partners across multiple healthcare delivery systems is the New York Citywide Coalition for Colorectal Cancer Control (C5).[39] In 2002, the city aimed to improve the colorectal cancer-screening rates as a means to reduce avoidable deaths. The agency created an advisory committee comprised of multiple stakeholders and led by co-chairs who could champion and encourage leadership across key stakeholder groups with the aim to change the way delivery systems work. While the steering committee was charged with overseeing all operations of the coalition, they also formed multiple subcommittees to implement activities to achieve goals set by C5. Health department staff provided project management for meetings, supported documentation and logistics of initiatives for meeting coalition goals, and organized and hosted an annual summit.

Some of these activities required coordination across multiple segments of the healthcare delivery system, examples of which include professional education, academic detailing of care providers, patient navigation programs, direct referral to endoscopy centers, and assurance of the quality of colonoscopies performed. In addition, the Health

Department worked with subcommittees to develop public education efforts and targeted programs to address inequities in colonoscopy screening, including language translation for Russian- and Chinese-speaking communities.

The healthcare delivery system, while something to study, is part of a growing, vibrant community. Engaging public health agencies can help broaden the types of partners and entities involved in research and policy development.

Policy

Another of the ten essential functions identified by the CDC is public health's role in developing policies and plans that support individual and community health efforts,[21] such as creating minimum thresholds in environmental standards and promoting preventive services that everyone should receive.[40] Public health institutions and their networks have developed processes and mechanisms that can act on research findings in order to help spread and scale evidence-based interventions broadly.

In 2012, the Million Hearts campaign was launched, aiming to save a million lives across the United States in five years by preventing heart attacks and strokes.[41] The campaign was a collaboration between two federal government agencies: one focused on public health, the CDC, and the second focused on care delivery, the Centers for Medicare and Medicaid Services (CMS). Based on extensive modeling, expert interviews, and literature reviews, the initiative generated a selected set of evidence-based public health and clinical goals and strategies that were promoted and promulgated by 120 official partners, 20 federal agencies, and all 50 states and the District of Columbia. The framework, informed by healthcare research, included strategies for the following:

- **Population action**—Reduce sodium intake by 20%, decrease tobacco use by 20%, and increase physical activity by reducing inactivity by 20%
- **Healthcare delivery**—Increase the delivery of ABCS (Aspirin/antithrombotic therapy, blood pressure control, cholesterol management, and smoking cessation intervention) to 80% of the eligible population, increase the use of cardiac rehabilitation to 70% for patients who have had a heart attack or stroke, and engage patients in heart-healthy behaviors (e.g., medication adherence, nutrition counseling, physical activity)
- **Improving outcomes for priority populations**—Blacks/African Americans with hypertension, 35–64-year-olds, people who have

had a heart attack or stroke, and people with mental and/or substance use disorders

These healthcare-directed recommendations were based on analysis that determined how that system would best contribute to reducing deaths from heart attack and stroke.[42] Across the country, local and state governments and collaborating partners were mobilized through funding opportunities, which in turn stimulated additional opportunities for related policy and programming developments. By partnering with public health agencies early in the program or policy design phase, the likelihood of implementation, action, policy, and impact based upon research findings from related fields, like healthcare delivery science, is enhanced.

APPROACHES TO SUCCESSFUL PARTNERSHIPS

Because the public health and healthcare delivery systems often operate quite separately, engagement requires thoughtful action. Here are some basic considerations for healthcare delivery researchers that may help guide the launch of successful public health department partnerships and are relevant across a variety of nonhealthcare delivery organizations:

- **Meet and be familiar with health departments at both the local and state levels.** Healthcare delivery system leaders often are familiar with their state health departments because regulatory guidance most commonly comes from this level. Healthcare delivery systems anchored in academic intuitions may have relationships with local health departments, as they are increasingly collaborating on population health research. Take the time to develop those relationships across the breadth of potentially relevant departments or divisions early so that you're starting from a position of mutual understanding of mission and interests when time-limited opportunities for collaboration arise or urgent research questions emerge.
- **Do your research before you meet.** Understand the mission of public health agencies and/or organizations of interest before you reach out. Consider what the public health agencies, CBOs, or other entities have to gain from the relationship when exploring the collaboration. Identify shared metrics of interest (e.g., prevalence and control of diabetes, controlling blood pressure, nicotine replacement therapy treatment, reducing premature mortality, or

enrollment in evidence-based intervention programs) ahead of time to help guide the conversation.
- **Appreciate that there may be differences in the way that specific words are used.** For example, for those working in public health agencies, the term *population health* commonly refers to the health of the entire community that is within its jurisdiction, while to a healthcare system, *population health* may refer to the health of their populations of patients; still large, but often a subset of the geographic area included by a public health agency. When speaking of population health, the intended denominators and priorities may differ.
- **When designing research, invite non-healthcare delivery systems to engage early as meaningful partners in idea development, and research production.** This means including them as co-principal investigators and coauthors in related manuscripts, as appropriate. However, unless you're responding to a formal opportunity for funding, don't rely upon them for resources. They are often operating under resource-constrained conditions, and existing funding is often earmarked for specific purposes and can't be redirected. To support partnership in your work, you might consider how your funding may allow them the human resources to participate in your research interests.
- **Offer to engage in formal data-sharing agreements when data are not publicly available, and establish formal expectations with outlined divisions of labor before undertaking projects.** This is particularly advantageous in long-term projects because staffing, leadership, and government priorities may change over time.
- **When research is complete, take the time to translate the findings into information that is actionable.** It will build goodwill going forward and make more likely that your findings can be acted on expeditiously.

CONCLUDING THOUGHTS

By bringing together healthcare operations and social, economic, environmental, and political factors that affect health, health systems science can apply research-quality methods to study healthcare delivery operations that take into account real-life issues for patients, populations, and their communities to innovate and improve care. Public health systems, through their many and varied partnerships, can help broadcast important discoveries, implement interventions, and create lasting changes in health.

> **KEY POINTS**
>
> - Healthcare and community organizations are partnering more and more, and these partners are essential to creating systems that link clinical and nonclinical environments with population health.
> - Key stakeholders in these relationships include all public, private, and voluntary entities that contribute to the delivery of essential public health services, such as government agencies, CBOs, advocacy groups, payers, and private industry.
> - Public health departments have access to data that can benefit healthcare delivery systems research from conception, to design and implementation to interpretation of findings. In addition, public health departments have staff with specific skills to meaningfully compile, analyze, and interpret these data sources.
> - Healthcare delivery systems researcher collaboration with public health agencies early in the research design phase may increase the likelihood of policy and action based upon research findings.

ACKNOWLEDGMENTS

Shadi Chamany, MD, MPH; Director of Science, Division of Prevention and Primary Care, New York City Department of Health and Mental Hygiene

Matthew Silverstein, MPH; Special Assistant, Primary Care Information Project, Division of Prevention and Primary Care, New York City Department of Health and Mental Hygiene

Katherine Sutkowi, MSW; Director of Special Initiatives, Division of Prevention and Primary Care, New York City Department of Health and Mental Hygiene

REFERENCES

1. McGinnis JM, Williams-Russo P, Knickman JR. The case for more active policy attention to health promotion. *Health Aff (Millwood)*. 2002;21(2):78–93.
2. Schroeder SA. We can do better—improving the health of the American people. *N Engl J Med*. 2007;357:1221–1228.
3. Centers for Disease Control and Prevention (CDC). *Social Determinants of Health: Know What Affects Health;* 2018. Accessed April 17, 2019, from https://www.cdc.gov/socialdeterminants/.
4. U.S. Department of Health and Human Services, Office of Disease Prevention and Health Promotion. *Social Determinants of Health;* 2018. Accessed July 29, 2018, from https://www.healthypeople.gov/2020/topics-objectives/topic/social-determinants-of-health.

5. The contribution of social and behavioral research to an understanding of the distribution of disease: a multilevel approach. In Smedley BD, Syme SL (eds.). *Promoting Health: Intervention Strategies from Social and Behavioral Research*. Washington, DC: National Academies Press; 2000.
6. Bracy NL, Millstein RA, Carlson JA, et al. Is the relationship between the built environment and physical activity moderated by perceptions of crime and safety? *Int J Behav Nutr Phys Act*. 2014;11(1):24.
7. Centers for Disease Control and Prevention (CDC). *Common Asthma Triggers*. 2012. Accessed April 19, 2019, from https://www.cdc.gov/asthma/triggers.html.
8. Seligman HK, Schillinger D. Hunger and socioeconomic disparities in chronic disease. *N Engl J Med*. 2010;363(1):6–9.
9. Power C, Graham H, Due P, et al. The contribution of childhood and adult socioeconomic position to adult obesity and smoking behaviour: an international comparison. *Int J Epidemiol*. 2005;34:335–344.
10. Mujahid MS, Diez Roux AV, Cooper RC, Shea S, Williams DR. Neighborhood stressors and race/ethnic differences in hypertension prevalence (The Multi-Ethnic Study of Atherosclerosis). *Am J Hypertens*. 2011;24(2):187–193.
11. Kamal R, Cox C. *How has U.S. spending on healthcare changed over time?* 2017. Accessed December 20, 2017, from https://www.healthsystemtracker.org/chart-collection/u-s-spending-healthcare-changed-time/?_sf_s=changed#item-start.
12. Thorpe KE. The rise in health care spending and what to do about it. *Health Aff (Millwood)*. 2005;24(6):1436–1445.
13. Berwick DM, Nolan TW, Whittington J. The triple aim: care, health, and cost. *Health Aff (Millwood)*. 2008;27(3):759–769.
14. Chee TT, Ryan AM, Wasfy JH, Borden WB. Current state of value-based purchasing programs. *Circulation*. 2016;133(22):2197–2205.
15. Centers for Medicare and Medicaid Services (CMS). *CMS' Value-Based Programs;* 2018. Accessed July 25, 2018, from https://www.cms.gov/Medicare/Quality-Initiatives-Patient-Assessment-Instruments/Value-Based-Programs/Value-Based-Programs.html.
16. Centers for Medicare and Medicaid Services (CMS). *Shared Savings Program;* 2018. Accessed January 5, 2018, from https://www.cms.gov/Medicare/Medicare-Fee-for-Service-Payment/sharedsavingsprogram/index.html.
17. McGinnis T, Crumley D, Chang DI. *Implementing Social Determinants of Health Interventions in Medicaid Managed Care: How to Leverage Existing Authorities and Shift to Value-Based Purchasing;* 2018. Washington, DC: AcademyHealth. Accessed May 31, 2019, from https://www.academyhealth.org/sites/default/files/implementing_sdoh_medicaid_managed_care_may2018.pdf.
18. Tipireni R, Vickery KD, Ehlinger EP. Accountable communities for health: moving from providing accountable care to creating health. *Ann Fam Med*. 2015;13(4):367–369.
19. Austen BioInnovation Institute in Akron. *Healthier by Design: Creating Accountable Care Communities: A Framework for Engagement and Sustainability*. Akron: Austen BioInnovation Institute; 2012.
20. Ammon N, Curry MB, Fratantonio M, et al. *Health in All Policies: Community Engagement Report*. Summit County, OH; 2015.

21. Centers for Disease Control and Prevention (CDC). *The Public Health System and the 10 Essential Public Health Services;* 2017. Accessed September 20, 2017, from https://www.cdc.gov/stltpublichealth/publichealthservices/essentialhealthservices.html.
22. Summers Holtrop J, Luo Z, Alexanders L. Inadequate reimbursement for care management to primary care offices. *J Am Board Fam Med*. 2015;28(2):271–279.
23. Bruen B, Docteur E, Lopert R, et al. *The Impact of Reimbursement Policies and Practices on Healthcare Technology Innovation*. U.S. Department of Health and Human Services. 2016. Accessed July 31, 2018, from https://aspe.hhs.gov/pdf-report/impact-reimbursement-policies-and-practices-healthcare-technology-innovation.
24. U.S. Department of Health and Human Services, Office of Disease Prevention and Health Promotion. *Public Health Infrastructure;* 2018. Accessed July 31, 2018, from https://www.healthypeople.gov/2020/topics-objectives/topic/public-health-infrastructure.
25. Angell SY, Silver LD, Goldstein GP, et al. Cholesterol control beyond the clinic: New York City's trans fat restriction. *Ann Intern Med*. 2009;151:129–134.
26. Wright M, McKelvey W, Curtis CJ, et al. Impact of a municipal policy restricting trans fatty acid use in New York City restaurants on serum trans fatty acid levels in adults. *Am J Public Health*. 2019;109(4):634–636.
27. Angell SY, Cobb LK, Curtis CJ, Konty KJ, Silver LD. Change in trans fatty acid content of fast-food purchases associated with New York City's restaurant regulation. *Ann Intern Med*. 2012;157:81–86.
28. Brandt EJ, Myerson R, Perraillon MC, Polonsky TS. Hospital admissions for myocardial infarction and stroke before and after the trans-fatty acid restrictions in New York. *JAMA Cardiol*. 2017;2(6):627–634.
29. Restrepo BJ, Rieger M. Trans fat and cardiovascular disease mortality: Evidence from bans in restaurants in New York. *J Health Econ*. 2016;45:176–196.
30. U.S. National Library of Medicine. *National Information Center on Health Services Research and Health Care Technology;* 2018. Accessed May 31, 2019, from https://www.nlm.nih.gov/hsrinfo/datasites.htm l#489.
31. Luck J, Chang C, Brown ER, Lumpkin J. Using local health information to promote public health. *Health Aff (Millwood)*. 2006;25(4):979–991.
32. Adler-Milstein J, Landefeld J, Jha AK. Characteristics associated with Regional Health Information Organization viability. *J Am Med Inform Assoc*. 2010;17(1):61–65.
33. Agency for Healthcare Research & Quality, Innovations Exchange Team. *Trends in Health Information Exchanges*. 2014. Accessed May 31, 2019, from AHRQ Health Care Innovations Exchange: https://innovations.ahrq.gov/perspectives/trends-health-information-exchanges.
34. Chamany S, Silver LD, Bassett MT, et al. Tracking diabetes: New York City's A1C Registry. *Milbank Q*. 2009;87(3):547–570.
35. Wu WY, Jiang Q, Di Lonardo SS. Poorly controlled diabetes in New York City: mapping high-density neighborhoods. *J Public Health Manag Pract*. 2018;24(1):69–74.

36. Wu WY, Jiang Q. *Variability of High Blood Sugar Levels Among Adults with Diabetes in New York City, 2006–2015*. New York City: New York City Department of Health and Mental Hygiene; 2017.
37. Hill AB. The environment and disease: association of causation? *Proc R Soc Med*. 1965;58(5):295–300.
38. Turner S, Merchant K, Kania J, Martin E. Understanding the value of backbone organizations in collective impact: Part 2. *Stanford Social Innovation Review*. 2012;18. Accessed July 31, 2018, from https://ssir.org/articles/entry/understanding_the_value_of_backbone_organizations_in_collective_impact_2#
39. Itzkowitz SH, Winawer S, Krauskopf M, Huang K, Weber T, Jandorf L. New York Citywide Colon Cancer Control Coalition (C5): a public health effort to increase colon cancer screening and address health disparities. *Cancer*. 2016;122(2):269–277.
40. Committee for the Study of the Future of Public Health. *The Future of Public Health*. Washington, DC: National Academies Press; 1988.
41. Centers for Disease Control and Prevention (CDC). *About Million Hearts*. Accessed July 31, 2018, from Million Hearts: https://millionhearts.hhs.gov/about-million-hearts/index.html.
42. Million Hearts. *Million Hearts: Meaningful Progress 2012–2016, A Final Report*. U.S. Department of Health and Human Services; 2017. Accessed July 31, 2018, from Million Hearts: https://millionhearts.hhs.gov/files/MH-meaningful-progress.pdf.

PART III

Seeing the Truth—Analytics in Healthcare

DATA IN HEALTHCARE
Where It Comes From, How It Is Structured, How to Govern It, and How to Get Your Hands on It

Michael J. Wall and Joseph Dudas

In the healthcare of today, we have a parallel universe of data. Increasingly, everything we do has a data trail, with more and more records to be kept and knowledge to be gleaned. However, some activities still aren't recorded electronically. For those still-untracked activities, we often spend extensive resources to bring them into the larger data matrix. We believe that more data will catalyze the data-information-knowledge process and knowledge holds the promise of improved outcomes. Healthcare data are among the most complicated in the world. When handled improperly, they can dangerously misdirect patient care and resources. On the other hand, when done well, healthcare analytics (the output needed to drive analysis and insight) opens a window so we can understand and improve performance—and see into the future.

The optimal use of healthcare data flows from identifying data needs, preprocessing data, adding value, and then applying information is illustrated in Figure 11-1. But using data in healthcare is rarely this simple. Until the last few decades, working with healthcare data had been limited to aspiring researchers and their small teams. Now, we have widespread data workers throughout the healthcare system. But data scientists and clinicians do not always understand one another: things sometimes get lost in translation. Not only does the nonclinician have the responsibility to learn clinical operations, but clinicians need to be conversant with the onslaught of technical requirements and terminology required to transform high-quality data into knowledge.

Poorly constructed analytics causes embarrassment, incorrect conclusions, wasted resources, and potentially patient harm. This chapter will cover ways that we can guard ourselves against bad data and what is required for a health system to develop and maintain reliable data analytics.

Caution

Healthcare data are among the most complicated in the world. When handled improperly, they can dangerously misdirect patient care and resources.

Key Point

When done well, healthcare analytics (the output needed to drive analysis and insight) opens a window so we can understand and improve performance—and see into the future.

PART 1: FUNDAMENTAL ISSUES IN HEALTHCARE DATA

Healthcare data and analytics challenges start with a major fundamental problem: healthcare has a very fragmented business model. Consider

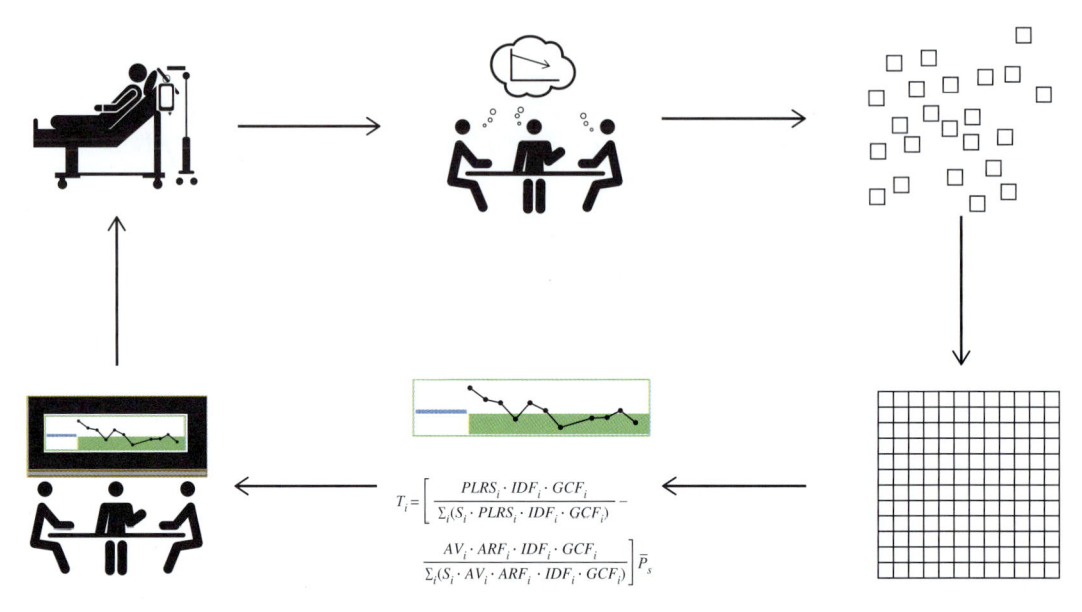

Figure 11-1 • A model of data flow in healthcare.
This figure above shows the flow of data in healthcare: beginning with the patient, who is the focus of the flow; the team specifying needs is guided by a data expert; data experts, connected to the best data, determine what is possible using these data; the data experts then organize, and validate data in a reproducible manner; then the data experts assemble, visualize, and/or model data as information; and then we journey back to the team who, using the information, creates action plans and knowledge to improve care to the patient.

$$T_i = \left[\frac{PLRS_i \cdot IDF_i \cdot GCF_i}{\Sigma_i(S_i \cdot PLRS_i \cdot IDF_i \cdot GCF_i)} - \frac{AV_i \cdot ARF_i \cdot IDF_i \cdot GCF_i}{\Sigma_i(S_i \cdot AV_i \cdot ARF_i \cdot IDF_i \cdot GCF_i)} \right] \bar{P}_s$$

> **Key Point**
>
> Healthcare data and analytics challenges start with a major fundamental problem: healthcare has a very fragmented business model.

where patients get their healthcare. If we focus only on hospitals in the United States, there are over 6,000, of which only 50% are in systems or networked, according to the American Hospital Association. Patients also seek services outside hospitals, through clinics, physician offices, retailers, and now even online services. In fact, there are almost a billion outpatient visits each year in the United States alone. These other points of care represent data gaps if they aren't highly coordinated (and they aren't). Further complicating healthcare data, most resources and services are not paid for directly. Instead, there are intermediaries such as insurance providers, third-party administrators, group-purchasing organizations, specialty-service providers, and distributors. This by itself starts to paint a pretty daunting picture for the average database developer trying to answer a simple question, such as how much does something cost or how many patients a healthcare provider is treating.

Beyond the fragmented nature of the healthcare business model, consider the role of electronic health records (EHRs) in generating healthcare data. EHRs, now ubiquitous in healthcare systems, emerged in the 1990s. At that time, the Institute of Medicine sponsored several studies that pointed the way toward the modern concepts that we have in place today for EHRs.[1,2] The EHR was intended to put a core system in place that would unwind the complexity of care at the time (e.g., facilitating communication and coordination across providers).

However, 30 years later, many EHRs remain fragmented and poorly integrated, particularly among health systems created by large system mergers.[3,4] Even when systems consolidation does occur, users quickly discover that much of the functionality of the EHR has been designed and developed to support an ordering and billing function, as opposed to providing and assessing care (and/or capturing care improvement data). As a result, clinically relevant information is often left in text dictation; distributed among disparate custom user fields; held within clinical support systems such as laboratory, imaging, pharmacy, and supply-chain systems; and/or captured outside the healthcare system altogether (such as social and economic data).

Healthcare information technology (IT) vendors often lead executives and physicians to believe that a great wealth of data and analytics will be possible with their particular EHR system. However, often the EHRs are limited both functionally and from a data aggregation and integration perspective. EHRs that support day-to-day tasks are not designed to handle complex queries; in fact, attempting to do so can add risks to an operation (in the form of severe performance degradation). Other industries, faced with a similar challenge, have fueled the growth of data warehouses. Big retailers do not run complex queries on their point-of-sale systems, but instead move the data into a database especially suited for analytics.

So with all these challenges, how would we build the ideal data and analytics program for healthcare? There are no short cuts. The first step is to focus on the analytics that are truly needed. Unfortunately, many healthcare organizations skip this step. Many healthcare data warehousing projects start with a focus on data as opposed to analytics. Starting with a list of prioritized questions (often referred to as "use cases"), the metrics needed can often reduce complexity and increase opportunities for reuse. For example, a question might be generalized from "Who is prescribing and administering sofosbuvir (a drug to treat hepatitis C)?" to "What drugs are providers prescribing and administering?"

Second, a data analytics program requires a strong governance function to keep the data quality high and standardized. *Garbage in, garbage out (GIGO)* was a popular saying in the early days of computing, but it applies even more today, when powerful computers can produce large amounts of data or information faster than ever before. A formal data quality program can guarantee quality at the source, as well as ensuring that the cost of capturing highly standardized data at the point of care is justified.

Caution

Many EHRs remain fragmented and poorly integrated, a problem that can be worsened with large system mergers.

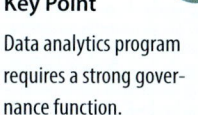

Key Point

Data analytics program requires a strong governance function.

Finally, consider how to build and make the best use of the skills and talents of a healthcare analytics team. Most institutions use healthcare analytics teams to "data wrangle" and develop endless numbers of reports and dashboards. Over time, analysts will develop and hone these skills but then not have anyone to actually do analysis. For example, analytic tools can be developed to automate the retrieval and summary of information for a cohort of patients, but someone connected to the activity is needed to apply insights in formulating a valid recommendation. The same is true for finance, supply chain, planning, quality, and other areas of the healthcare organization.

Programs and certifications are now advancing training for healthcare analysts such as the AMIA Clinical Informatics program (which is widely available) or private programs such as that of the University of Pittsburgh Medical Center. Finally, executive leadership should clearly establish a leader of their healthcare analytics function (such as a chief analytics officer, chief data officer, or medical director of analytics). Some progressive organizations have also gone so far as to employ a product management approach wherein a portfolio of analytics products is managed, as well as tactics that directly link to an enterprise's strategic plan.

PART 2: THE IMPORTANCE OF UNDERSTANDING DATA LINEAGE, AND HOW THIS LEADS MATURE ORGANIZATIONS TO BOTH INFORMAL AND FORMAL DATA GOVERNANCE

Good healthcare data come from caregivers and nonclinical staff, who capture their work via a complex system of electronic applications. Good data have been defined as those that are "fit for their intended uses."[5] Similarly, healthcare delivery is a highly specialized and fragmented system. Patients navigate among uncoordinated visits and providers. Patients often serve as the interpreter and historian to their providers, explaining their experiential and treatment histories, regardless of a plethora of electronic applications intended to do just this. Today, it is not uncommon for patients to be the primary connection between multiple providers, hand-delivering clinical documentation from one to the other. In fact, many healthcare facilities have departments that are designated to manage this process of scanning papers, or transcribing data, into their local electronic system.

Due to this same fragmentation, healthcare workers navigate through their own confusing, disjointed environment. Workers wend their way through disconnected electronic systems, clinical activities, and priorities.

Healthcare is now delivered through countless software applications that are sometimes connected to, and sometimes disparate from, the patient's primary electronic medical record. Consider these very possible situations, and the downstream consequences, to set the stage for the incredible need for solid data governance and structure:

- A senior executive receives two reports of inpatient lengths of stay. One shows improvement and the other, in sharp disagreement, indicates worsening. A root cause analysis (RCA) finds that this is due to differences that are deliberate and well-intentioned—but neither well articulated nor understood by decision-makers.
- Blood pressure is being reported from an EHR-sourced blood pressure field, but physicians document in a different, newly launched, and disconnected custom flowsheet field. The performance is shared with the clinicians as considerably lower than the benchmark.
- Heart attack patients are being undercounted for a regulatory report because the data are focused on the patient's problem list (which is inconsistently filled out) rather than the billing data field (which is uniformly used).
- As a member of the patient safety team, you receive a list of patients who had a procedure for which some received a product recalled for safety. The specific details are not available through billing data and require a database table that is not yet activated in your local system.
- The report being used for staff budgeting is unintentionally figuring averages at certain points in the calculations, leading to inaccurate results.
- You are unintentionally given access to your colleague's mortality performance because of an out-of-date master employee list. Or perhaps you receive a report that includes the narrative comments from a coworker's recent patient experience survey report.
- The readmission risk prediction for a patient you are treating is overestimating the risk by 300% because of a recent change made to a field in the EHR.

Nearly every U.S. healthcare system has created its own unique environment of applications during its journey to digitize medical records. Each has acquired and assembled its own IT ecosystem over many years, based on local clinical judgment, leadership preferences, consultant recommendations, and standing technical landscape and capabilities. Today, it would be quite remarkable if two systems were found to have identical ecosystems of applications and installations of those tools.

With every new software application and module, connections and interfaces are forged from one application to the next. Given the uniqueness of each health system, we don't always have a guarantee that systems can be implemented as described by the software vendor, and once these connections are made, they may run smoothly or be problematic. Sometimes interfaces are too resource-intensive or technically implausible to make sense, and they are left as independent systems. Some programs have licensing restrictions that disallow connecting to certain applications.

Once applications are operational, some software companies restrict direct access to the databases behind their software, while others charge additional (sometimes quite large) fees to access the raw data. This obviously adds to the complexity and costs of working with healthcare data. Successful navigation among semiconnected systems is an often under-recognized value of the IT department because the readily visible shininess of the latest cutting-edge software and the marketing materials of the software vendor often overshadows the complex technical underpinnings they deploy. IT teams are charged to manage these challenges to enable electronic and caregiver success.

While all this is happening on the electronic front, medical knowledge continues to grow, giving hospitals a continuous stream of new discoveries and process redesign needs for healthcare delivery. Nearly every discovery requires a change to the electronic system, affecting the downstream systems and the data used by clinicians and administrators.

With potentially hundreds of applications interacting, it's not surprising that we can end up with ten different ways to enter a patient's pain score or weight. Within a single healthcare system, it's not uncommon to have several sources for what appears to be the same data element. As healthcare systems remain in a constant state of change, the change management and communication processes supporting updates to the EHR are critical.

How do we make sure that our data are fit for use? Formal data governance is driven to increase the value of data throughout an organization, maximizing that data's value to its users through standards and policies. Informal data governance is the precursor to the formal version; it's done at a local level, focusing on a specific project, usually without thought of extensible processes, with the value dissipating upon delivery.

Data governance can be compared to the way that food is certified as organic by the U.S. Department of Agriculture (USDA). Although anyone can produce organic food, the official USDA certification communicates that specific standard processes have been followed. A healthcare

Caution

Within a single healthcare system, it's not uncommon to have several sources for what appears to be the same data element. This will require digging to what is the truth.

organization that has a fully implemented data governance strategy will have these guidelines available to producers and consumers of data.

Clear data lineage and data quality are perhaps the most important products of successful data governance and effective data management processes responding to data governance. *Data lineage* is an activity in which we trace the data journey from production to consumption according to clear steps supported by vetted domain experts. The process of documenting data lineage is not about ensuring perfect data so much as investigating and communicating the journey that the data have taken from production to the consumer. This transparency allows the user to judge the data's quality. Knowing where and how data originated and were handled afterward is essential to understand before they are consumed. High-quality data lineage can trace data to the source, identify who entered the data, and similar details. A data analyst who can wrap a deliverable in context like "These data include results from the flowsheet row, which is the only discrete location in our EHR where nurses can document postoperative pain scores; and this data set includes all results within 6 hours of surgery end time for inpatients, whose surgery end time was last month, except for those that were deleted or corrected in the EHR" imparts confidence in the appropriate use of the data. Translating the journey that data take, including filters and transformations, from entry to analysis solidifies one's reputation with almost any audience.

If you don't have formal data governance, then you are responsible for data lineage and data quality. Many resources may be needed to ensure that you are using your data safely. Departments like IT, quality, strategy, research, and health information management are often the best place to begin because these departments are typically highly dependent on understanding data. In the absence of a well-matured system, these departments can help you navigate your questions about data lineage, data transformations, and data experts in order to determine if your data are fit for use.

We are now in an age where bad data is quickly recognized, and the cost of bad data is high. Users of data today extend far beyond the IT department, quite commonly to the areas of quality, strategy, finance, and research. It is also common to have staff beyond these main hubs building their own data reports, supported by the availability of tools like desktop spreadsheet software and data visualization suites. Organizations now create formal structures to support these fragmented data activities, in a step toward ensuring that the data are fit for their intent across an entire enterprise.

Industry experts agree that data governance is a critical piece of successful data programs by providing authority and control mechanisms to maximize the value of data. Accepted definitions for data governance vary from basic to comprehensive governance and data management structures. Basic data governance will govern through policymaking and approval of data management activities, providing oversight of the organization's data operations. Comprehensive data governance includes oversight and support structures for data management. Many of these domains are often led or strongly supported by IT teams, but depending on local cultures, many can be intentionally embedded into teams outside of IT. The following are domains commonly connected with data governance:

- **Access management:** A function to ensure that each user has correct access
- **Algorithm development:** Algorithms and value sets for definitions (e.g., defining what is meant by the term *stroke patient*)
- **Business intelligence:** A presentation layer of reports
- **Data quality management:** Understanding data and preparing it for use
- **Data request assignment:** Ensuring that data requests are handled by the most capable and appropriate staff
- **Data warehousing/unified data platform:** Data are organized and readily available for use and reuse
- **Data steward community:** Organizational data experts (Business owners who can answer specific questions such as: What field is the 837i discharge date? How is this field used in the cardiology clinic?)
- **Interventional model review:** Ensuring that predictive and optimization models provide the most benefit to the patient
- **Master data management:** Providing one maintained source of truth for high-priority data (e.g., there is one list of patients with clearly documented nonreal patients, duplicates, overlays, and overlaps)
- **Security, privacy, and compliance:** Ensuring that data processes and tools meet appropriate standards

As organizations begin to deploy models that are aimed to add value by doing things like predicting cardiac arrests or optimizing patient throughput, there is a balancing need to confirm the accuracy and appropriateness of these interventions. Rolling out and maintaining the processes around these models requires an approach that is connected to other efforts for managing data and analytics, with clear governance.

Data governance is a tricky activity. Too much governance stifles growth and creativity, whereas too little leads to instability and vulnerabilities. As technology continues to evolve and the use and reuse of data in healthcare expands, the need to protect organizations from bad data becomes more imperative than ever. In mature environments, data governance supports consumers through formal standard processes and policies. Without formal governance, these same standards need to be discussed between the producer and consumer with each initiative.

PART 3: BASIC UNDERSTANDING OF RELATIONAL DATABASE STRUCTURES

In 1970, Codd demonstrated that information of any level of complexity could be described using a few simple rules, developing the *relational database*.[6] Relational databases dominate healthcare; the language of relational databases is Structured Query Language (SQL). Relational databases divide data into tables of rows and columns, with a unique *key* identifying each row. The tables themselves are one entity (e.g., microbiology results). Columns represent different attributes (e.g., date, time, specimen type, and result). Rows can be linked across tables. The keys between tables are essential for linking them and being able to trace a patient's path through the data.

Relational databases can exist within unified data platforms. A *unified data platform* consists of three distinct layers: the data lake (raw data that are extracted directly from the source), data integration (series of topical data warehouses), and data marts (series of analytics databases specific to the needs of data consumers).

Heavy cleansing of data within the data warehouse due to poor quality at the source system must be minimized for the system to be sustained as well as be understood. If "magic" occurs within the data warehouse, the data will not be credible or trusted. Key data are critical to joining and comparing data. Many try to fabricate keys (derive keys from nonkey data), which is referred to as a *fuzzy join*. Avoid fuzzy joins whenever possible; instead, standardize key data that are to be integrated. Fuzzy joins produce fuzzy results.

As the field of machine learning comes to healthcare, database technology has evolved to accommodate big data (i.e., data sets that are too large for traditional relational databases) and large in-memory databases that make queries that used to take hours run in seconds. Online analytics processing (OLAP) moves the data from a relational model to a cube, very similar to that of a very large spreadsheet pivot table. It can provide response times that are very fast, particularly when slicing and dicing a particular, defined set of data.

Key Point

Relational databases dominate healthcare; the language of relational databases is Structured Query Language (SQL).

Caution

Avoid fuzzy joins whenever possible; instead, standardize key data that are to be integrated. Fuzzy joins produce fuzzy results.

PART 4: REVIEW OF COMMON APPROACHES TO ACTUALLY ACCESSING HEALTHCARE DATA

With a well-executed data warehouse and data governance strategy, an organization can be expected to have streamlined paths to point consumers to good data. If your organization isn't there yet, there are some basic approaches to access good data.

Starting with the simplest solution, most organizations that don't have central analytics teams often have at least one data guru or data czar (and possibly several). These individuals might be analysts, or they might be vice presidents. One thing that is sure, though, is that they typically have amassed a good deal of data experience and access over many successful initiatives. They are often the source of data-related oral lore that a more mature organization would vet and document in a standardized fashion. These experts often have been authorized to work with data from many sources, and they know how to "work magic," like intermingling data from multiple systems. You can often find these people in departments like quality, strategy, managed care, and, of course, IT. Many began their careers as data gurus working on projects ranging from quality to strategy to operations to research, and we believe that the independently successful data guru is an incredible resource for organizations to have and keep safe. These individuals are a gold mine to your data journey—if you can find them.

A great starting point for healthcare data is billing data, which often can be sufficient for a variety of requests. Managed care and finance departments are typically the gatekeepers for these data. Facility billing data consist of what the organization invoices for services like an inpatient stay or a clinic appointment, whereas professional billing data are generated from professional services like a physician's visit or procedure. These data drive revenue for the organization, and so they are subject to standards and quality assurance performed by your organization, as well as payors. Billing data also allow you to compare results beyond your organization, and the comfort of the quality assurance allows increased confidence in the accuracy. The majority of quality measures that are publicly reported utilize facility billing data to construct their populations, and often those data are used to measures the outcomes as well.

Once you connect with your data provider, you should discuss with them what data you need and what you intend to do with it. To begin with, a conversation about your data provider's data processes is usually valuable. This echoes the data lineage discussion earlier in this chapter, in that you should fully understand how these data were created and then what happened to them afterward. In ideal situations, the analysts will already have standards that are documented with respect to data lineage, data-quality assurance, and data-steward involvement. In other situations, you will need to prepare for a discussion to assess the limitations of the data, addressing these questions:

- What do you know about the process of these data from production to consumption?
- What system will these data come from? (Some possible answers include EHRs, cost-accounting systems, state associations, and external benchmarking vendors.)
- Are there any suitable alternatives for any of these data, and if so how are they different? For instance, is a diagnosis available from another source?
- What are the caveats you suggest as I use these data?
- How will you validate this data set's accuracy?
- What should I do to validate the data?

In your consultation, sketch out what you want to receive and define all terms. Often, data analysts receive a verbal request that they have to translate into a data table or a visualization. Being less specific might feel like you are providing the analyst professional autonomy, but often that translation step is difficult for the data analyst, and more specific direction can be helpful to both parties. Communicating clearly can save many hours and much frustration; if you know what you want, just ask for it.

Advanced organizations will offer data sets, visualizations, and even advanced analytics supported by more standard processes; however, most organizations are more limited in capabilities and can provide only data sets and summary statistics. With the latter description, you will be responsible for more complicated analytics, further emphasizing the need for understanding the data. In either situation, though, it is helpful to design *a priori* the data set and final deliverable (that is, the final table, graph, report)—even if the design is just an informal sketch. This exercise will help you recognize which data fields are necessary and which are optional, which could save substantial rework and ensure that you are respecting the time of your data provider.

When you receive your data, you should trust but verify. Ensure that there is clear documentation related to data lineage, filters applied, and people who supported the work. Ideal documentation would enable a second, similarly equipped analyst to recreate the report; if you struggle to confirm this, you should ask questions and supplement the documentation. Soon after receipt, review the data and communicate anything that is out of line with your expectations to determine if changes are necessary. Working with your data analyst soon after delivery will be helpful

Key Point
Be specific and concrete when working with your data analyst. Communicating clearly can save many hours and much frustration.

> **Key Point**
> Usually, getting the data set right requires several iterations.

to ensure that the work, and decisions made during the report creation, are fresh in their minds. Recognize that getting the data set right often requires several iterations.

Some organizations move beyond the call-your-favorite-analyst design. Many of these organizations have one main data team, while others have systems to connect your request to a specific, decentralized team based on scope and complexity. Although there is likely a more advanced system at these organizations, with oversight of data operations, your attention to being a requester in the process should be no less vigilant. Understanding data quality and data lineage should remain your top priority.

Some of the items in this section are extremely basic, but they are often overlooked or skipped, even by the most senior leader, clinician, or researcher. Considering this section during your data processes will be critical, regardless of the stage of the analytics evolution at which your organization is.

CONCLUSION

Having a healthy skepticism of data quality is appropriate before diving into analytics work. Targeting perfect data is directionally correct, but recognizing the complexity of the data systems that exist in healthcare and the low likelihood of having perfect data is important. Good results depend on your understanding, and the transparency, of the gap that lies between your data and perfection.

Healthcare is being flooded with data. We collect more information than ever, and we now use that data to create still more data through algorithms and models. This onslaught has great potential to dramatically overwhelm and distract healthcare providers. However, when used well, these same data will actually increase resources to healthcare effectively by showing providers where to focus their attention and energy.

REFERENCES

1. Institute of Medicine Committee on Improving the Patient Record. In: Dick RS, Steen EB, Detmer DE, eds. *The Computer-Based Patient Record: An Essential Technology for Health Care*. 1st ed. Washington, DC: National Academy Press; 1997.
2. Institute of Medicine Committee on Improving the Patient Record. In: Dick RS, Steen EB, eds. *The Computer-Based Patient Record: An Essential Technology for Health Care*. Washington, DC: National Academy Press; 1991.

3. Jha AK, Ferris TG, Donelan K, et al. How common are electronic health records in the United States? A summary of the evidence. *Health Aff (Millwood)*. 2006;25(6):w496–w507.
4. Jha AK, DesRoches CM, Campbell EG, et al. Use of electronic health records in U.S. hospitals. *N Engl J Med*. 2009;360(16):1628–1638.
5. Redman TC. *Data Driven: Profiting from Your Most Important Business Asset*. Boston, MA: Harvard Business Press; 2008.
6. Codd EF. A relational model of data for large shared data banks. 1970. *MD Comput*. 1998;15(3):162–166.

12 MEASURING QUALITY AND SAFETY

The chapters that follow, including this one, focus on how to analyze data—on how to turn data into information, and information into knowledge. One of the most important kinds of data that you will find yourself analyzing is about the quality of care that health systems deliver. Because quality of care is so important, a substantial amount of research has gone into how to measure the quality, safety, and experience of care. This research has led to common approaches for measuring quality—but it also has revealed numerous challenges in measuring quality fairly and consistently. Finally, Medicare, Medicaid, and private payers have moved increasingly to paying for performance on certain quality and safety measures. Because substantial amounts of hospitals' and physicians' revenue is now dependent on quality measures, healthcare delivery scientists should be familiar with some of the major measures involved in measuring quality and safety. This chapter reviews these issues.

QUALITY MEASUREMENT FRAMEWORKS

The Donabedian Model

Avedis Donabedian is widely regarded as the founder of the study of healthcare quality. In 1966, Donabedian published a seminal paper, "Evaluating the Quality of Medical Care."[1] This paper (worth reading in its entirety) laid out what has become known as the Donabedian Model (Table 12-1). The Donabedian Model is now the standard approach for assessing quality. It includes three categories of measures: structural, process, and outcome. Conceptually, this makes sense: The structure of the health system creates and constrains the processes of care that the health system delivers. The process of care interacts directly with patients to create outcomes. Structure leads to process, and process leads to outcome.

Structural measures assess aspects of the health system that help it deliver high-quality care. Is the infrastructure adequate for care? Do

> **Key Point**
> Donabedian's Structure-Process-Outcome-(Balancing) framework is a core approach to healthcare quality measurement.

Table 12-1 STRUCTURE, PROCESS, OUTCOME: THE DONABEDIAN MODEL AND SOME EXTENSIONS

	Type of Measure	Characteristics	Example
Donabedian Model	Structural measures	Characteristics of the healthcare system or provider organization	Does the hospital have a community-acquired pneumonia (CAP) management pathway?
	Process measures	Specific, measurable actions that are theorized to have an impact on outcome measures	Percent of eligible CAP patients who receive appropriate antibiotics within 4 hours
	Outcome measures	Represent the goal of healthcare: the impact on the patient and the outcome that patients care about	Risk-adjusted 30-day survival rate of patients with CAP
Other Common Measure Categories	Balancing measures	Monitors for potential unintended consequences of improvements	Percentage of congestive heart failure patients treated with antibiotics[27]
	Intermediate outcomes	Commonly measured clinical markers that are usually associated with outcomes but do not themselves affect patients' outcomes or quality of life	Time to defervescence in pneumonia HbA1c in diabetes Blood pressure control in hypertension

the right policies and procedures exist? Examples might include whether a hospital has a cardiac catheterization lab (which is important for the treatment of acute myocardial infarction), or whether it has a mechanical ventilation guideline for acute respiratory distress syndrome. Structural measures are most commonly binary—something is either present or absent.

Process measures reflect what happens in the performance of care. Are evidence-based medications delivered? How long does a patient wait to be admitted to the hospital? Are vital signs checked at a defined frequency? Does a child receive vaccines at a recommended schedule? Process measures have several advantages. First, they require that an evidence-based (or at least consensus-based) optimal care pathway be defined. The very act of specifying a care pathway often improves it. Second, process measures usually do not require patient-level risk adjustment. While a patient's outcome depends on their underlying severity of disease, whether a hospital provides aspirin when a patient presents with a heart attack is relatively independent of patient severity. This also means that process measures are good targets for assessing whether care is being delivered equitably. However, process measures are unequivocally *not* the goal of healthcare. Rather, we should care about outcomes, the final category of Donabedian's framework.

Outcome measures reflect what healthcare is actually trying to achieve: better quality of life and longer quantity of life. The most common outcome measures focus on mortality, patient harm/patient safety, or patient experience. Examples of these measures might be 30-day mortality following a hospitalization for acute myocardial infarction, quality of life at 1 year after heart failure diagnosis, or the percentage of patients who would definitely recommend a hospital. (It is worth saying explicitly that the experience of care is an outcome in and of itself, independent of clinical outcome.) Therefore, we should generally strive to improve outcome measures when we are trying to improve quality. Outcome measures, though, have some downsides. Perhaps the most important is that, when used for comparison between providers or hospitals, they require risk adjustment (see Chapter 18). Risk adjustment is always imperfect—sometimes markedly so. Second, the timeline until the outcome that we really care about is sometimes quite prolonged. For example, after cancer care we might care about 5- or 10-year disease-free survival. This makes it impractical to use these kinds of measures for most improvement programs. Finally, sometimes adverse outcomes are quite rare. For example, a common patient-safety measure, "Death rate in low-mortality diagnosis related groups" occurs at an average rate of about 0.45 times per 1,000 discharges.[2] Why is this important? It means that determining whether a particular intervention improved or worsened outcomes can require very large numbers of patients, sometimes prohibitively so. For example, detecting a 20% reduction in this patient safety measure would take upward of 1.6 million discharges, depending on the analytic method.

Patient-reported outcomes (PROs) are an important category of outcome. These measures tend to focus on items such as functional status and quality of life. For example, while a process measure for congestive heart failure might be angiotensin-converting-enzyme (ACE) inhibitor use, and an outcome measure might be survival, a PRO might include the Rose Dyspnea Scale or the Seattle Angina Questionnaire. An important resource for PROs is the Patient-Reported Outcomes Measurement Information System (PROMIS) program of the National Institutes of Health (NIH). PROMIS includes PROs in numerous domains, with a searchable, web-based repository of measures.

External Resource

The NIH's PROMIS measures include numerous patient-reported outcome measures and are available at http://www.healthmeasures.net/explore-measurement-systems/promis.

Extension of the Donabedian Framework: Balancing Measures and Intermediate Outcomes

Balancing Measures

Balancing measures are an important extension of the Donabedian framework. Quality improvement programs are interventions in complex systems (see Chapter 2), and they have the potential to cause unintended harm. Balancing measures are designed to detect these unintended consequences early, so that the unintended consequences can be minimized. Designing good balancing measures takes creativity and understanding of how what is being implemented might inadvertently cause harm. For example, programs to improve rapidity of anticoagulation might be accompanied by an increase in bleeding. Interventions to hasten antibiotics for patients with sepsis might unintentionally worsen antibiotic stewardship; likewise, programs to prevent falls could worsen efforts at early mobility.

> **Key Point**
>
> Balancing measures—those that detect potential unintended consequences of quality improvement—are an important extension of Donabedian's framework.

Balancing measures are important because there are numerous examples where quality improvement programs have—empirically—created unintended consequences. For example, public reporting of cardiac outcomes in New York reduced physicians' willingness to do procedures for the sickest patients.[3-5] A national program that focused on rapid antibiotics for emergency department (ED) patients with pneumonia inadvertently led to the increased use of antibiotics in patients **without** infections.[6,7] Efforts to improve blood sugar control in intensive care unit (ICU) patients became the national standard of care largely due to a single-center, nonblinded randomized trial published in 2001 in the *New England Journal of Medicine*. A multicenter study, Normoglycemia in Intensive Care Evaluation–Survival Using Glucose Algorithm Regulation (NICE-SUGAR), was eventually done and published in 2009; it found that tight glycemic control *increased* the odds of death by 14%,[8] as discussed in Chapter 1. Kavanaugh summarized the potential amount of harm done by quality improvement programs: "If the multinational data are indeed broadly applicable to mechanically ventilated ICU patients, then implementation of protocols directing glucose normalization might potentially have been responsible for approximately 26,000 additional deaths per year in the United States alone (assuming approximately 1 million ventilated ICU patients per year in the United States)."[9] While the actual number is probably substantially lower, this episode clearly demonstrates the importance of balancing measures.

Intermediate Outcomes

In clinical trials, intermediate outcomes are sometimes called *surrogate end points*. They are measurements that are believed to be on the causal pathway to the outcome that we care about. Examples might be hemoglobin

A1c (HbA1c) in diabetes, blood pressure control in hypertension, or low-density lipoprotein (LDL) cholesterol in hyperlipidemia. Why are these not outcome measures? They do not directly affect the outcome that a patient cares about. In these examples, the outcome we might care about could be major adverse cardiac events, such as myocardial infarction. High HbA1c, out-of-control-hypertension, and elevated cholesterol all surely contribute to the risk of the outcome—but they are not outcomes in and of themselves. However, they are useful surrogates for the outcome that we care about because other evidence (usually from randomized trials) shows us that if we improve the intermediate outcome, we improve the outcome we care about. In the language of causal modeling (see Chapter 20), they are mediators of the outcome. This makes them pragmatically useful because we can see responses in these factors (e.g., in HbA1c) much sooner than in the outcome itself (e.g., acute MI). However, it is important to remember that sometimes the intermediate outcome does not perfectly predict the outcome we care about. For example, some drugs lower cholesterol but do not reduce coronary artery disease (and some have even worsened outcomes).[10] Still, intermediate outcomes form the basis for numerous important quality measures.

Another Framework: The Institute of Medicine's Six Aims for Improvement

The Institute of Medicine released *Crossing the Quality Chasm*, its landmark report on how we should think about improving the quality of care, in 2001.[11] This report laid out a way of thinking about high-quality care that was broad enough to be conceptually attractive, but specific enough to be practically useful. High-quality healthcare should be safe, effective, efficient, timely, patient-centered, and equitable (Table 12-2). Today, these Six Aims for Improvement are widely used in quality measurement.

Using Donabedian's Framework and the Six Aims Together

We recommend thinking of the Structure-Process-Outcome-(Balancing) framework and the Six Aims as complementary to each other. For each of the Six Aims, it is possible to have structural, process, and outcome measures. When developing a robust quality measurement program, you can think of Donabedian's framework and the Six Aims as a matrix (Table 12-3). This is a way to assess quickly whether you have gaps in your approach. For example, it is common to find that you may have few equity measures, or that you have overweighted process measures. While this approach is more complex than you will wish to use for simple quality

Table 12-2 SIX AIMS OF A HIGH-QUALITY HEALTHCARE SYSTEM

Aim	Description from Crossing the Quality Chasm[11]
Safe	Avoiding injuries to patients from the care that is intended to help them
Effective	Providing services based on scientific knowledge to all who could benefit, and refraining from providing services to those not likely to benefit
Efficient	Avoiding waste, including of equipment, supplies, ideas, and energy
Timely	Reducing waits and sometimes-harmful delays for both those who receive and those who give care
Patient-centered	Providing care that is respectful of and responsive to individual patient preferences, needs, and values, and ensuring that patient values guide all clinical decisions
Equitable	Providing care that does not vary in quality because of personal characteristics such as gender, ethnicity, geographic location, and socioeconomic status

Table 12-3 USING THE SIX AIMS AND DONABEDIAN FRAMEWORK TOGETHER

Aim	Donabedian Measure Category		
	Structure	Process	Outcome
Safe			
Effective			
Efficient			
Timely			
Patient-centered			
Equitable			

improvement projects, it is a useful way to assess an organization's quality measurement strategy as you are thinking through potential gaps.

WHAT ARE YOU TRYING TO ACHIEVE? IMPROVEMENT, COMPARISON, OR ACCOUNTABILITY

When setting out to use or analyze quality measures, it is important to think through what you are trying to achieve because this defines many of the requirements for your measures. If you are focused on internal improvement, you often just need measures to be stable over time. It is still important to avoid overreacting to common-cause, random variations in your data (see Chapter 14). However, risk adjustment usually plays only a very minor role within a single practice or facility over a few months or a few years, because average patient characteristics tend to remain stable over these time periods.

On the other hand, if you intend to use quality measures to compare performance—between doctors, floors, or hospitals—then both the stakes and the methodological requirements increase substantially. In these cases, risk adjustment is tremendously important because patients with different inherent risks tend to end up at different facilities. Even with very careful attention to risk adjustment, the adjustment may well remain inadequate.[12] Relatively esoteric statistical issues (like clustering and whether you determine confidence intervals using parametric or bootstrap approaches) can play an important role in which physicians or which hospitals are judged to be outliers.[13] This is even more important when measures are being used for accountability: for determining payment, or for publicly declaring a hospital or surgeon as high or low quality.

WHAT MAKES A GOOD MEASURE?

Quality measures are commonly evaluated based on their importance, scientific soundness, feasibility, and usability.[14] The National Quality Forum has developed substantial procedures for implementing these criteria in the evaluation of measures.[15]

What does *importance* mean in this context? It means that assessing the proposed measure must have a meaningful potential clinical impact. First, there must be a compelling reason that what is being measured is related to a meaningful health outcome. This can be a conceptual relationship (like biological plausibility), through clinical evidence, or from a combination of the two.[14] Second, there must be a gap between ideal performance and the current state: If everyone is already performing at 100%, there is not a lot to gain from the measure. Third, if performance improved by a reasonable amount, would there be a meaningful clinical improvement in the outcome that you care about?

Scientific soundness, or *scientific acceptability,* has to do with the measure itself. Does the measure produce reliable, consistent, and valid estimates of the quality of care? A few common problems arise in the scientific acceptability of measures. First, there may be problematic variation in the source data used for measures. For example, variation in ICD-9 or ICD-10 coding accounted for up to 63% of the improvement seen in a readmission reduction program;[16] an apparent national decline in pneumonia mortality rates was explained by shifts in diagnostic coding.[17] Second, another common problem in quality measures has to do with interobserver reliability. For example, ventilator-associated pneumonia was a common quality measure in the 2000s but, even when standardized vignettes were used, there was little agreement between hospitals about whether individual patients had the condition.[18] Similarly, a study of a national sepsis measure found that abstractors agreed on time zero (when the measure's clock started) in only 36% of cases.[19] Third, sample sizes for individual hospitals or physicians are commonly too small to allow meaningful comparisons. This is exacerbated by statistical approaches that fail to take into account clustering of patients within providers.[20] Fourth, a common category of measures is composite measures (i.e., those that combine various single measures into an aggregate measure of performance). The measures are attractive because they provide easy-to-interpret measures of quality (e.g., five stars versus three stars), but many of these measures today have significant conceptual and statistical flaws.[21]

Feasibility focuses on whether the data that are needed to calculate the measure are easily and readily available. What is the burden required for the measure? Do the data exist at all, or do they require new collection? Are the data electronic? Easily extractable? Or does the measure require substantial, manual, expensive extraction? As noted below, data collection can be startlingly expensive. *Usability* refers to how well the results of the measure are understood—by patients, providers, the public, and others. Can they be used for public reporting? Accountability? Performance improvement?

Problems in *usability* and *interpretability* can greatly reduce the impact of a quality measure. Some quality measures may be too complicated for straightforward understanding by patients and clinicians. In other cases, the visual presentation of data can obscure the underlying meaning. Recent studies of infection-prevention measures are instructive in this regard. These studies found that generalists misinterpreted central-line infection measures 39% of the time, and experts made errors 27% of the time. Performance was substantially worse in both groups when risk-adjusted data were involved.[22,23] These are examples of challenges with the usability of metrics.

> **Caution**
> Coding variation, low interobserver reliability, small sample sizes, and issues with composite measures are common problems with the scientific acceptability of measures.

CHALLENGES

There are numerous challenges in appropriately measuring quality and patient safety. We detail a few of them next.

It's Conceptually Hard

In his seminal 1966 paper defining the Structure-Process-Outcome framework, Donabedian himself issued the following warning:

> The assessment of quality must rest on a conceptual and operationalized definition of what the "quality of medical care" means. Many problems are present at this fundamental level, for the quality of care is a remarkably difficult notion to define.[1]

If Donabedian thought this, we should all recognize that there are substantial challenges in fundamental aspects of quality measurement.

In Some Cases, It's Statistically Impossible

We all want a simple answer to the straightforward question, "Who is the best doctor?" In an important 2003 *JAMA* paper, Landon and colleagues laid out the practical and methodological challenges of individual physician quality measurement. While many of these were pragmatic (e.g., having to do with data availability), some were more fundamental:

> We conclude that important technical barriers stand in the way of using physician clinical performance assessment for evaluating the competency of individual physicians. Overcoming these barriers will require considerable additional research and development. Even then, for some uses, physician clinical performance assessment at the individual physician level may be technically impossible to accomplish in a valid and fair way.[20]

Some of these fundamental limitations have to do with sample size and with the diversity in the types of patients that an individual physician sees. For example, if a highly specialized surgeon only does one or two procedures, then measures are more likely to be reliable. A primary care physician, on the other hand, may see patients with hundreds of diverse conditions—thus lowering the sample size for any individual measure to a point where signal is drowned out by noise. For example, one study of diabetes measures found that each physician's panel would need >100 patients with diabetes just to get to 80% reliability in physician comparisons. However, >90% of physicians in the study had fewer than 60 patients with diabetes.[24] This example points out that sometimes it may be impossible to compare physicians' quality fairly.

Goodhart's Law: It Used to Work, Now It Doesn't

One of the most frustrating aspects of quality measurement is that the act of measuring can change the relationship between what you're measuring and the patient's outcome. This is often called *Goodhart's Law*. Strathern summarized Goodhart's Law as: "When a measure becomes a target, it ceases to be a good measure." Applied to educational examinations (which is the case in Strathern's paper), this means that "[t]he more ... examination performance becomes an expectation, the poorer it becomes as a discriminator of individual performances."[25]

The same is often true of quality measures. What is the pattern that has played out repeatedly? Initial studies show that particular process measures predict patient outcomes. These measures become quality measures, with public reporting or pay-for-performance implications. Subsequent studies then show that the original measure is no longer correlated with patient outcomes. This has been the case, for example, with numerous cardiology measures over the years,[26] and also with pneumonia measures,[6,7,27] among others.

> **Key Point**
>
> Goodhart's Law has been summarized as "When a measure becomes a target, it ceases to be a good measure."[25]

Measurement Isn't Free

We often treat quality measurement as if it is free. It isn't. Costs for data collection can be substantial. One paper described quality-reporting costs for two required quality-reporting programs (sepsis and surgery) from three hospitals. Annual costs for data collection ranged from $114,000 per program to $2 million.[28] In the outpatient setting, Casalino et al. estimated that U.S. physician practices spend $15.4 billion per year on quality-measure reporting.[29] This led to a *JAMA* commentary calling measuring the cost of quality measurement the "missing link" in our national quality strategy.[30]

COMMON MEASURE SETS AND MAJOR PAY-FOR-PERFORMANCE PROGRAMS

Quality measures have proliferated significantly in recent years, now numbering in the hundreds.[31] Today, they are routinely used by Medicare, Medicaid, and private payers for both payment and public display of provider performance. Because increasing amounts of providers' revenue is now dependent on the performance on these measures, U.S. healthcare delivery scientists should be familiar with some of the key measure sets and the programs that use them.

Although the actual measures have changed, Panzer et al. (2013) remains an outstanding read for understanding just how many measures the U.S. payment and public reporting framework can require.[31] In particular, the supplementary appendix to this article is a compendium of the more than 300 potential payment measures in 2014, and it helps demonstrate the potential burden to providers.

Measure Databases and Aggregators

> **External Resource**
> The National Quality Forum maintains its QPS at https://www.qualityforum.org/QPS.

The National Quality Forum maintains its Quality Positioning System (QPS) at https://www.qualityforum.org/QPS. This web-based tool allows identification of measures endorsed by the National Quality Forum across a wide variety of domains.

> **External Resource**
> Medicare's MIPS program quality measures are available at https://qpp.cms.gov/mips/explore-measures/quality-measures.

Medicare's Merit-based Incentive Program System (MIPS), also known as the *Quality Payment Program,* maintains a list of approved quality measures at https://qpp.cms.gov/mips/explore-measures/quality-measures. A description of MIPS is given later in this chapter.

Between January 2001 and July 16, 2018, the Agency for Healthcare Research and Quality (AHRQ) also maintained the National Quality Measures Clearinghouse. This resource was taken down because there was no longer federal funding to support it. Whether this important resource will be brought back is unknown at this time. AHRQ's updates on the matter are at https://www.ahrq.gov/gam/updates/index.html.

Composite Scorecards

> **External Resource**
> HANYS' *Report on Report Cards: Understanding Publicly Reported Hospital Quality Measures* is available at https://www.hanys.org/quality/data/report_cards/2013/.

Hospitals and health systems are subject to numerous (and proliferating) scorecards, including many proprietary scorecards. Many of these report cards are quite poor, and most of them are conflicting: A hospital will frequently have an "outstanding" rating in one report card and a "poor" rating in another. This issue is significant enough that the Healthcare Association of New York State developed a "Report on Report Cards" that reviews many of these issues (and gives grades to many of the report cards).[32]

> **External Resource**
> The Leapfrog Group's Hospital Safety Score is available at http://www.hospitalsafetygrade.org/.

Two prominent hospital scorecards are the Leapfrog Group's Hospital Safety Grade and the overall hospital quality rating from the Centers for Medicare and Medicaid Services (CMS), known as Hospital Stars. Each of these is a composite indicator, with easy-to-understand summaries of quality/safety data—though both of them also have the inherent challenges of composite indicators discussed previously. While neither of these programs is directly linked to payment, each uses measures that are part of numerous payment programs. Leapfrog assigns letter grades (A, B, etc.) to hospitals based on a combination of 25–30 measures representing infection data, coding-based patient safety indicators, and self-reported data about safety practices, staffing, and other issues.

The Hospital Star rating combines more than 60 measures into a single one- to five-star score. While many applauded CMS's attempt to make quality ratings more interpretable, its methods received significant and widespread criticism,[33] at least in part because the Hospital Stars appear to detect the high socioeconomic status of hospitals' ZIP codes as much as they do innate hospital quality.[12] CMS continues to iterate on the methods for this rating, which is likely to improve over time. CMS also has important aggregate quality rating systems for Medicare Advantage plans (https://www.medicare.gov/find-a-plan/), which is also (confusingly) commonly called Medicare Stars, and nursing homes (https://www.medicare.gov/nursinghomecompare/).

External Resource

Medicare's Overall Hospital Star Rating is available at https://www.medicare.gov/hospitalcompare/.

Common Payment Programs and Measure Sets

While a full elicitation of pay-for-performance programs and measure sets is beyond the scope of this chapter, healthcare delivery scientists should be familiar with at least some of the key national programs. The descriptions given here (including the amount of financial risk) represent the current status in 2018, but Medicare routinely changes both the measures and the specific amounts at risk:

- **Hospital Inpatient Quality Reporting Program:** Hospitals who do not participate in this program lose one-quarter of Medicare's annual payment update. Data reported under the program become the basis for many other pay-for-performance programs. Patient experience surveys such as the Hospital Consumer Assessment of Healthcare Providers and Systems (HCAHPS), participation in the National Healthcare Safety Network (NHSN) infection-reporting system and submission of chart-abstracted Clinical Process of Care Measures (sometimes called *Core Measures*), and electronic Clinical Quality Measures (eCQMs) are required.
- **Hospital Outpatient Quality Reporting Program:** Hospitals who do not submit data to this program will lose 2% of their Outpatient Prospective Payment System payments. This program requires submission of data related to emergency department measures, radiology measures, outpatient procedural and outpatient surgery measures, and others. Most of these measures require chart abstraction.
- **National Healthcare Safety Network (NHSN):** The NHSN is run by the Centers for Disease Control and Prevention (CDC). It uses highly specified abstraction criteria to perform surveillance for a number of healthcare-associated infections such as central-line-associated bloodstream infections, *Clostridium difficile* infections, etc. It is used in numerous payment programs and public reporting venues.

- **Hospital Consumer Assessment of Healthcare Providers and Systems (HCAHPS):** HCAHPS is a survey-based assessment of patient experience following a hospitalization. It is used in numerous payment programs and public reporting venues. Similar instruments exist for ambulatory visits and other venues. The ambulatory version of this survey is called Consumer Assessment of Healthcare Providers and Systems (CAHPS).
- **Hospital Readmissions Reduction Program (HRRP):** This program aims to reduce hospital readmissions. Hospitals may lose up to 3% of Diagnosis-Related Group (DRG)–based payments from CMS. The program has historically targeted specific disease states for readmission. As of 2018, these include acute myocardial infarction, heart failure, pneumonia, chronic obstructive pulmonary disease, coronary artery bypass graft surgeries, and elective primary total hip and/or total knee arthroplasty.
- **Hospital-Acquired Conditions (HAC) program:** This program aims to reduce harm from medical care. Hospitals may lose up to 1% of DRG-based revenue based on performance. This program aggregates coding-based patient-safety indicators (via the PSI-90) and NHSN-based measures of healthcare-associated infections.
- **Hospital Value-Based Purchasing:** This program aims to improve the quality of care while reducing cost to Medicare. Hospitals have 2% of DRG-based revenue at risk in this program. Hospitals with better performance may receive a bonus under this program (unlike under HAC and HRRP). Hospital Value-Based Purchasing aggregates NHSN-based measures of healthcare-associated infections, coding-based patient-safety indicators (via the PSI-90), claims-based 30-day mortality rates, Medicare spending per beneficiary, and measures of patient experience (via HCAHPS).

The items listed here largely focus on governmental, hospital-based programs. Many private payers have similar types of programs, though often with different measures. Several important programs and measure sets are primarily focused on physician practices, payers, and new payment models, as well:

- **Healthcare Effectiveness Data and Information Set (HEDIS):** This set of measures is maintained by the National Committee for Quality Assurance and used by the vast majority of health plans for quality assessment. Its more than 90 measures are also incorporated into numerous payment programs.
- **MIPS:** This Medicare program is designed to improve quality and reduce costs for physicians receiving fee-for-service Medicare payments. By 2020, it may create up to an 18% swing in a physician's

Part B revenue—there is the possibility of a 9% penalty or a 9% bonus. The actual calculation of the payment impact is quite complicated and includes quality measures, as well as other factors. Many of the eligible quality measures are HEDIS measures.

- **ACO measures:** Accountable Care Organizations (ACOs) are an important mechanism to incent value-based, rather than volume-based, care. Many ACOs are measured on a similar set of measures that include measures of patient experience, several HEDIS quality measures, ambulatory-sensitive admissions (calculated from claims data), and readmission rates. Details of these measures for 2018 are available at https://www.cms.gov/Medicare/Medicare-Fee-for-Service-Payment/sharedsavingsprogram/Downloads/2018-reporting-year-narrative-specifications.pdf. The Center for Medicare and Medicaid Innovation has also announced and launched several other new payment programs with similar types of measurement approaches.
- **Medicare Stars.** Confusingly, there are several programs colloquially known as "Medicare Stars." Previously, we discussed Hospital Stars, which is not linked to payment. However, the Medicare Stars program that is linked to Medicare Advantage programs is tightly linked to payment. Results on these measures may account for a 5% bonus in revenue for Medicare Advantage plans (as well as other potential benefits). Medicare Stars includes numerous HEDIS measures, the CAHPS patient experience survey, items from the Medicare Health Outcomes Survey (https://www.hosonline.org/), and other measures.

KEY POINTS

- The Donabedian Structure-Process-Outcome-(Balancing) framework is a practical and useful framework for thinking about quality measures, as is the Institute of Medicine's Six Aims, which state that high-quality healthcare should be safe, effective, efficient, timely, patient-centered, and equitable.
- Measures that are used for provider comparison, or for accountability, almost always require much more attention to complex statistical issues than measures used for internal improvement.
- Quality measures should be evaluated based on their importance, scientific soundness, feasibility, and usability.
- There are numerous, serious pitfalls in developing good quality measures and deploying them successfully.
- Increasing amounts of provider revenue are determined directly by performance on quality measures, and the number of measures in these programs may reach into the hundreds.

REFERENCES

1. Donabedian A. Evaluating the quality of medical care. *Milbank Mem Fund Q.* 1966;44(3):Suppl:166–206.
2. Owens P, Limcangco R, Barrett M, Heslin K, Moore B. *Patient Safety and Adverse Events, 2011 and 2014.* HCUP Statistical Brief No. 237. 2018. Accessed August 19, 2018, from https://www.hcup-us.ahrq.gov/reports/statbriefs/sb237-Patient-Safety-Adverse-Events-2011-2014.jsp.
3. Apolito RA, Greenberg MA, Menegus MA, et al. Impact of the New York State Cardiac Surgery and Percutaneous Coronary Intervention Reporting System on the management of patients with acute myocardial infarction complicated by cardiogenic shock. *Am Heart J.* 2008;155(2):267–273.
4. Waldo SW, McCabe JM, O'Brien C, Kennedy KF, Joynt KE, Yeh RW. Association between public reporting of outcomes with procedural management and mortality for patients with acute myocardial infarction. *J Am Coll Cardiol.* 2015;65(11):1119–1126.
5. Joynt KE, Blumenthal DM, Orav EJ, Resnic FS, Jha AK. Association of public reporting for percutaneous coronary intervention with utilization and outcomes among Medicare beneficiaries with acute myocardial infarction. *JAMA.* 2012;308(14):1460–1468.
6. Welker JA, Huston M, McCue JD. Antibiotic timing and errors in diagnosing pneumonia. *Arch Intern Med.* 2008;168(4):351–356.
7. Kanwar M, Brar N, Khatib R, Fakih MG. Misdiagnosis of community-acquired pneumonia and inappropriate utilization of antibiotics: side effects of the 4-h antibiotic administration rule. *Chest.* 2007;131(6):1865–1869.
8. Investigators N-SS, Finfer S, Chittock DR, et al. Intensive versus conventional glucose control in critically ill patients. *N Engl J Med.* 2009;360(13):1283–1297.
9. Kavanagh BP, Nurok M. Standardized intensive care. Protocol misalignment and impact misattribution. *Am J Respir Crit Care Med.* 2016;193(1):17–22.
10. Canner PL, Berge KG, Wenger NK, et al. Fifteen-year mortality in Coronary Drug Project patients: long-term benefit with niacin. *J Am Coll Cardiol.* 1986;8(6):1245–1255.
11. Institute of Medicine. *Crossing the Quality Chasm: A New Health System for the 21st Century.* Washington, DC: National Academies Press; 2001.
12. Reidhead M, Kuhn H, Orlowski J. My favorite slide: Why five-star hospitals may be more closely related to five-star restaurants than innate quality. *NEJM Catalyst*, October 25, 2016. Accessed August 19, 2018, from https://catalyst.nejm.org/five-star-hospitals-five-star-restaurants/.
13. Glance LG, Dick A, Osler TM, Li Y, Mukamel DB. Impact of changing the statistical methodology on hospital and surgeon ranking: the case of the New York State cardiac surgery report card. *Med Care.* 2006;44(4):311–319.
14. McGlynn EA, Adams JL. What makes a good quality measure? *JAMA.* 2014;312(15):1517–1518.

15. National Quality Forum. *Measure Evaluation Criteria and Guidance for Evaluating Measures for Endorsement.* 2016. Accessed August 20, 2018, from http://www.qualityforum.org/Measuring_Performance/Submitting_Standards/2016_Measure_Evaluation_Criteria.aspx.
16. Ibrahim AM, Dimick JB, Sinha SS, Hollingsworth JM, Nuliyalu U, Ryan AM. Association of coded severity with readmission reduction after the Hospital Readmissions Reduction Program. *JAMA Intern Med.* 2018;178(2):290–292.
17. Lindenauer PK, Lagu T, Shieh MS, Pekow PS, Rothberg MB. Association of diagnostic coding with trends in hospitalizations and mortality of patients with pneumonia, 2003–2009. *JAMA.* 2012;307(13):1405–1413.
18. Stevens JP, Kachniarz B, Wright SB, et al. When policy gets it right: Variability in U.S. hospitals' diagnosis of ventilator-associated pneumonia. *Crit Care Med.* 2014;42(3):497–503.
19. Rhee C, Brown SR, Jones TM, et al. Variability in determining sepsis time zero and bundle compliance rates for the centers for medicare and medicaid services SEP-1 measure. *Infect Control Hosp Epidemiol.* 2018;39(8):994–996.
20. Landon BE, Normand SL, Blumenthal D, Daley J. Physician clinical performance assessment: prospects and barriers. *JAMA.* 2003;290(9):1183–1189.
21. Barclay M, Dixon-Woods M, Lyratzopoulos G. The problem with composite indicators. *BMJ Qual Saf.* 2018;28(4).
22. Govindan S, Wallace B, Iwashyna TJ, Chopra V. Do experts understand performance measures? A mixed-methods study of infection preventionists. *Infect Control Hosp Epidemiol.* 2018;39(1):71–76.
23. Govindan S, Chopra V, Iwashyna TJ. Do clinicians understand quality metric data? An evaluation in a Twitter-derived sample. *J Hosp Med.* 2017;12(1):18–22.
24. Hofer TP, Hayward RA, Greenfield S, Wagner EH, Kaplan SH, Manning WG. The unreliability of individual physician "report cards" for assessing the costs and quality of care of a chronic disease. *JAMA.* 1999;281(22):2098–2105.
25. Strathern M. "Improving ratings": audit in the British University system. *European Review.* 1997;5(3):305–321.
26. Chatterjee P, Joynt KE. Do cardiology quality measures actually improve patient outcomes? *J Am Heart Assoc.* 2014;3(1):e000404.
27. Nicks BA, Manthey DE, Fitch MT. The Centers for Medicare and Medicaid Services (CMS) community-acquired pneumonia core measures lead to unnecessary antibiotic administration by emergency physicians. *Acad Emerg Med.* 2009;16(2):184–187.
28. Wall MJ, Howell MD. Variation and cost-effectiveness of quality measurement programs. The case of sepsis bundles. *Ann Am Thorac Soc.* 2015;12(11):1597–1599.
29. Casalino LP, Gans D, Weber R, et al. US physician practices spend more than $15.4 billion annually to report quality measures. *Health Aff (Millwood).* 2016;35(3):401–406.
30. Schuster MA, Onorato SE, Meltzer DO. Measuring the cost of quality measurement: a missing link in quality strategy. *JAMA.* 2017;318(13):1219–1220.
31. Panzer RJ, Gitomer RS, Greene WH, Webster PR, Landry KR, Riccobono CA. Increasing demands for quality measurement. *JAMA.* 2013;310(18):1971–1980.

32. Healthcare Association of New York State (HANYS). *HANYS' Report on Report Cards: Understanding Publicly Reported Hospital Quality Measures*. 2013. Accessed August 21, 2018, from https://www.hanys.org/quality/data/report_cards/2013/docs/2013_hanys_report_card_book.pdf.
33. Xu S, Grover A. CMS' hospital quality star ratings fail to pass the common sense test. *Health Affairs Blog* 2016. Accessed August 21, 2018, from https://www.healthaffairs.org/do/10.1377/hblog20161114.057512/full/.

OVERVIEW OF ANALYTIC TECHNIQUES AND COMMON PITFALLS

13

The rest of this section of the book focuses on specific approaches to analyzing healthcare data: that is, how to use analytics to see the truth in the world so that you can improve patients' health and healthcare. All these approaches, though, build on an understanding of several core principles about healthcare data. That is the focus of this chapter: These principles are important across all analytic techniques, and they represent issues that are easy to miss but can cause you to get the wrong answer if you don't pay attention to them. Understanding these core concepts will help you select the right analytic method for the problem at hand. This chapter will introduce these core concepts, including data types (e.g., binary versus continuous), why missing data are critical, and the Four Horsemen of Mistaken Conclusions (chance, confounding, and bias — and violating the assumptions of your analytic method). It will also provide a brief overview for the analytic methods that will come in the following chapters.

DINOSAUR FOOTPRINTS AND WHAT THEY TELL US ABOUT DATA ANALYSIS IN HEALTHCARE

The electronic record created as part of a healthcare encounter is not a patient. Rather, the record is made up of the electronic footprints that the patient leaves behind from her or his interactions with the health system. That sounds obvious, but it is remarkably easy to forget. What's left in the record is a pale, sparse reflection of the complexity of a human being ... a reflection that is transformed, diluted, and adulterated by the environment, by financial considerations, and by clinical interfaces that sometimes are difficult to use.

That doesn't mean that we can't learn anything from patient data generated as part of routine care—exactly the opposite! We often think of this like dinosaur footprints, which have been tremendously important to modern paleontology[1] (Figure 13-1). A dinosaur footprint isn't a dinosaur, but rather it represents a dinosaur's interactions with the world

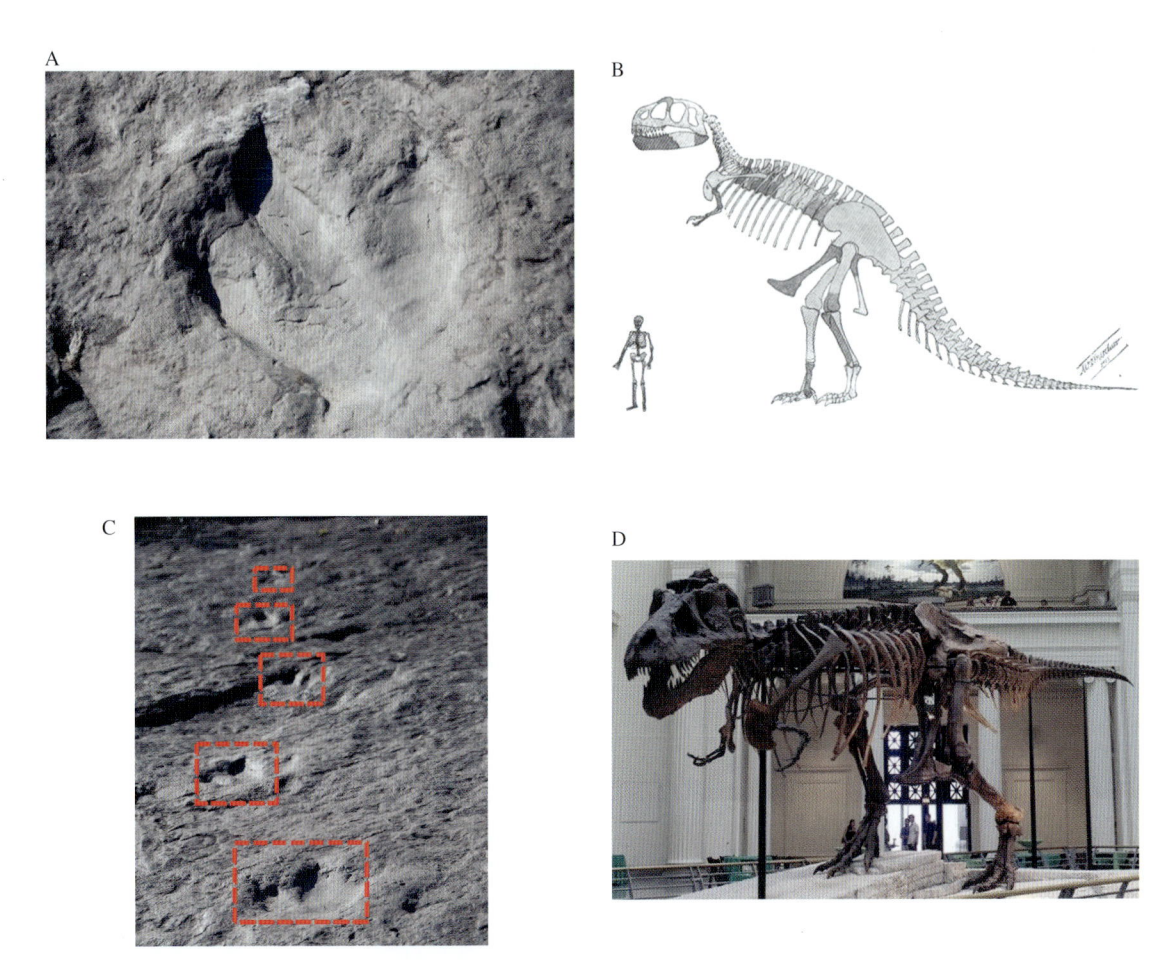

Figure 13-1 • Dinosaur footprints as a metaphor. (A) Dinosaur footprint in the Connecticut River Valley in Massachusetts. The three toes identify it as a theropod. (B) 1905 sketch of *T. rex*, showing incorrect hip orientation. (C) A trackway of dinosaur footprints, showing no markings consistent with a tail being dragged. (D) Current understanding of the orientation of a *T. rex*'s hips and pelvis, based partly on examination of dinosaur footprints and trackways (this is *Sue*, in Chicago's Field Museum).
Image credits: (A), (C) photos by Michael Howell (B) From 1905, the first publication of a reconstructed *T. rex* skeleton, drawn by William D. Matthew, in Osborn, Henry Fairfield. "Tyrannosaurus and other Cretaceous carnivorous dinosaurs," in *Bulletin of the American Museum of Natural History*, vol. 21 (1905), pp. 259–265. Via Wikipedia https://en.wikipedia.org/wiki/Tyrannosaurus#/media/File:Tyrannosaurus_skeleton.jpg.) (D) (From Wikipedia, by Connie Ma. https://en.wikipedia.org/wiki/Sue_(dinosaur)#/media/File:Sues_skeleton.jpg. License CC BY-SA 2.0.)

around it … mitigated and transformed over the subsequent millions of years. Most of the information about the dinosaur is lost, but we can still make inferences from what's left behind. In panel A of Figure 13-1, a single dinosaur footprint has three toes, which is a characteristic of a set of dinosaurs called *theropods* (a group which includes the largest land-dwelling carnivores ever discovered, like *Tyrannosaurus rex*). Panel B shows how—for many decades—scientists thought the *T. rex*'s skeleton looked ... standing upright, dragging its tail. Based on many pieces of evidence, though, paleontologists revised how they thought *T. rex* stood and how its skeleton was put together—with a much more horizontal orientation (panel D). One of the pieces of evidence was studying trackways—fossil records of multiple dinosaur footprints as they walked across the land (panel C shows a trackway of the same theropod shown in panel A). It turns out to be remarkably rare to find traces of tails in dinosaur trackways, suggesting that dinosaurs rarely dragged their tails, and thus paleontologists' original orientation of *T. rex* was wrong.[2] Paleontologists have also made inferences about dinosaurs' gate, speed, hip height, and pack behavior from trackways.

There are a number of lessons for us here. Electronic footprints are important sources of data, they but mustn't be mistaken for the actual patient. Carefully handled with expertise, they can provide a tremendous amount of information. Even more important, seeing how these electronic footprints evolve over time, like trackways, can teach us a lot about the patient that created them.

THE FOUR HORSEMEN OF MISTAKEN CONCLUSIONS

It's really important to get the right answer in healthcare because you will make clinical or policy decisions that affect real people's lives. There are three categories of classic threats to the validity of your conclusions: chance, bias, and confounding. These threats apply to all analytic methods. Many of the more sophisticated analytic methods are specific attempts to mitigate the likelihood of getting the wrong answer because of chance, bias, or confounding. To these threats, we add a fourth—violating the assumptions of your analytic method. As you consider the following chapters, keep these issues in the front of your mind.

> **Key Point**
>
> Chance, bias, and confounding are the classic threats to the validity of your analyses. Violating the inherent assumptions of your analytic method is another.

Chance

Chance amounts to randomness. Imagine that you wanted to know what the most common eye color is of patients in your clinic. You decide to look at your next patient (who has green eyes). What's the likelihood that green is the most common eye color in your clinic? What if you look at 2 patients, or 10, or 100? Does your confidence increase?

Similar problems apply to both randomized and observational studies. Sometimes a finding is just noise, not signal. Statisticians have developed tools to help us estimate when a conclusion is likely to be due to

> **Key Point**
>
> *Chance* is random error. Tests like P values and confidence intervals help assess the likelihood that chance is a threat to the validity of your conclusions.

chance alone. This is the fundamental purpose of statistical tools like *P values* and *confidence intervals* (and their Bayesian counterpart, *credible intervals*).

It is important to know that a P value of <0.05 doesn't mean that a finding is "definitely true." It means—if your null hypothesis is true—that you have a <5% chance of getting a sample as extreme or more extreme than what you saw in your data. An important implication of this is that the more statistical tests you do, the more likely you are to get a false positive by chance alone. When you perform large numbers of tests of significance, you are almost guaranteed to get at least a few low P values, just by chance alone. We will spend even more time discussing the pitfalls of P values in Chapter 14.

A particular kind of chance is nondifferential *misclassification error*. For example, imagine that you are interested in whether nutrition counseling reduces the risk of developing diabetes. Imagine also that it turns out that 10% of patients with diabetes are not diagnosed. So long as this underdiagnosis is randomly distributed between patients who get nutrition counseling and those who don't, then this is just an issue of power and sample size (nondifferential misclassification dilutes your study results, making it harder to find an association). However, you will often find that misclassification is *differential*: that is, that it happens in one group with a higher probability than in another. Maybe nutrition counselors increase the rate at which diabetes is diagnosed. You might mistakenly conclude that nutrition counseling causes diabetes. That is no longer a problem of chance, so it means that there is bias in your study, which will be discussed next.

Bias

> **Key Point**
>
> In this context, *bias* means that data are collected or analyzed in a way that systematically differs from the truth.

> **Caution**
>
> Bias can be a lethal problem for your analyses because it may be impossible to use statistical techniques to correct it.

The word *bias* has many meanings, but in this context, it means that data are collected in a way that systematically misrepresents the truth in the world—or that the way the analysis is constructed introduces this systematic misrepresentation. This happens when patients or outcomes of one type or another are systematically overrepresented or underrepresented when the data are collected or analyzed. For example, a landline phone-based survey of food insecurity would dramatically underrepresent the homeless. (This is an example of the problem called *selection bias*.) These problems will often be invisible in a data set because they happen before the data are created or collected. Therefore, bias inherent in the data are often impossible to correct by statistical methods, no matter how sophisticated. Not difficult or complicated—*impossible*. Therefore, always be alert for bias in the way that your data are collected.

CHAPTER 13 | ANALYTIC TECHNIQUES AND COMMON PITFALLS

Bias can also be introduced as you formulate the analytical problem. This might happen because you define cohort inclusion/exclusion criteria in a way that is somehow dependent on the outcome that you care about or are investigating. A common way that this can happen is to base inclusion/exclusion criteria on coded diagnoses (using ICD-9 or ICD-10 codes), on discharging service, or on discharge destination, for example. Because these codes are created *after* a patient is discharged, they can sometimes conflate future and past events. For example, it is common for administrators to grade performance of service lines based on the discharging hospital service (e.g., medicine, surgery). Because patients are transferred between services based on clinical events, this approach will sometimes give dramatically wrong answers.

For example, you might be interested in one measure of quality (looking at deaths among full-code patients, stratified by physician service). You might make a report on the topic and share it with your hospital's leadership. If you did this analysis, you might find that the oncology service has very low mortality rates, while the pulmonary service has very high mortality rates. But it would turn out that this is a very misleading answer. Why? Because you've conflated exposure ("hospital service") and outcome ("mortality") by the way that you've specified the problem. Full-code patients who are on an oncology service, when they develop life-threatening problems, are almost always transferred to the intensive care unit (ICU). When they transfer to the ICU, they also change physicians and become part of the pulmonary service. This means that—if true performance is equivalent between oncology and pulmonary—mortality will appear (artifactually) much higher on the pulmonary service because of selection bias. A similar analysis holds for the cost of patient care when attributed to discharging services.

A related problem is the Will Rogers effect. This phenomenon acquired its name from the humorist Will Rogers, who supposedly remarked, "When the Okies left Oklahoma and moved to California, they raised the average intelligence in both states." That sounds like a paradox, but turns out not to be. This problem can happen whenever a group of patients moves between one category and another. When hospitals increase ICU capacity, less sick patients may be moved from the regular floor to the ICU.[3] This will reduce the mortality rate in the ICU, and it will reduce the mortality rate on the regular floor … but the overall mortality rate will remain unchanged. The same thing happens when a new diagnostic test or criteria moves patients between stages in a disease.

An example of this is shown in Figure 13-2. In this hypothetical scenario, a new diagnostic test identifies a number of stage 1 patients as

> **Caution**
> Selection bias can be introduced as the data are collected, or as you design inclusion/exclusion criteria for your cohorts.

> **Caution**
> Be careful to avoid accidentally conflating outcomes and exposures, which can be easy to do when using administrative or billing data.

Original Disease Classification

Stage	Number of patients	Deaths	Mortality Rate
1	2,000	100	5%
2	1,000	200	20%
3	800	240	30%
4	200	100	50%
Overall	4,000	640	16%

A new diagnostic test identifies 1,000 patients with stage 1 disease who actually have stage 2 disease.

In these 1,000 patients, there are 90 deaths (a mortality rate of 9%).

New Disease Classification

Stage	Number of patients	Deaths	Mortality Rate
1	1,000	10	1%
2	2,000	290	14.5%
3	800	240	30%
4	200	100	50%
Overall	4,000	640	16%

Apparently, mortality rates in stage 1 and stage 2 dropped (by a startling relative 80% and 28%!)

But, overall mortality remains **exactly unchanged.** This is the Will Rogers effect in action.

Figure 13-2 • A hypothetical example of the Will Rogers effect.

Caution

The Will Rogers effect, which also manifests as stage migration, is the epidemiological manifestation of a quotation attributed to the humorist: "When the Okies left Oklahoma and moved to California, they raised the average intelligence in both states."

actually having stage 2 disease. An example might be a more sensitive computed tomography (CT) scan that now better detects adenopathy in cancer patients. These patients migrate to stage 2. Because their mortality rate is higher than that of the average stage 1 patient, but lower than that of the average stage 2 patient, both stages' mortality rates fall—while the overall mortality rate remains unchanged. This is also called *stage migration* and is a well-documented effect of new-technology use in disease staging.[4]

Sometimes how potential variables are collected and recorded differs between groups of patients. This is called *information bias*. For example, maybe you decide that you want to compare performance between primary care physicians. You decide to risk-adjust using billing codes (such as ICD-10 codes). However, one practice has a much higher coding intensity than another—the same patient who goes to one practice will get more ICD-10 codes than if the same patient went to a different practice. This would result in lower estimated risks for one practice than another and would introduce an apparent performance difference which does not actually exist.[5] An interesting demonstration of this kind of bias was shown with the "weekend effect" in acute stroke—the idea that patients admitted on the weekend have worse outcomes due to lower quality of care. Investigators found that a substantial portion of this effect was related to lower coding intensity on the weekend, which introduced biases that could not simply be adjusted away.[6]

A common and important type of information bias is *surveillance bias*. Imagine that you are interested in venous thromboembolism (VTE) rates in hospitalized patients, and that you intend to publicly compare hospitals based on these rates. (By the way, this is actually a real measure in many public reporting programs.) Because many patients with VTE are asymptomatic, one hospital has an active program that proactively screens for VTEs. Patients there will have a higher observed rate of deep venous thrombosis (DVT) than those at a hospital without a screening program. This was studied by Billemoria and colleagues, who found that hospitals that used more VTE imaging had worse performance on this measure of quality. In fact, risk-adjusted VTE rates went up from 5.0 per 1,000 discharges (in the lower quartile of imaging use) to 13.5 in the highest quartile ($p < 0.001$) ... almost triple the rate.[7]

Numerous other types of bias exist. The commonality between them is that they *differentially* affect the groups you are interested in (e.g., control versus intervention groups). It is important to be inquisitive and critical about the possibility of bias in the data because bias can fundamentally alter the conclusions of your analysis, no matter how sophisticated the rest of your methods.

Caution

Information bias occurs when data are collected differently between one group of patients and another. This can happen when there are different intensities of coding or different approaches to surveillance for disease.

Confounding

Confounding happens when another factor distorts the apparent relationship between an exposure (or a predictor) and an outcome. This third factor—the confounder—increases or decreases the frequency of both the exposure and the outcome (Figure 13-3). If you don't know to measure the confounder (and to adjust for it), you will think that the exposure is what's driving the outcome you care about.

Just like bias, confounding can cause you to get the wrong answer in your analysis. Unlike bias, confounding can often be straightforward to handle if you (1) recognize that it might be a problem, and (2) measure the right data to let you adjust for the confounders. The purpose of many of the more advanced statistical methods is to let you adjust for confounders.

Key Point

Confounding happens when the apparent relationship between an exposure (or predictor) and an outcome is distorted by a third variable—the confounder.

What you think is happening is

A thing you observed —Seems to increase (or decrease)→ The outcome you're interested in

But what's actually going on is ...

A thing you didn't observe (or at least, didn't include in your analysis) — Increases (or decreases) both → The outcome you're interested in and → A thing you observed

This makes it look like the thing you observed is associated with the outcome you're interested in, but the truth is that something else (the confounder) is what's causing the apparent relationship.

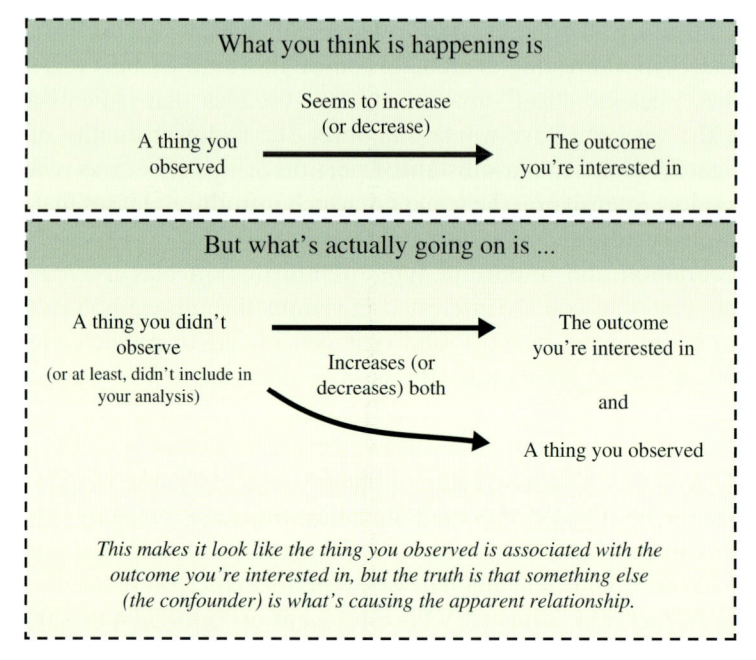

Figure 13-3 • Defining confounding.

> **Key Point**
> Confounding can cause you to get the wrong answer in an analysis, but it can often be handled by statistical techniques.

For a confounder to exist, there are three conditions that must be present:

- The confounder must be associated with *both* the exposure *and* the outcome (i.e., it must be associated with both the independent and the dependent variable).
- The confounder must be unequally distributed between the groups that you are comparing.
- The confounder cannot be a step on the causal pathway.

This last point is important. But what does it mean? For example, high levels of low-density lipoprotein (LDL) cholesterol are on the causal pathway to coronary disease. If you found that a particular diet lowered the risk of coronary disease but also lowered LDL cholesterol, you should not adjust for LDL—it's on the causal pathway. (Also see Chapter 20, "Causal Methods" section.)

Theoretical discussions about confounding can sometimes be difficult to follow. For this reason, Figure 13-4 shows a somewhat silly, but very concrete, hypothetical example. In this scenario, you're trying to figure out why people go into one store over another. A consultant suggests that perhaps height is the reason—the key driver of choice between stores. You set out to find out whether that's true, so you observe 100 people going into the stores, 50 into each. You find that height is indeed very strongly associated with choice of store (p <0.0001). However, it turns out in this case that self-reported sex is a confounder because one store sells clothes targeted toward men, and the other sells clothes targeted toward women. The Centers for Disease Control and Prevention (CDC) reports that the median height for U.S. males is about 70 inches, and the median height for U.S. females is about 65 inches.[8] (In fact, the heights for Figure 13-4 were randomly sampled out of this distribution.) Thus, the apparent relationship between height and choice of store is *confounded* by sex.

When your data captures all the potential confounders, you can usually adjust for them statistically. There are still some challenges (e.g., collinearity and interactions), but it is typically a tractable problem. However, it is very rare that you've captured all the confounders. When this happens (which is most of the time), you are left with some *residual confounding*. This is the underlying reason why randomized, controlled trials are so powerful. Because a flip of a coin (or generation of a random number) cannot be associated with patient-level characteristics, randomization tends to balance out both known and unknown confounders.

A particularly thorny and difficult type of confounding with which you should be familiar is *confounding by indication*.[9] This occurs when the reason that a treatment is given is also a risk factor for the outcome that is being studied. For example, patients at high risk of gastrointestinal (GI) bleeding are often given acid-suppressive medications like proton pump inhibitors. In unadjusted analyses, these acid-suppressive medications are associated with a 50% increase in the likelihood of GI bleeding. That is obviously incorrect because acid-suppressive medications are used to treat GI bleeding. But, because physicians give these medications to patients at higher risk of GI bleeding, they suffer from confounding by indication. (When sophisticated methods are used to handle confounding by indication, acid-suppressive medications reduce the odds of GI bleeding by about 37%.)[10] A subtype of confounding by indication is *confounding by severity*, where different treatments are given to those with different prognoses.

Be very wary of confounding by indication and confounding by severity. These kinds of confounding are particularly difficult, and it is frequently impossible to adjust for them fully because physicians make decisions based on many prognostic signals that are never captured in the data.

Caution

Confounding by indication (or severity) is a particularly difficult type of confounding that often cannot be fully handled by adjustment methods.

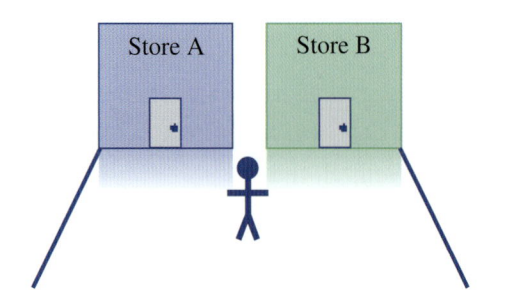

III | UNDERSTANDING HEALTHCARE DELIVERY SCIENCE

You are trying to figure out the key drivers that cause people to go into store A or store B. You observe 100 people entering the stores, and you observe the following heights (measured in inches):

Store A	Store B
76.5	68.6
72.4	67.2
67.6	66.2
70.4	66.8
70.9	66.8
...	...

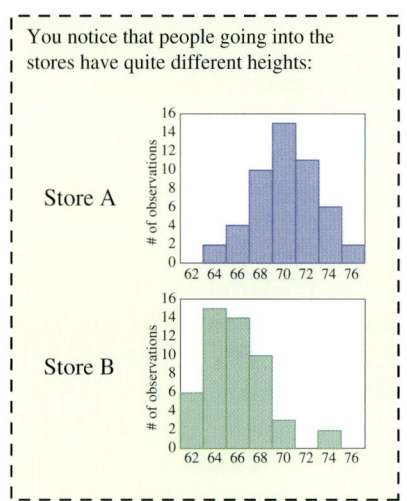

You notice that people going into the stores have quite different heights:

Store A

Store B

Because the distributions are normal, you calculate means and standard deviations.*

	Store A	Store B
Mean	69.5	64.6
Std Deviation	2.7	2.4

Next, you do a *t test* because this is the right test of difference for normally distributed, continuous data.

P <0.0001 (!!!)

So, you conclude that height is the main factor causing people to choose one store or another.

But ... it turns out that Store A is store that makes clothes designed for men, and Store B makes clothes designed for women.

People who self-identify their sex as male are more likely to go to store A. Those who self-identify as female are more likely to go to store B.

	Store A	Store B
Male	47	3
Female	3	47

When you perform a stratified analysis, you find out:

	Height (Mean)			Height (SD)	
	Store A	Store B		Store A	Store B
Male	69.5	69.1	Male	2.7	3.6
Female	64.9	64.6	Female	0.4	2.5

That looks like height is not very different between stores once you stratify by sex.

In fact, if you adjust for sex, the relationship you saw between height and choice of store is driven just by self-reported sex (p <0.0001, not height (P ~0.74).

*Note that you observe 100 people, but only 10 are shown here. You may notice that the means and SDs of the 100-person population differ from the 10 shown. This is an example of chance, discussed earlier in this chapter.

Figure 13-4 • A hypothetical, concrete example of confounding.

Violating the Assumptions of Your Method

We should acknowledge that, traditionally, people talk about only three major threats to your analyses (chance, bias, and confounding). We prefer to add a fourth: violating the assumptions of the analytic method you've chosen. We elevate this problem because it is startlingly common and it can result in entirely incorrect conclusions.

All statistical and epidemiological methods have inherent assumptions built into them. For the methods to work—for them to give you unbiased, reliable estimates of effect or tests of difference—those assumptions must be met. For example, a *t test* expects data to be normally distributed. A logistic regression expects that a continuous predictor is linearly related to the log of the odds of the outcome. And so on. Many assumptions that are built into statistical models have to do with the type of data that the model expects to see. For this reason, we devote a fair amount of the rest of this chapter to an overview of the shapes and types of data.

> **Key Point**
> All statistical methods make assumptions. You need to know what these assumptions are, and make sure that your data fulfill them.

THE CRITICAL IMPORTANCE OF MISSING DATA

You should first think about whether some of your data might be missing. The reason that this is so important is that missing data can introduce a type of bias into your analysis that *cannot* be corrected statistically. Missing data are ubiquitous, and even in research published in top-tier journals, these data are often not methodologically well handled.[11–13]

A few examples of how missing data can arise include the following, adapted from Altman and Bland:[14]

- Vital signs and labs are checked with different frequencies for different patients.
- Some people do not respond to a survey.
- Some patients are lost to follow-up in a randomized trial.
- In a hospital system, some hospitals collect data that others do not.
- A lab machine fails for some samples, or some are lost in transit.

Except for the final example, these all have the potential to introduce bias into your analysis.

How you should handle missing data depends on the *mechanism of missingness*—the reason that the data are missing. The standard terminology is described next.

> **Key Point**
> Missing data are common and an important source of bias.

Missing Completely at Random (MCAR)

With Missing Completely at Random (MCAR) missing data, the data that are missing have no relationship whatsoever to any observed or unobserved patient characteristics. These data just randomly fell off the truck—perhaps due to corruption of a file, information lost in transit, or other event. This means that you can basically just ignore the problem. For example, you could use complete case analysis (dropping any patient with any missing data) and you would get unbiased estimates. Unfortunately, this is almost never the situation in real analyses.

Missing at Random (MAR)

The name for this kind of missingness is pretty misleading. Missing at Random (MAR) does not assume that data are missing completely at random. Instead, it assumes that the missingness can be explained by values that you've observed and recorded, and that you can use those observed variables to predict what the missing data would have been. This is the mechanism that most modern methods for handling missing data assume is going on.

Missing Not at Random (MNAR)

Data are often missing because of reasons you haven't captured in your data set. When this happens, it is called *missing not at random (MNAR)*. Specifically, there is a relationship between the likelihood that a variable is missing and its value. For example, imagine that you wanted to do a survey to predict depression. People who are depressed might be less likely to fill out your survey. This introduces MNAR missingness into your data and will typically lead to biased results. Missing data that are MNAR are missing because of variables not observed in your data, so you can't deal with them in an easy statistical way. In fact, here's what Newgard and Lewis wrote in their 2015 *JAMA* review of missing data:

Caution

When data are missing not at random (MNAR), statistical correction of bias may be impossible.

> *When MNAR is present, statistical adjustment for missing information is virtually impossible.*[11]

Approaches to Handling Missing Data

A full treatment of missing data methods is beyond the scope of this chapter, but you should be familiar with a few key points. First, the best way to handle missing data is to avoid it in your study design and execution. But it often arises anyway.

The most common approach to handling missing data is called *complete case analysis*. In fact, this is the default approach in many statistical software packages' regression routines. In this approach, you simply drop patients from the data set if they have any missing variables. Perhaps your regression model has 20 variables. If a patient only had 19 (i.e., one was missing), you would drop them from the data set. Complete case analysis is almost always a poor way to handle missing data. It tends to drop a large number of cases (reducing power), and it will often yield biased results. You should avoid doing this if you have much missing data.

The next most common way missing data are handled is through a variety of simple imputation techniques. For example, if blood pressure is missing in some patients, you might fill it in with the mean blood pressure from other patients. Or, in time series data, you might fill in missing data with whatever the value was when it was previously measured ("last observation carried forward"). These techniques are problematic because they do not handle variance correctly. When we impute a value, we aren't certain about it—and we need to handle that uncertainty when we calculate confidence intervals, P values, and other elements. You should avoid simple imputation if you have much missing data.

Sensitivity analyses are sometimes used to handle missing data. Imagine that you are assessing a program focused on readmissions, but for 5% of patients, you don't know whether they got readmitted. These data are missing. You can do two separate analyses: one in which you assume that all of the 5% of patients were readmitted, and another in which you assume that none of the 5% of patients were readmitted. Did your analysis change enough that it matters? Or did you get essentially the same answer? If you got essentially the same answer, then you are confident that your analysis is robust to these missing data.

Finally, there are more sophisticated methods to handle missing data, such as multiple imputation and maximum likelihood. For many of these techniques, you may wish to obtain specialist statistical help. *Multiple imputation* is the most common robust technique for dealing with missing data. It assumes that missing data are MAR. Multiple imputation builds a predictive model for the data that are missing, and then it makes several copies of the data set in which it fills in the missing data using the prediction. However, it randomly samples from the distribution of predicted values, so each new data set differs a bit from the other. (This helps it account for variance correctly.) You then do your analyses (e.g., building a regression model) simultaneously on all the data sets. The final step is combining the parameter estimates back into a single estimate, using a technique that preserves the uncertainty in the original imputations. Multiple imputation gives unbiased parameter estimates when the data are missing at random, though it still has several limitations that can be tricky in practice.[15]

> **Caution**
> Complete case analysis and other naïve, simple methods of imputation usually do not adequately handle missing data ... and may lead to biased and incorrect analyses.

> **Key Point**
> Multiple imputation is a stronger method for handling missing data than complete case analysis, imputation of the mean, and other simpler methods.

THE SHAPE OF DATA: CATEGORIES OF DATA AND WHY THEY MATTER

Why This Is Important

The techniques that you will use to analyze your data make assumptions about the data themselves. It is easy to get a P value, or an odds ratio, out of an analysis and not realize that it is wrong. Understanding the shape of your data will help you pick the right analytical tools out of your toolbox.

Structured Versus Unstructured

Structured data usually refers to data that comes out of a database; these kind of data are made up of numbers or a small set of categories. These data consist of the kinds of information that traditional statistical techniques are good at handling. Examples include age, gender, heart rate, blood pressure, and lab values like hemoglobin or creatinine. Billing codes like ICD-10 are useful because they are structured-data representations of complex concepts.

The term *unstructured data* usually refers to things that don't fit these characteristics. A physician's history and physical, typed in traditional form, is a good example of unstructured data. Photographs or videos of procedures, x-rays, and pathology studies are also usually considered unstructured. These data, of course, have underlying structures, but they aren't analyzable by traditional statistical techniques. Modern machine-learning techniques (covered in Chapter 17) can handle many of these kinds of data.

The rest of this section will focus on structured data. Several of these concepts will also be taken up in Chapter 14.

Types of Structured Data

The first question is whether your data are continuous or categorical.

Continuous Versus Categorical

Age, blood pressure, labs like sodium and hemoglobin, and rate of fluid administration are all continuous data. *Continuous data* are numbers that can occupy any value over their range. You might measure blood pressure as 120, or 121, or 122 … but it could be measured at 120.3, or 120.35, and so on, if you had an accurate enough measurement device.

Another characteristic of continuous data is that the conceptual "distance" between two values is determined just by their numerical difference. A hemoglobin of 10.0 is the same distance from 9.0 as from 11.0. You can see an important contrast here if you think about *survey data,* which are often confused with continuous data. These are often measured on a 5-point Likert-type scale. For example, a common scale might be "Strongly disagree" = 1, "Disagree" = 2, "Neutral" = 3, "Agree" = 4, and "Strongly agree" = 5. It is very important to realize that—even though numbers are used—this is not a continuous variable. First, responses such as "1.5" or "4.7" are not possible. Second, the distance between values is not likely to be constant. That is, there is no guarantee that the difference between "Strongly disagree" and "Disagree" is the same as the distance between "Disagree" and "Neutral" — even though they are each separated by exactly one category.

Continuous Data: Normally Distributed (Gaussian)

Continuous data can have many different distributions. Many statistical tests work only for certain distributions. One of the most important of these is the *normal distribution*, the classic "bell curve"; this is sometimes called the *Gaussian distribution* after Carl Friedrich Gauss, who introduced it in 1809.

Data that are normally distributed have some handy properties. The *mean* is a good measure of the central tendency of the data—the mean and the *median* are identical in a perfectly normal distribution. The *standard deviation (SD)* is also useful for normal data: About 68% of values are within 1 SD of the mean, about 95% are within 2 SDs, and about 99.7% are within 3 SDs. Because the normal distribution is well understood, statistical tests that use the normal distribution often have more power than tests that don't assume normality. For example, the *t test* is a common test of difference used for normal data.

Continuous Data: Data that Aren't Normally Distributed—Much of the Data You'll Deal With!

Many of the continuous data you'll deal with are not normally distributed. For example, hospital length of stay is almost always quite right-skewed (Figure 13-5). Similarly, costs of care are usually quite right-skewed.

When your data aren't normally distributed, there are a few things you can do. First, you can use a *nonparametric* analytic method. Examples

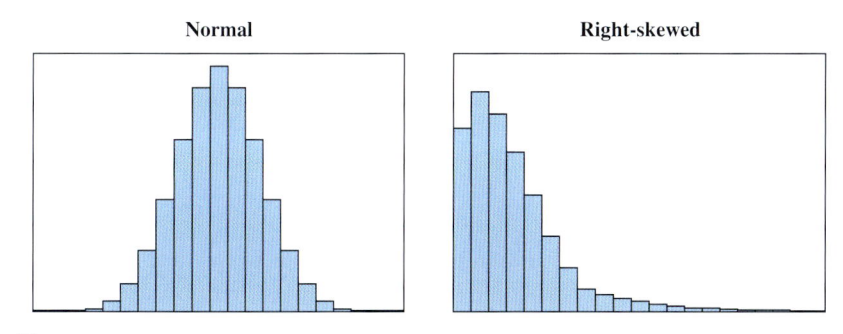

Figure 13-5 • Normal and right-skewed distributions. In healthcare, many common targets of analysis (such as length of stay and costs of care) are almost always right-skewed, which has important implications for the kinds of statistical tests that are appropriate.

of these tests include the Wilcoxon rank-sum test or the Mann-Whitney U test. These kinds of tests don't require a normality assumption, though they lose a bit of power. Second, you can sometimes make the data close enough to normal with a transformation. A common approach to this is to take the log of the data, and then do your analyses on the log-transformed data. If your data are from the log-normal distribution (which is reasonably common), they will be transformed into the normal distribution. Third, if you have a large-enough sample, then tests like the *t test* will be robust to data that are not normally distributed. (This is because of something called the *central limit theorem,* and it seems to work when you have several dozen observations or more.)

Categorical Data

Categorical data are data that are naturally divided into groups, rather than representing a continuum of values. Race, ethnicity, sex, diagnoses (e.g., "CHF versus not CHF"), and many outcomes (including mortality) are all types of *categorical data.* Other types of data that, on first glance, may appear to be continuous turn out to be categorical. The survey data example (from a Likert scale) discussed previously is one common example. Another has to do with counts—for example, you might use a patient's number of hospitalizations in the prior year as a predictor variable. This will have values like 0, 1, 2, and so on (and actually comes from an important distribution called a *Poisson distribution*).

Binary Data
One of the most important kinds of data you will deal with are binary data. Did a patient live, or die? Were they readmitted, or not? Did they develop cancer, or remain cancer-free? These are all *binary data,* which often represent the absence of an outcome as a 0, and its presence as a 1. The binomial distribution has some interesting properties: if you know the number of positive cases, then you also know the distribution's mean and its variance. Binary data are analyzed using tools like the chi-square or Fisher exact (for unadjusted analyses) and logistic regression (for multivariable analyses). These tools are discussed in Chapters 14 and 16.

Multicategory Data
Many kinds of data are multicategory: race, state of birth, and number of siblings are all multicategory because they have many more possible values than 0 and 1. In addition, there are many times when you will categorize (or discretize) a continuous variable. One of the most common ways that this comes up is when you find that a continuous predictor is not linearly related to the outcome you're interested in.

CHAPTER 13 | ANALYTIC TECHNIQUES AND COMMON PITFALLS

An example may be helpful here. It turns out that the shock index (systolic blood pressure divided by heart rate) has a U-shaped relationship with mortality in trauma patients. That is, a low shock index is associated with higher mortality, as is a high shock index ... but values in the middle have lower mortality rates.[16] Many types of analyses require a *monotonic* relationship between predictor and outcome: that is, they can't deal with the relationship changing directionality (Figure 13-6). Even when there is a monotonic relationship, one of the assumptions of logistic regression (see Chapter 16) is that there is a linear relationship between the predictor and the beta coefficient (the log of the odds of the outcome), which often doesn't exist. People often deal with this by breaking the continuous predictor into a set of discrete, categorical values—and you will see this quite often in reported studies. Even though there are more sophisticated ways of handling this issue that maintain better statistical power, discretizing continuous predictors is common and perhaps has benefits of improved interpretability.

Data that are categorical sometimes have no directional relationship between the categories. Eye color might be an example of that kind of data. Sometimes, however, there is a defined, ordinal relationship. For example, when you discretize a continuous variable, as described previously, there is an inherent order between the categories. Similarly, survey response items may have an inherent order. When data have this property, they are called *ordinal categorical* data. The reason for knowing this distinction is that there are some modeling techniques that specifically take advantage of this order.

A Few Other Points About the Shape of Your Data

There are a few other very common assumptions of analytic methods that you'll use. It's important to be able to tell whether your data meet these assumptions or not.

Linear? Monotonic? What Does all that Mean, Anyway?

Many methods make a fundamental, core assumption that your data are *monotonic* ... and they may go further, assuming that they are *linear*. Figure 13-6 shows what these terms mean graphically. To be a bit more precise, both of these terms refer to the relationship between two variables (although the concepts could extend to more dimensions). *Monotonic* means that the direction of change is always in the same direction. For example, if age is on your *x*-axis, and blood pressure is on the *y*-axis, the scatterplot between them always move up or down (not both!) as you move left to right across the *x*-axis. *Linear* is a subtype of *monotonic;* it means that as you move by equal amounts on the *x*-axis, the change on

Linear and Monotonic   **Monotonic but not Linear**   **Neither Monotonic nor Linear**

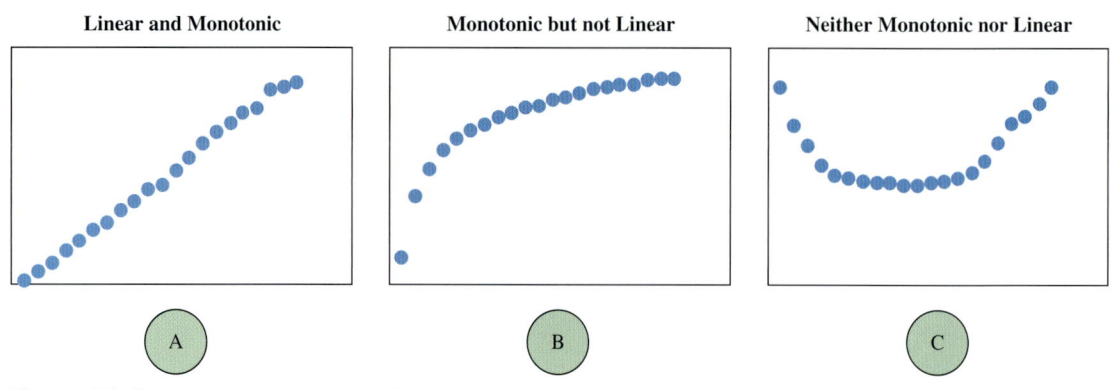

A   B   C

Figure 13-6 • Identifying data that are linear, monotonic, both, or neither.

the *y*-axis is constant every time. For example, if systolic blood pressure is 120 at age 50, 130 at age 55, and 140 at age 60, the relationship is linear (with a slope of a 2-mmHg increase per year).

How important is this? Really, really important. Let's use Figure 13-6 for an example. Let's imagine that we will use linear regression to model the relationship between whatever variables are on our *x*- and *y*-axes. A common measure of the goodness of fit of linear regression is R^2, which tells you how much of the variance in what's on your *y*-axis is accounted for by the variable on the *x*-axis. (A value of 0.0 is perfectly random, and 1.0 is perfectly correlated.) A linear regression on Figure 13-6A has an R^2 of 0.99. When looking at Figure 13-6B, it is obvious to your eye that these data aren't a straight line—and you also see that with a linear regression, which has an R^2 of 0.75. A slightly more sophisticated model (which doesn't make the linear assumption) has an R^2 of 0.99. (That specific model assumes a log-linear relationship, which is what these data are.) Figure 13-6C is interesting because the data change *direction*—that is, they aren't monotonic. There's a visually obvious pattern, but your eye tells you that it's also obviously not a linear pattern. This is borne out in the linear regression, where $R^2 = 0.06$. Only 6% of the variance is captured in this model—if you ran this analysis, you would just conclude that there's no pattern! A slightly more sophisticated model (which again doesn't assume linearity) has an $R^2 = 0.96$ … clearly documenting the relationship that's obvious to your eyes, but invisible to linear regression.

You often see this particular failing when people present slides of data in operational meetings. With modern spreadsheets, it is really easy to fit a linear trend line to the data. But always look at this skeptically. Are the data really linear? If they aren't, be skeptical of any conclusions that are getting drawn from them.

Key Point

Many methods assume that data are *linear* and *monotonic*. When your data don't fulfill these assumptions, avoid those kinds of methods.

CHAPTER 13 | ANALYTIC TECHNIQUES AND COMMON PITFALLS

Are Your Data Made Up of Independent Observations, or Are They Clustered?

Most simple statistical tests (e.g., *t tests*) assume that every observation in your data set is independent of every other one. Similarly, many fairly sophisticated analytic tools (e.g., logistic regression) make this same assumption. What does "independent" mean? It means that the value of a variable in one patient doesn't influence the value in another. The opposite of this is *clustered*.[1] For example, if you randomly selected patients and measured their creatinine levels, one person's creatinine value is unlikely to influence another patient's. This can be a reasonable assumption to make—but you have to be careful because it is often false. For example, if you randomly selected households but interviewed everyone in a household, those data would be said to be "clustered within households." Similarly, in routine data, patients are usually clustered within doctors, and doctors within hospitals. Another kind of clustering can happen over time (here, it is called *autocorrelation*): For example, the most important predictor of the hospital census on Wednesday is probably the hospital census on Tuesday. Finally, issues like crowding can cause correlation of risks between patients. For example, patients are more likely to be discharged from the ICU when it is full, independent of the severity of their own condition.[17,18]

Why is this important? It matters because there are specific kinds of analyses that can handle clustering correctly (see Chapter 16). Failing to use these methods can sometimes result in getting the wrong answer. This is usually less important when you care only about the point estimate of a relationship, but it can be extremely important if you're trying to compare between providers, hospitals, and other areas of healthcare. This is commonly done in quality measures, where these methods can be quite important.

Key Point

Many methods assume that every observation in your data set is *independent* of each other. When this isn't true, data are *clustered* and you need to use more sophisticated methods.

OVERVIEW OF ANALYTIC METHODS

Much of the rest of the book provides a deeper dive into important analytic methods. We provide an overview here to help you navigate the following chapters.

---

[1] Here, *clustering* means that values tend to be more like each other across patients than you would find if they were randomly distributed. When you make a model or prediction, it means that the variances and error terms are correlated, and that you need special handling for them. In machine learning, *clustering* means something different; it is a form of unsupervised learning that is intended to find structure and patterns in data. Same word, different meaning.

Chapter 14, "Everyday Analytics"

This chapter covers types of analytics that are easy to implement, even if they are somewhat more sophisticated than those used in many healthcare operations today. Topics include run charts, univariable tests and when to use them, and statistical process control charts. This chapter will also include core principles and pitfalls of visual display of data, as well as examples when poor visual choices obscure important messages.

Chapter 15, "Survey-Based Data: Pitfalls and Promises"

Surveys sometimes seem like simple, straightforward tools to get a handle on a problem. But it turns out to be remarkably easy to get it wrong when you use them. This chapter will help you avoid these common pitfalls by introducing principles of surveys, survey administration, and analysis of survey results.

Chapter 16, "Predictive Modeling 1.0 and 2.0"

This chapter will provide foundational tools that encompass most predictive modeling done today, such as linear and logistic regression. This second section will review approaches to predictive modeling that handle limitations of the 1.0 methods, such as what to do when the data are clustered. Tools such as generalized estimating equations and hierarchical linear models are needed to deal with common situations in healthcare (such as patients being clustered on a hospital ward), and will be introduced here.

Chapter 17, "Predictive Modeling 3.0: Machine Learning"

This chapter introduces emerging techniques in healthcare predictive modeling that are generically termed *machine learning,* such as support vector machines and random forest models. It also reviews recent developments in neural networks with healthcare applications, including deep-learning models.

Chapter 18, "What Everyone Should Know About Risk Adjustment

Risk adjustment is commonly used in healthcare (e.g., by Medicare for pay-for-performance programs) but is less commonly understood. The math underlying risk adjustment and predictive modeling is essentially identical, so you are well positioned to apply the principles from the prior three chapters to practical issues of risk adjustment and predictions. This

CHAPTER 13 | ANALYTIC TECHNIQUES AND COMMON PITFALLS

chapter will introduce how to compare the accuracy of risk-adjustment and predictive models (e.g., area under the receiver operating characteristics curve).

Chapter 19, "Modeling Patient Flow: Understanding Throughput and Census"

This chapter introduces three key concepts from the discipline of operations research/operations management: Little's Law, queuing theory, and discrete event simulation. These are effective tools for making decisions under conditions of significant uncertainty in complex systems like healthcare.

Chapter 20, "Program Evaluation: How to Tell If Something Worked in the Real World"

This chapter provides tools for sophisticated evaluations of whether a program produced a change in patient (or system) outcomes. These tools build off of Chapter 14 (run charts, statistical process control) and include interrupted time-series techniques (perhaps the single most important method in healthcare delivery science) and their extensions. The chapter will also review methods recently imported into healthcare from economics, including instrumental variable approaches, regression discontinuity, and causal modeling.

KEY POINTS

- Chance, bias, and confounding are the three classic threats to the validity of your analyses.
- Violating the inherent assumptions of your analytic method is another threat. All statistical methods make assumptions. You need to know what these assumptions are, and make sure that your data fulfill them.
- Bias can be a lethal problem for your analyses because it may be impossible to correct bias in the data using statistical techniques. In this context, *bias* refers to the collection or analysis of data in a way that systematically differs from the truth.
- Missing data can introduce a bias that is particularly difficult to deal with, especially if the data are not missing completely at random.
- Many common analytic methods assume that data are linear and monotonic. When your data don't meet these assumptions, avoid those kinds of methods.

REFERENCES

1. Svoboda E. The paleontology of footprints. *Discover*. December 2005. Accessed November 29, 2018, from http://discovermagazine.com/2005/dec/paleontology-dinosaur-footprints.
2. A Tale of Tail Traces. *National Geographic*. September 4, 2013. Accessed November 29, 2018, from https://www.nationalgeographic.com/science/phenomena/2013/09/04/a-tale-of-tail-traces/.
3. Howell MD, Stevens JP. ICUs after surgery, mortality, and the Will Rogers effect. *Intensive Care Med*. 2015;41(11):1990–1992.
4. Dinan MA, Curtis LH, Carpenter WR, et al. Stage migration, selection bias, and survival associated with the adoption of positron emission tomography among Medicare beneficiaries with non-small-cell lung cancer, 1998–2003. *J Clin Oncol*. 2012;30(22):2725–2730.
5. Iezzoni LI, Foley SM, Daley J, Hughes J, Fisher ES, Heeren T. Comorbidities, complications, and coding bias. Does the number of diagnosis codes matter in predicting in-hospital mortality? *JAMA*. 1992;267(16):2197–2203.
6. Li L, Rothwell PM, Oxford Vascular S. Biases in detection of apparent "weekend effect" on outcome with administrative coding data: population based study of stroke. *BMJ*. 2016;353:i2648.
7. Bilimoria KY, Chung J, Ju MH, et al. Evaluation of surveillance bias and the validity of the venous thromboembolism quality measure. *JAMA*. 2013;310(14):1482–1489.
8. Centers for Disease Control and Prevention (CDC). *Cumulative Percent Distribution of Population by Height and Sex: 2007 to 2008*. 2011. Accessed November 29, 2018, from https://www2.census.gov/library/publications/2010/compendia/statab/130ed/tables/11s0205.pdf.
9. Kyriacou DN, Lewis RJ. Confounding by indication in clinical research. *JAMA*. 2016;316(17):1818–1819.
10. Herzig SJ, Vaughn BP, Howell MD, Ngo LH, Marcantonio ER. Acid-suppressive medication use and the risk for nosocomial gastrointestinal tract bleeding. *Arch Intern Med*. 2011;171(11):991–997.
11. Newgard CD, Lewis RJ. Missing data: how to best account for what is not known. *JAMA*. 2015;314(9):940–941.
12. Wood AM, White IR, Thompson SG. Are missing outcome data adequately handled? A review of published randomized controlled trials in major medical journals. *Clin Trials*. 2004;1(4):368–376.
13. Burton A, Altman DG. Missing covariate data within cancer prognostic studies: a review of current reporting and proposed guidelines. *Br J Cancer*. 2004;91(1):4–8.
14. Altman DG, Bland JM. Missing data. *BMJ*. 2007;334(7590):424.
15. Sterne JA, White IR, Carlin JB, et al. Multiple imputation for missing data in epidemiological and clinical research: potential and pitfalls. *BMJ*. 2009;338:b2393.

16. Odom SR, Howell MD, Gupta A, Silva G, Cook CH, Talmor D. Extremes of shock index predicts death in trauma patients. *J Emerg Trauma Shock*. 2016;9(3): 103–106.
17. Profit J, McCormick MC, Escobar GJ, et al. Neonatal intensive care unit census influences discharge of moderately preterm infants. *Pediatrics*. 2007;119(2):314–319.
18. Strauss MJ, LoGerfo JP, Yeltatzie JA, Temkin N, Hudson LD. Rationing of intensive care unit services. An everyday occurrence. *JAMA*. 1986;255(9):1143–1146.

14 EVERYDAY ANALYTICS

Make sure to read this chapter carefully: The tools presented here are the basic building blocks for all of our future work in this book. We will cover how to describe data, how to begin to compare data, how to look at data over time, and some fundamental principles of the display of data. Each of these steps are the first steps toward more complex data analytics presented in subsequent chapters. Every time we move from a single piece of data to some method of summarizing a collection of data, we make assumptions. If our assumptions are wrong, the truth may be lost in the noise. Even worse, if we make inappropriate assumptions at this level, in our building-block summary statistics and preliminary comparisons, these errors will get compounded when we begin to employ the kind of larger and more complex models described in the later chapters of this part of the book.

The first step in any analysis is to look at the data. This cannot be emphasized enough. You need to plot the data, and look at them. Look at the raw data. Examine your data, before you do any more-sophisticated analysis. Looking at the data will shine a light on *outliers,* defined as values in the data that are very different and more extreme than others. Sometimes outliers are real, like a length of stay of 220 days or a systolic blood pressure of 60 mmHg. Sometimes outliers are errors in recording, like a true length of stay of 22 days (but recorded as 220 days) or a systolic blood pressure of 160 mmHg (but recorded as 60 mmHg). Looking at the data themselves and understanding in detail how they were collected, as discussed in Chapter 12, can help us understand what might lead to the data we see. Do we need to correct the data or change our assumptions?

Perhaps more important is that the findings in our data—the truth in what lies in the numbers—are rarely discovered just with more advanced analytics. Rather, more advanced analytics usually help confirm the findings of simpler analyses. In the previous chapter, we discussed *confounding,* the concept that a third variable has a relationship with both our exposure and our outcome. When we account for confounding in our analyses, most often our findings become attenuated. For example, if we

Key Point

Look at your data, with your own eyes and in their rawest form. It is tempting to skip this step, but don't. You'll catch many problems that get obscured by later analyses.

CHAPTER 14 | EVERYDAY ANALYTICS

are interested in the effect of gender on the risk of ischemic heart disease, we must make sure to take age into consideration. But even before we do that, if there really is a difference between men and women, our comparison of rates of ischemic heart disease between the two groups make this clear. The truth should already start to emerge when we make even the most straightforward of comparisons. Look carefully at your data when you begin your analytics. Your answers will usually already be there.

Key Point

The truth is already in your data. You usually don't need advanced analytics to find it.

In this chapter, we will start with how to summarize your data, including means, medians, and ranges. These are essential to giving us words to describe large amounts of data all at once. We will then move into how to display data and how to turn our data into a story. In particular, we will highlight run charts. We will then move to concepts that let us describe changes in summary statistics between two exposures, which let us take our first steps toward tests of association. We will conclude with statistical process control charts (putting the foundation of our run charts and our tests of difference together!) to look at the role of time and variation on our healthcare interventions.

SUMMARIZING YOUR DATA

All summary measures should contain two pieces of information: *central tendency* and *spread*. In Figure 14-1, the two lines both have the same measures of central tendency (mean, in this case Box 14-1), but very different

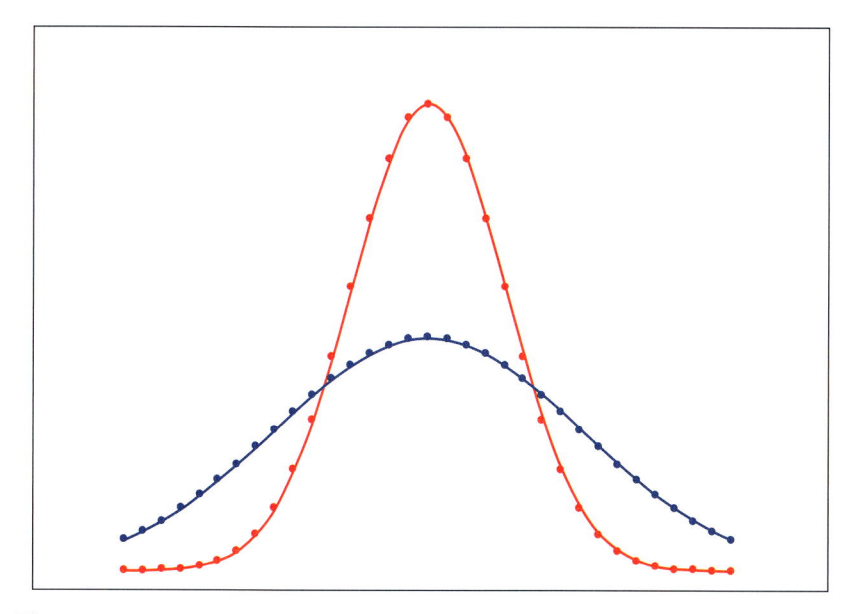

Figure 14-1 • Two series of data with the same mean, but different SDs, both normally distributed.

distributions of data. Occasionally, even this information isn't sufficient, as it fails to communicate that the distribution of some data (like length of stay) is not equally weighted on either side of the measure of central tendency, or skewed. We will review how to calculate these measures and a few land mines to consider. These summary measures will then allow us to compare information, understand whether we've made a significant change, and look at that information over time.

We will present a case at the end of the chapter which can be used as a worked example to move through these methods of describing data, and can then be used in the next section to present data. In this case, Maria, the chief medical officer at the Arbitrary Regional General Hospital (ARGH), is interested in measuring and improving staff satisfaction. Feel free to work through these concepts with her data.

Mean

The *mean*, or average, is the most common method of reporting central tendency. The mean is the sum (Σ) of all values x divided by the total number of values (n). Frequently, the value is described with a bar over the sample ($\bar{x}$). The equation is then written as

$$\bar{x} = \frac{\Sigma x}{n}$$

with the units of the answer being the same as the units of each of the individual values. Most of the time, we will communicate our results in terms of means. The major land mine to the mean is that it can be changed substantially by a small number of outlying values. As an example, assume that we are interested in reducing the average length of stay of patients after an intervention. Prior to our intervention, five patients have lengths of stay of 5, 4, 6, 5, and 4 days, respectively, for a mean length of stay of 4.8 days ($\bar{x} = (5 + 4 + 6 + 5 + 4) / 5 = 4.8$ days). After our intervention, five new patients stay 3, 3, 4, 4, and 12 days, for an average of 5.2 days. The long-length-of-stay patient, who stayed 12 days, makes the mean in the post-intervention period greater than the pre-intervention period, making any conclusions about the benefit of our intervention hard to understand or rely on.

Median

The *median*, or the middle of the data at the 50th-percentile mark, gets around this issue of outliers. The median of the pre-intervention period in the example given here is 5 days, and in the post-intervention period, it is 4 days; as we can see, because the median is the middle value, the patient

Pre-intervention	Post-intervention
4	3
4	3
5 ← median	4 ← median
5	4
6 days	12 days

with a 12-day length of stay has no influence on it. In an odd number of samples, as we have here, the median is the middle one.

In the case of an even number of values, the median becomes the average of the two middle values. For example, if we made six measurements of length of stay, we would take the average of the third and fourth values when the data are in ascending or descending order. While not at risk of outliers, the median provides us with no information about the spread of the data itself. We can know that when the mean and median are different, the distribution of data on either side of the mean is not symmetric and the data may be skewed. When the median > mean, the tail of the data lies in the lower values (termed *left-skewed*) and when the median < mean (as in this example), the tail of the data lies in the upper values (termed *right-skewed*). Means, rather than medians, are used more often in the univariable tests of difference that we will discuss later in this chapter.

Mode

The third and least-used measure of central tendency is the *mode*, defined as the most frequent value seen in the data. In small populations, like our length-of-stay values, the mode is often unhelpful, with the repeated values offering little insight as to the distribution of the data. Further, none of our statistical comparisons will use the mode. But examining the mode may provide further insights into how your larger data sets are skewed, particularly in the context of the means and medians, and is an element of the diagnostics of any set of data that you will want to perform to understand the inherent patterns.

Range

The *range*, which consists of the maximum and minimum values of your data set, is also helpful as you start to understand the patterns in your data. By understanding the span of values, you will begin to understand the variability of your data. Further, you will see if there are any outlying values that are likely incorrect (e.g., a systolic blood pressure of 1560 mmHg rather than 156.0 mmHg). The range of values, however, does not provide you with information about how those data are distributed.

While the full range encompasses all of the available data, the *interquartile range* begins to help a reader discern what the full range actually looks like. Interquartile range is based around the median and includes the quarter of the data below (Q2) and the quarter of data above (Q3) the median. Put another way, the interquartile range is the 25th–75th percentile.

Standard Deviation (SD) and Standard Error

The standard deviation (SD) calculates the spread of our data in our sample around the mean and uses a value called the *variance*. To calculate the variance, we first find the distance of each value of x from the mean $\bar{x}$. The sum of the squares of each of these distances (to eliminate the signs on each variance figure) divided by $n-1$ equals the variance, and the square root of the variance is the standard deviation. We can see that in Figure 14-1, while the mean was the same (centered at 0), the standard deviation was different (red, SD = 1; blue, SD = 2). When median = mean, the distribution is roughly symmetric above and below the mean. The normal distribution is the most common type of distribution with this property. In a normal distribution, 68% of values will fall within 1 standard deviation and 95% of values will fall within 2 standard deviations of the mean.

The standard error is often confused with the standard deviation. The standard deviation is a measure of the distribution of the data within the sample population, which makes it another tool to describe the study population. The standard error, however, is a measure of how precise our sample mean is to our population mean. The standard deviation tells us what the data look like around our mean. The standard error tells us how confident we can be that mean we calculated is close to the mean in the population. It is calculated as the $SD/\sqrt{n}$ where n is the sample size. When the sample, n, is very small, the standard error becomes large, suggesting that we cannot say very precisely that our sample mean is the same as the population. We will see in Chapter 16 that if we take multiple samples from a single person (e.g., multiple lab draws from the same patient), we could increase n falsely and make the standard error smaller than it is, thereby making our estimated mean look more precise than it is. We will discuss methods of dealing with

Caution

If repeated measures are not accommodated in the analysis, the standard error will be wrong, and it probably will tell you that you have a significant finding when you don't.

values that are clustered in our study population subsequently, but the definition of the standard error highlights the importance of using research methods correctly to draw conclusions about healthcare delivery. Repeated measures from the same patient that aren't accounted for in the analysis will distort the standard error.

DISPLAYING DATA

Now that we have some tools to describe our data, how can we think about how to turn those data into our story? What have we learned and how can we share that in the most clear, effective, and intentional way possible?

When we move to communicating our findings using graphical representations of data or developing easy-to-read tables, we should consider the creation of each graph a paragraph. The move by news organizations like *The New York Times* to have entire divisions of graphical reporters highlights the critical value of displaying your data well. Tell a visually compelling story, and you've not only conveyed your research message, but you have won the respect of your listeners. Toward the end of this section, we will establish a number of first principles in the visual display of data. Return to these when the temptation is great to stray into lazy displays. Keep in mind that there are multiple available tools available that will let you run statistics and then to create more compelling data displays, including some that even use movement to move beyond two-dimensional constraints. However, even classical, horizontal graphs can convey substantial amounts of information if they are created with care—we will see the power of one of these with a run chart in our next section.

Methods of Data Presentation

Data can be presented either in table form or graphically. The table form can be distinctly powerful, despite the dry appearance of a series of numbers. One choice for table presentation is a frequency distribution, which describes as how many of the population fit into each category. Alternatively, you may display your data using relative frequencies, which gives the proportion of the population in each category. The same set of data is displayed in Tables 14-1A and 14-1B.

Graphs also come in multiple forms. Several common examples, including the bar graph and the line graph, are outlined in Table 14-2, each with examples and using the same data presented in Tables 14-1A and 14-1B. Again, the types of data and the message of interest should determine the way that those data are presented to the reader.

Table 14-1A A FREQUENCY DISTRIBUTION OF HOSPITAL LENGTH OF STAY, BY GENDER

Length of Stay (days)	Number of Women	Number of Men
1	8	7
2	6	4
3	3	3
4	5	9
5	5	4
6	5	2
7	2	2
8	1	1
9	3	1
10	2	0
11	3	1
12	1	0
13	1	0
14	2	0
17	1	0
18	2	1
19	4	0
20	3	0
21	1	0
22	2	0
23	2	0
24	0	1

Tufte's Principles of Graphical Excellence

Displaying data well is one of the hardest things we can do as data scientists, but it is also one of the most powerful tools available. One influential writer, artist, and statistician in data display is Edward Tufte, a cutting critic of the dominance of computer slide software over presentations, and a careful thinker about the central principles of graphical representation of

Table 14-1B	A RELATIVE FREQUENCY DISTRIBUTION OF HOSPITAL LENGTH OF STAY, BY GENDER	
Length of Stay (days)	Women (%)	Men (%)
1	12.9	19.4
2	9.7	11.1
3	4.8	8.3
4	8.1	25.0
5	8.1	11.1
6	8.1	5.6
7	3.2	5.6
8	1.6	2.8
9	4.8	2.8
10	3.2	0.0
11	4.8	2.8
12	1.6	0.0
13	1.6	0.0
14	3.2	0.0
17	1.6	0.0
18	3.2	2.8
19	6.5	0.0
20	4.8	0.0
21	1.6	0.0
22	3.2	0.0
23	3.2	0.0
24	0.0	2.8

data.[4] Central to all of his thoughts about data presentation is this: We must fundamentally respect the intellect of the reader. To support his position, Tufte cites E. B. White's statement that "no one can write decently who is distrustful of the reader's intelligence, or whose attitude is patronizing."[1] This includes Tufte's recommendations to present complex ideas (and

Table 14-2 TYPES OF AVAILABLE CHARTS, ALL USING THE DATA IN TABLES 14-1A AND 14-1B

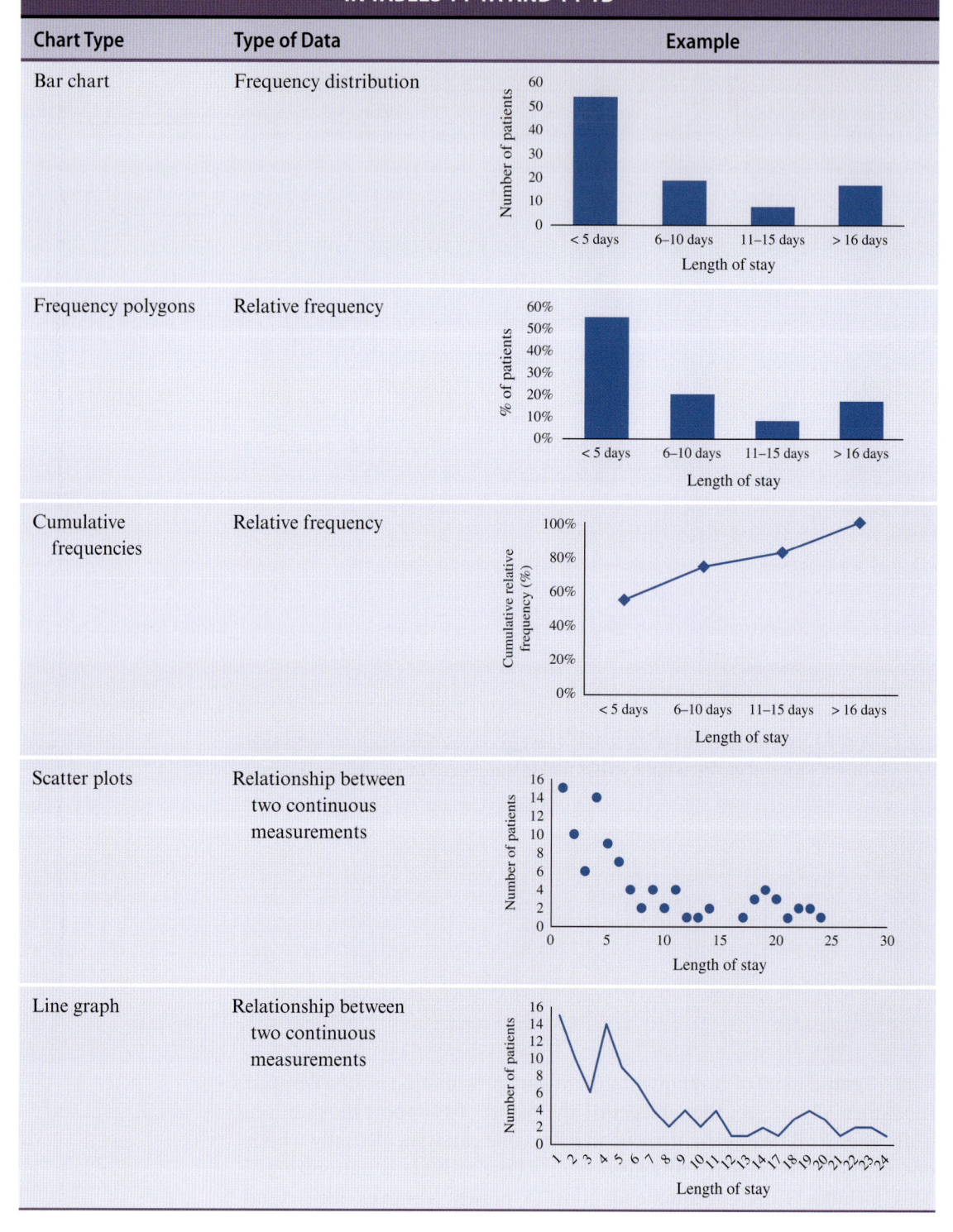

Chart Type	Type of Data	Example
Bar chart	Frequency distribution	Bar chart of Number of patients (0–60) vs Length of stay (< 5 days, 6–10 days, 11–15 days, > 16 days)
Frequency polygons	Relative frequency	Bar chart of % of patients (0%–60%) vs Length of stay (< 5 days, 6–10 days, 11–15 days, > 16 days)
Cumulative frequencies	Relative frequency	Line chart of Cumulative relative frequency (%) (0%–100%) vs Length of stay (< 5 days, 6–10 days, 11–15 days, > 16 days)
Scatter plots	Relationship between two continuous measurements	Scatter plot of Number of patients (0–16) vs Length of stay (0–30)
Line graph	Relationship between two continuous measurements	Line graph of Number of patients (0–16) vs Length of stay (1–24)

respect a reader's ability to comprehend them), to read and integrate multiple layers of data into a single display, and to move away from graphics as substitutes for small tables.[2]

Tufte defines the following Principles of Graphical Excellence:

Graphical excellence is the well-designed presentation of interesting data—a matter of substance, of statistics, and of design.

Graphic excellence consists of complex ideas communicated with clarity, precision, and efficiency.

Graphical excellence is that which gives to the viewer the greatest number of ideas in the shortest time with the least ink in the smallest space.

Graphical excellence is nearly always multivariate.

And graphical excellence requires telling the truth about data.[2]

These central principles should guide all the efforts that we do to communicate our work clearly to readers: high-quality data that does not obfuscate the truth, presented carefully without excess information or annotation and that integrates multiple variables.

Four Common Mistakes in Displaying Data

Tufte coined the term *chartjunk* to identify unhelpful, simplistic, and unintentionally (or intentionally) confusing statistical graphics. Relying again on Tufte's work, we put forward several examples of common mistakes to avoid.

1. **Avoid illustrations that trigger a *Moire effect*, the effect of one's eye signaling movement when none exists due to autocorrelation.** Several examples of the Moire effect in simplified graphs are given in Figure 14-2. Figure 14-2A uses the contrast between dark and light with too small of a gap between bars, making the resulting graph difficult to look at. The pattern in Figure 14-2B causes the same effect.
2. **Use three-dimensional graphics sparingly.** Most of the time, they serve only to obscure data and make identifying clear messages from that data unnecessarily complex. In the example in Figure 14-3, consider a graph of three hospital floors interested in the average number of admissions per day in each month. While the data are all present, the information behind the first set of bars is lost. Even worse, the three-dimensional element of the graph is unnecessarily complex and distracting, with the depth itself adding no information.
3. **Never use pie charts.** Pie charts are rarely used correctly, which is to say the proportions are frequently off, they often sum to greater than 100%, they cannot convey more than a single variable clearly, and

> **External Resource**
> Seek out the collection of books by Edward Tufte for multiple beautiful examples of displays of data. His work is available at his own website: https://www.edwardtufte.com/tufte/

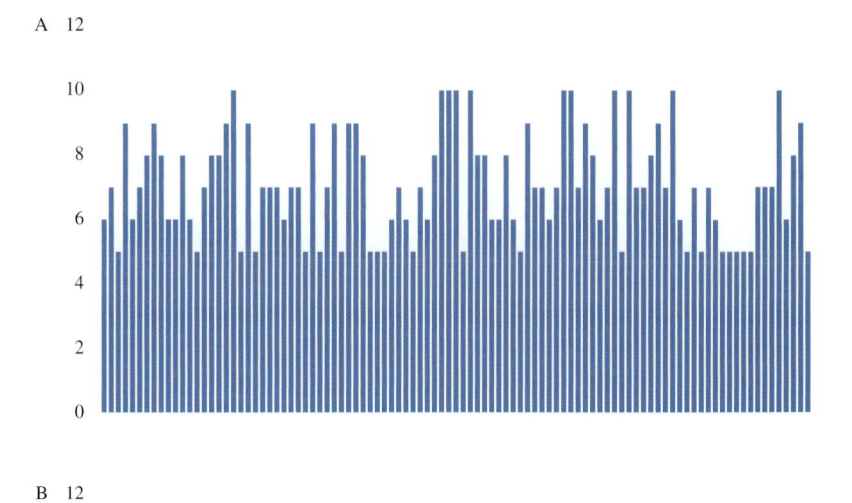

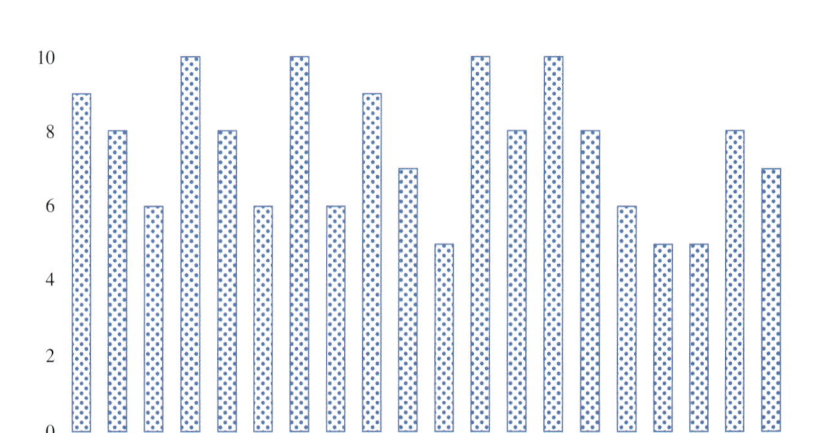

Figure 14-2 • Two examples of bad graphs that fail the Tufte test due to disconcerting Moire effects. A. A bad graph with Moire effects. B. A bad example of a bar graph.

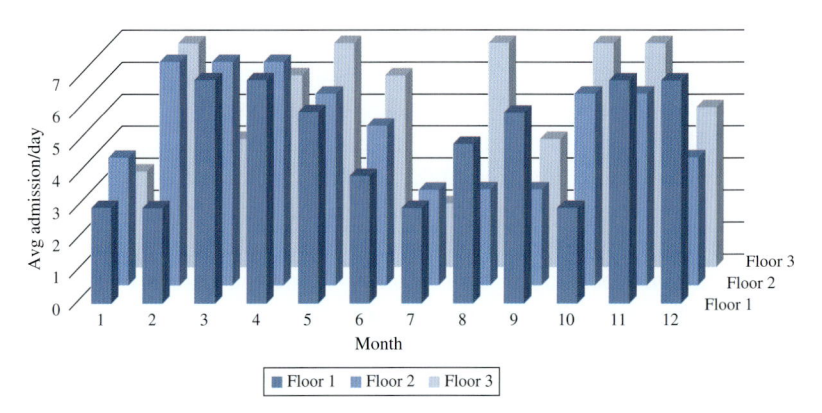

Figure 14-3 • Another bad example of a way to display data: a three-dimensional graph of the average number of admissions per day, by month, across three hospital floors. Much of the data is not visible to the reader.

a substantial amount of data is often lost or unreadable when any proportion falls below 25%. That said, even when they are used correctly, they rely on our ability to discern subtle differences in angles, something that humans typically are not skilled at. Tufte writes simply, "Given their low data-density and failure to order numbers along a visual dimension, pie charts should never be used."[2]

4. **Don't waste space with annotations or other unnecessary information such as chart lines.** Background chart lines and annotations are frequently distracting from the graphic itself. Take the two examples in Figure 14-4; recognize where your eyes are drawn and which example is easier to read. Unless useful information is gained by

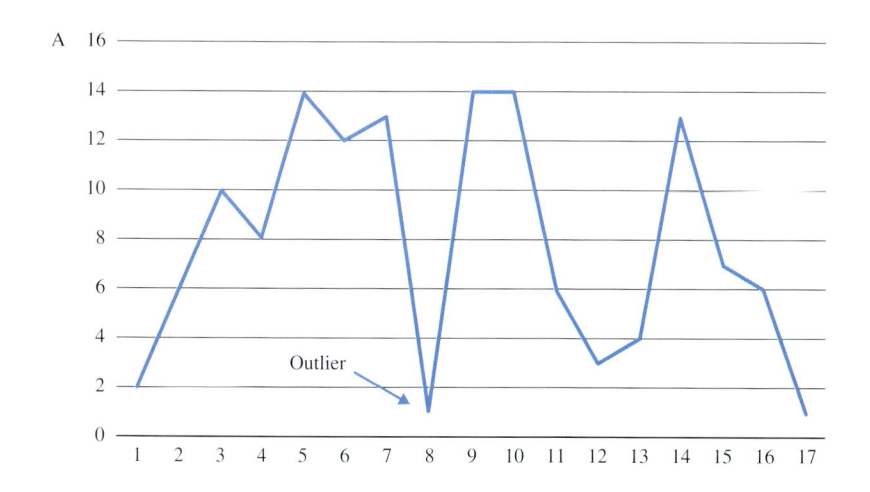

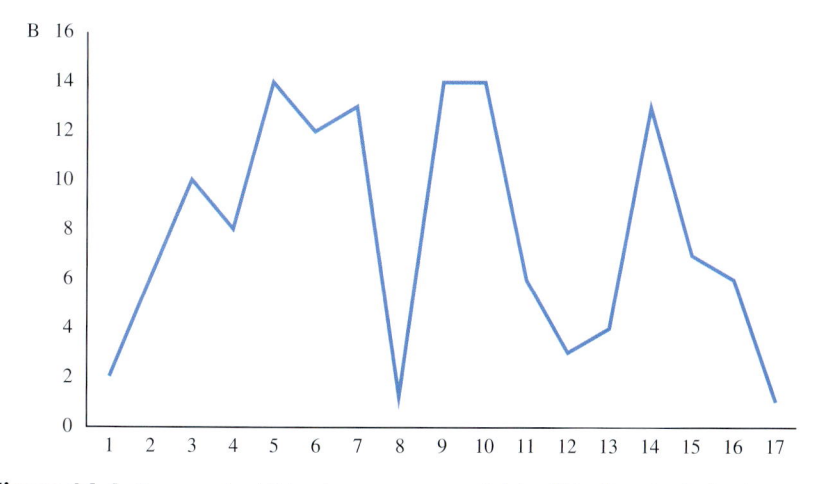

Figure 14-4 • Two graphs, (A) having unnecessary ink in all the lines in the background and labels, and (B) showing just the necessary information.

background chart lines, remove them. Similarly, text should be easy to read, not rotated or excessive; and it should be in a font and size that allows easy readability, without distraction.

OUTCOMES OVER TIME, PART I – RUN CHARTS

Next, let's take these tools we have learned to summarize data and present these over time. We will return to this concept at the end of the chapter with a more complex version of this, statistical process control charts, which will incorporate even more information. Run charts, though, are straightforward, clear, and informative ways to communicate our data, falling in line with our first principles above.

Run charts display data over a specific order (often time) and allow us to see all the data at once, while simultaneously preserving the relationship of the data to each other. Many statistical tests, like those described later in this chapter, aggregate the data at the expense of temporality.[3] Run charts get around this problem. They are particularly useful to answer the question of whether the change we want is actually happening and whether that change is likely to be sustained or is regressing back to a mean.

Run charts are simply designed. Figure 14-5 provides an example with sample data graphed around the median. As in this example, the *x*-axis should have accurately spaced time measurements; other examples could include individual patients. The *y*-axis shows the measure of study, such as rate of infections, percent compliance, and falls/patient-days. The

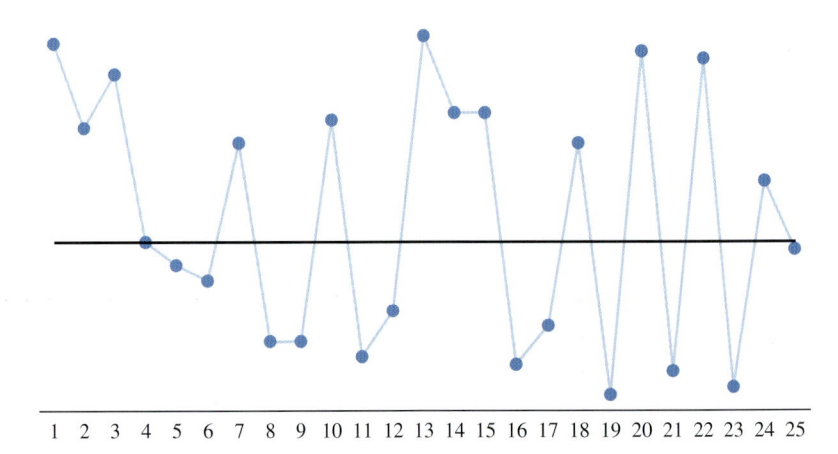

Figure 14-5 • A sample run chart. The data points and connecting lines represent plotted data. The solid line represents the sample median. The *x*-axis can be used for consecutive time periods or patients.

median is frequently included in order to orient the reader and limit the effect of outliers on the visual representation of the data. The chart can then be annotated to indicate the timing of various interventions.

Several terms indicate that a statistically meaningful change has taken place, as illustrated in Figure 14-6. First, a *shift* is when six or more consecutive data points fall on one side of the median. Second, a *trend* refers to five more consecutive data points moving in the same upward or downward direction. Third, *runs* are the number of data points on one side of the median or the other. If data randomly fall on either side of a median line, then we would expect a statistically estimable number of runs based on the number of data points included in the chart. To count the number of runs, count the number of times the line between data points crosses the median and then add 1. Then reference a critical-value table to identify whether the number of runs exceeds the range expected for the size of the data, based on a *P* value of 0.05, which is a concept we will explain more in the next section. Finally, an *astronomical point* is a value that subjectively appears well outside the range of all other data.[3]

Run charts are meant to identify early changes in data. Their rules for significance fall apart when there are ceiling or floor effects in the data (i.e., when much of the data sit at the minimum or maximum of the range). Understanding when the processes for delivering care are in or out of control relies on the topics that will be discussed with statistical process control (SPC) charts toward the end of the chapter. But first, we will now take our summary statistics and begin to compare them to each other. When is one mean about the same as another mean and when can

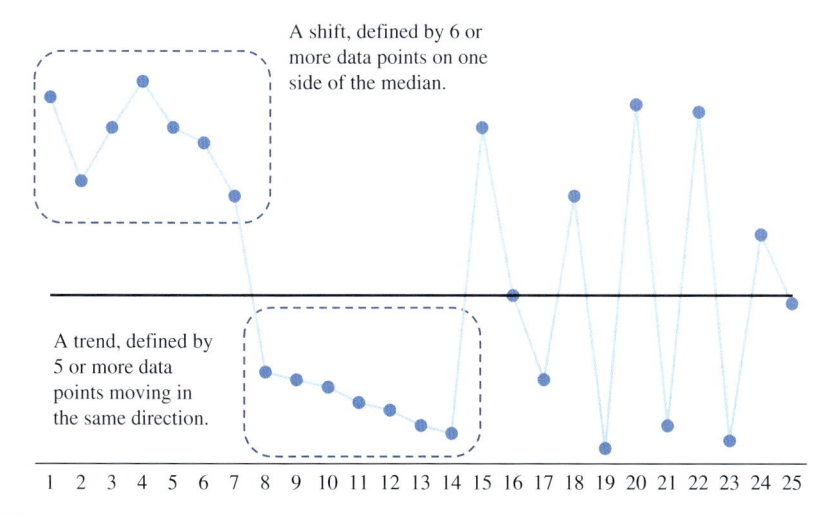

Figure 14-6 • A sample run chart with a shift and a trend illustrated.

we say with some confidence that they are different? When can we start to infer that, with a healthcare delivery intervention, we have identified some subsequent meaningful change in an outcome we care about? When have we made a difference?

HOW TO TELL IF TWO GROUPS ARE DIFFERENT: UNIVARIABLE TESTS OF DIFFERENCE AND MEASURES OF COMPARISON

Now that we are more conversant in summative measures of data, we can begin to compare measures. Fundamentally, we want to be able to ask if summative values are meaningfully different from one another. With the intervention introduced earlier in this chapter to change the length of stay of our patients, it is worth asking: Is an average length of stay of 4.8 days actually different from a length of stay of 5.2 days? Would our hospital care about that degree of difference? This returns to the challenges that underlie the work of healthcare delivery science: How do we know that we've made a meaningful change every time we work to improve care? How do we know that the results we find are not due simply to chance?

The most important test of difference is not a statistical test. Instead, it is to find what amount of change actually matters. Would it matter to a hospital to change the length of stay in the intensive care unit (ICU) by 8 hours, from 5 days to 4.7 days? It might when we averaged those 8 hours over all the beds of an ICU over a year. If our ICU has 10 beds, Little's law tells us that we could care for 1 patient more per week (more about this in Chapter 19).[4] We first have to ask ourselves what amount of change matters before we apply any test of statistical significance.

The *P* Value: Simple or Oversimplified?

Many tests of significance rely on a *P* value. Let's take our example from above. We've implemented our intervention in the ICU and reduced our length of stay from 5 days (pre-intervention) to 4.7 days (post-intervention). We perform a test of difference (more on how to do this below) and the result is a *P* value of 0.05. What does this mean? If we can assume that there is actually a relationship or association between the exposure we are testing and the outcome of interest, our intervention and our change in our length of stay, the *P* value tells us the probability of seeing our results, or a more extreme difference, due to chance alone.[5] A *P* value does **not** tell you there is a 5% chance that your answer is "wrong" (or put in statistical terms, it is not a measure of the likelihood that the null hypothesis is false)—a common misinterpretation of the probability.[6]

A small *P* value helps you minimize the chance of concluding there is a true association – when in fact one doesn't exist. This is also called a *Type I error*. But, as sample sizes get larger, *P* values get smaller—because the larger your sample size, the less likely you are seeing things by chance alone. As a result, very large studies may have very small absolute findings that are still mathematically unlikely to be due to chance alone. But the results may be too small to matter clinically.

Put another way, the size of the study determines our likelihood of making a *Type II error*, or the risk of assuming there is not a difference when there is (by convention, this probability is designated as β). In most medical and health journals and studies, we use a 1 in 20 probability of $P < 0.05$ as a cutoff to determine what statistically matters to us; and the risk of a type II error is 0.20 (the "power" of a study becomes 1-β, or 80%). We also must decide if want to learn if our exposure could be helpful or harmful, in which case we are interested in a two-tailed test of difference (testing for findings at the two extreme ends of the normal distribution, both high and low). If we are only interested in one direction, if the exposure causes harm only, as an example, then we would use a one-tailed test and study findings only on one side of the distribution. We have to decide in advance which one we want and, most of the time, a two-tailed test makes sense to give you the most information about your data.

We want to call attention to the downsides of *P* values. It is common, and potentially treacherous, to become overreliant on *P* values to determine our cutoffs for statistical significance in the medical literature. Debate about how to consider this problem has created two primary camps of statistical positions: frequentists and Bayesians.

Bayesians use Bayes' theorem, derived over two centuries ago, to use new data to alter their prior assumptions about truth.[6] We utilize the Bayes theorem in medicine and healthcare all the time. As an example, when we meet a patient, we have a prior assumption, whether acknowledged or not, that the patient does or does not have a specific disease. When we do a laboratory or radiology test, the result of that test should change what we estimate to be the likelihood a patient has a disease. This means that you interpret the same test result differently, depending on your pretest probability of disease. Imagine you are seeing two patients whom you are evaluating for whether they have a pulmonary embolism (PE). In patient A, your clinical sense is that they are low probability for PE. In patient B, your sense is that they are high probability for PE. Because the CT scanner is down, you order a ventilation-perfusion (VQ) scan to assess for pulmonary embolism in both. You get back a "low probability" result for both patients (VQ scans are reported as normal, low probability, intermediate probability, or high probability). Even though the test results are

Caution

P values tell you about statistical significance, but nothing else. They do not tell you about the magnitude of the difference, or how confident you can be in your result.

Key Point

Conventionally, the most common statistical thresholds used in the medical literature for statistical significance are a *p* value of 0.05 (alpha=0.05) and a power of 80% (beta=0.2). While these are arbitrary cut-points with many problems, it is worth knowing the approaches commonly used identical, the chance that patient B actually has a PE is 10-fold higher than patient A (40% vs 4%).[7]

During the 20th century, scientists turned to deductive reasoning and sought to understand scientific results only in the context of the statistical likelihood based on all possible outcomes, also known as the *frequency of all results*. This became known as the *frequentist* school of thought; in this way of viewing data, if the only thing that matters is the frequency of results, the *P* value becomes the measure of interest.[5]

Why should we be cautious of frequentist interpretations of data? The first and most fundamental reason is that frequentist theories run counter to human nature. Few of us embark on a healthcare delivery project without having some expectation or hope that our intervention will be helpful in some way. We have an intuition about the world, based on our experience and prior data. Bayesians would call this our prior probability. A second concern is that *P* values do not comment upon the magnitude of the result, something we have already discussed in this chapter. Other authors draw on the *P* value's historical place in statistics to challenge the concept that a single value can somehow reveal truth and that while we contextualize the *P* value itself in a series of repeated experiments to be repeated over time, the null hypothesis is rejected in a single sitting.[6]

We bring up this controversy for two reasons. First, it is worth recognizing that the scientific methods and rigor we bring to the measurement of healthcare delivery have their own controversies and history. Researchers who abhor the P value in clinical trials will be equally unconvinced in healthcare delivery science. Realistically, we will rarely rely on only one method of judging the truth of our intervention, but the confidence interval can also provide important context for people interpreting your results. The second reason to discuss a statistical controversy is that we are all Bayesians at heart. It is rare that we undertake a project (say, a method to limit excessive telemetry use[8] or an investigation into a state policy about healthcare delivery),[9] without at least some suggestion of what we expect to find, even if our actual results differ from our prior expectations.

Sensitivity and Specificity

To make further use of the power of Bayes' theorem, we bring up the measures of sensitivity and specificity. These concepts, while useful in thinking about how to interpret test results, will also be useful when we think about different measures of risk adjustment that we will describe in Chapter 18, and how to build prediction rules in Chapter 16. The values of sensitivity and specificity give us language to understand whether our test of interest (or prediction rule) correctly identifies those with the true disease.

To do this, we will use some common notation to explain probability. You may also find this to be a useful framework when looking at other descriptions of probabilities or thinking through how variables are related to each other. P(A) is read as "the probability of A", and P(A | B) is read as "the probability of A, conditional on B." What does that mean? Often, you care about one probability only in certain conditions. For example, maybe you care about the probability of being admitted to the hospital—P(hospitalization)—but only among patients with a diagnosis of congestive heart failure (CHF). This might be written as P(hospitalization | CHF), and read as "the probability of hospitalization, conditional on a diagnosis of CHF."

Sensitivity and specificity are concepts that are based on describing how well a test—like a lab test—performs. So to explain them, we will use these terms and think in terms of tests and diseases. T^+ will be a positive test result, T^- a negative test result, D^+ a person with true disease, and D^- a person without the disease. Another way to think about these concepts is that a test is something we create or design to give us an answer while a disease is the truth. We could use these same concepts for, as an example, a prediction rule that predicts whether a hospitalized patient will live or die. The prediction rule will be a test, which will give us an answer—yes, our prediction rule thinks this patient will die. But there is also a truth, the patient either will live or die that hospitalization (i.e., our "disease"). The prediction rule doesn't always get it right.

Tests can yield true positives, true negatives, false positives, or false negatives. If our prediction rule from above predicts the patient will live and she lives, the test is a true negative. If it predicts she will live and she dies, this is a false negative. *Sensitivity* is the probability of getting a positive test **among people who truly have the disease**, or P(T^+ | D^+). *Specificity* is the probability of getting a negative test result **among people who truly do not have the disease**, or P(T^- | D^-).

As another working example, let's imagine a test to identify patients with metastatic breast cancer. It is easier to actually think in terms of tests and diseases so let's abandon our earlier example for now. We apply the breast cancer test to 100 women, and we know who has metastatic cancer and who does not. We get the following results:

Disease	Test +	Test −	Total
+	17	3	20
−	10	70	80
Total	27	73	100

The total number of positive tests is 17 + 10 = 27, the total number of negative test results is 3 + 70 = 73, There are 17 + 3 = 20 women with metastatic breast cancer and 10 + 70 = 80 women without metastatic breast cancer. The sensitivity of the test is $P(T^+ \mid D^+) = 17/20 = 0.85$. The specificity of the test is $P(T^- \mid D^-) = 70/80 = 0.875$.

Returning to Bayes' theorem, we can now ask, "Based on our test characteristics, what is the probability that an individual woman with a positive test result has metastatic breast cancer?" This concept is neither the specificity nor the sensitivity but a new concept, the *positive predictive value*, or the probability of having the disease **among people who have a positive test**. There is also the *negative predictive value,* or the probability of not having the disease **among people who have a negative test.**

To answer our question, Bayes tells us that our probability of interest, which can also be written as $P(D^+ \mid T^+)$, is equivalent to the probability that a woman has the disease and a positive test/probability of a positive test, which is mathematically equivalent to

$$P(D^+ \mid T^+) = \frac{P(D^+)P(T^+ \mid D^+)}{P(D^+)P(T^+ \mid D^+) + P(D^-)P(T^+ \mid D^-)}$$

We know $P(T^+ \mid D^+) = 0.85$ and $P(T^+ \mid D^-)$ is 1 − the specificity, or 0.125. $P(D^+)$ is the prevalence of the disease. In our data, 20% of the population has the disease. So

$$P(D^+ \mid T^+) = \frac{0.20 \times 0.85}{0.20 \times 0.85 + 0.80 \times 0.125}$$
$$= 0.63, \text{the positive predictive value.}$$

Remember that in this example, we have used the terms *test* and *disease* literally, but let's return to using these concepts with to other aspects of healthcare delivery. Imagine that we want to create a prediction rule that will help us identify patients who will need additional services at home like a visiting nurse and home physical therapy when they are discharged from the hospital. Our prediction rule, which we will discuss more in our chapter on prediction (Chapter 16), incorporates a patient's age, gender, marital status, functional status on admission to the hospital (stratified into ambulatory, ambulatory with assistance, and bed-bound), and admission location (stratified into home, skilled nursing facility, long-term acute-care hospital, and all others). The output of our prediction rule in 100 consecutive patients is the same as our previous test result:

Needed home services on discharge	Predicted to need home services	
	+	−
+	17	3
−	10	70

The test characteristics of our prediction rule would be the same: a sensitivity of 0.85 and a specificity of 0.875. Put in the context of this study, when our prediction rule was positive, patients needed home services 85% of the time, which we could set up in advance during the stay so the hospitalization wouldn't be unnecessarily prolonged. However, because we set up services for 10 people who didn't need them, we would have wasted resources for these patients. To make sure that we don't set up services unnecessarily, we may want a prediction rule with a very low false-positive rate.

Prevalence, Incidence, Relative Risk (RR), and Odds Ratio (OR)

There are multiple ways to describe data that occur within a population (e.g., in-hospital mortality among trauma surgery patients or the number of filled prescriptions among new prescriptions for patients discharged from the hospital). The *prevalence* of an event is the number of people with the event divided by the number in the population. Put another way, the prevalence tells us what percentage of people have the disease or condition we care about *at a given time.* For example, we might find that the prevalence of diabetes in American adults was 12.2% in 2015.[10] Prevalence fails to take into consideration the survival time or people coming in and out of the group, so it can only be used to ask questions of association that are not biased by varying degrees of time in a given state. *Incidence*, however, solves this problem by making the denominator the population-time. Incidence tells us what rate at which people get the disease/condition/etc. of interest over a given period of time. For example, we might find that the incidence of diabetes among U.S. adults in 2015 was 1.5 million new cases, or 6.7 per 1000 people.[10] An example in healthcare delivery science could be the correct reporting of hospital-acquired infections, as number of infected patients/patient-hospital days (with the denominator here being total patient days, calculated as the number of patients, multiplied by the average length of stay).

Relative differences in rates and risks are useful in describing the difference between exposed and unexposed groups in a percentage change in outcomes associated with exposure. As an example, we can take two incidence ratios, one of those patients exposed to our intervention (I_E) and one of those unexposed (I_U), and divide them:

$$\text{Relative Risk} = RR = I_E / I_U$$

Let's use as our example an effort to reduce the risk of *Clostridium difficile* infection, a morbid hospital-acquired infection associated with antibiotic use, in our hospital.[11] We plan to use a special new cleaning product to clean the room of patients with known *C. difficile* infections in order to reduce the risk of transmission between infected patients and uninfected patients. We design our study as a pre/post study, looking at our rate of *C. difficile* prior to our cleaning strategy (3 infections per 3,000 person-days) and our rate after our cleaning strategy (2 infections per 3,000 person-days). If we divide the two values, we find that the post period has a relative risk (RR) of 0.67, which is to say that patients admitted to the hospital in the post-intervention period had a 33% decreased risk ($1.0 - 0.67 = 0.33 \times 100 = 33\%$) of infection compared to patients admitted in the pre-intervention period. (Whether we can then confidently attribute the change to the cleaning product is a more complicated question, which we will address in Chapter 20.) We can use a similar statistic, called the *odds ratio (OR)*, to calculate the relative difference in odds (the odds of one event divided by the odds a second event), often useful in case-control studies where we are estimating the odds of exposure rather than the risk of disease.

The challenge of statistics like RR and OR is that they are just that—relative. They remain agnostic to the *actual* change in disease occurrence between groups. If the underlying rate or risk of a disease is very small, the RR could seem quite large but reduce the absolute risk by only a small percentage. Let's say that the risk of falls in our hospital is 1 in 10,000 admissions, or 0.01%. The chief operating officer identifies special sticky bedsheets that, in well-conducted studies, reduce the risk of falling from bed by 25% (a RR of 0.75), so she asks you to implement this innovation in the hospital. A 25% reduction to an already-low risk amounts to dropping the risk of fall from 0.01% to 0.0075% (only a tiny absolute difference). Admittedly, if these bedsheet studies are to be believed, the chief operating officer has reduced the risk of a fall event from a rare event to an even rarer event. But the RR of 0.75 is probably not producing such a substantial difference in real-world outcomes as it first sounds.

Confidence Intervals (CIs)

Identifying confidence intervals is one useful way to counterbalance the shortcomings of the *P* value and to inform us if our null hypothesis (defined as there is no difference between groups) cannot be rejected.

Confidence intervals not only convey both a method of evaluating the effects of chance but they also add something new: they give us a sense of the underlying population size. The values of the confidence intervals describe the range in which the true outcome lies based on the underlying population of study, with some level of confidence. If we identify a 95% confidence interval around a mean $\bar{x}$, our estimate of the true population mean μ, we can say that we are 95% confident that the true value of μ lies within the two bounds of that interval. To calculate the 95% confidence intervals for an estimated mean, we use both the standard deviation σ and the study population n and calculate the value as follows:

$$\left(\bar{x} - 1.96\frac{\sigma}{\sqrt{n}}, \bar{x} + 1.96\frac{\sigma}{\sqrt{n}}\right)$$

To provide an example of how to interpret confidence intervals, let's briefly examine a study that we conducted, which assessed patient outcomes associated with being treated in the hospital by different types of medical physicians. We compared receiving care in the hospital from one's primary care provider (PCP), a physician who knows you well, as compared with a physician who only takes care of hospitalized patients, termed a *hospitalist* (a physician who knows the hospital system well).[12] We found that, after controlling for patient- and hospital-level factors, inpatient care by a PCP had an adjusted odds ratio for 30-day mortality of 0.94 with a 95% confidence interval of 0.91–0.97 and a *P* value of < 0.01. These results suggest that care by one's PCP decreased the odds of death at 30 days by 6% (because the odds ratio is 0.94, there is a 6% reduction). An odds ratio of 1.0 means that there is no effect—that the odds of the event in one group is equal to the odds in the other group. The same is true for risk ratios. That's called a 'null value.'

When the null value is included in the range of the confidence interval, then we know that the results are not statistically significant, which is not the case in this example. Put another way, if the confidence interval includes 1.0 in its range, then the results are not statistically significant. The *P* value also tells us that the results are statistically significant. But as this was a study on over half a million Medicare recipients, most differences were likely to be significant. The *P* value, cited alone, tells us nothing about whether PCPs reduce the average patient's risk of death at 30 days a lot or a little. However, the result (0.94) and the confidence interval (0.91–0.97) tells us a good deal more. Based on the confidence interval, which does not cross 1.0, we can conclude that the results are statistically significant without ever looking at the *P* value. Further, we can conclude that care by one's PCP may incur as little as a 3% benefit in 30-day mortality or as much as a 9% benefit, as compared to care by a hospitalist. We can also see, based on the width of the confidence interval, that the estimate itself is relatively stable. An alternative range not found in this study (of, say, 0.75–0.99) would tell us that we had a good deal less certainty in our outcome and that PCP care could either be very protective of death or relatively similar to hospitalist care. Ultimately, if these were our data, we couldn't be sure.

T Tests

Finally, to ask whether two values (e.g., two means or two proportions) are different from one another, we must identify the most appropriate test of difference. The correct test largely comes from the underlying type of data in question.

Continuous data are data that are not required to take on any identified values, like integers or 0 or 1. Examples could include heart rate, blood pressure, and temperature measurements. Continuous data are described using measures of central tendency and dispersion, as described previously. For continuous data, we are usually interested in whether two means differ from one another. Several statistical tests exist to help us answer this question. The most commonly used, especially with normal data or when sample sizes are large, is the t test. To answer this question, we use the t test, which itself uses the t distribution. The numerator of the t statistic uses the difference in means $\bar{x}_1$ and $\bar{x}_2$ for the two means, as compared with the null hypothesis (presumably that the means are equal). The denominator uses both the sizes of the two study groups (n_1 and n_2) and the overall variance of the study population (s^2_p). With the study size and variance in the denominator as outlined next, the larger the t statistic, the less likely it is that the difference in means that we observe is due to chance. To transform the t statistic into a P value, we require the *degrees of freedom,* or the number of independent pieces of information (which can be calculated by $n_1 + n_2 - 2$), and a t table, often found in the back of statistics texts or online. To calculate the pooled variance, we use the following equation:

$$s^2_p = \frac{(n_1 - 1)s^2_1 + (n_2 - 1)s^2_2}{n_1 + n_2 - 2}$$

and then the t statistic as follows:

$$t_{(df)} = \frac{(\bar{x}_1 - \bar{x}_2) - 0}{\sqrt{s^2_p \left(\frac{1}{n_1} + \frac{1}{n_2}\right)}}$$

Chi-squared Tests

Discrete data have measurable quantities where no intermediate values are possible, like counts or integers. An example in healthcare may be the number of women in a study. These values are usually described using proportions. To test whether two proportions are different from one another, we use the *chi-squared test,* which measures whether what we see (observe) differs from what we expected (our null hypothesis). To start with, we summarize our data in rows and columns—a 2 × 2 table at its simplest. As an example, we start with the following:

Exposure	Disease Yes	Disease No
Yes	a	b
No	c	d

The chi-squared statistic is calculated as

$$X^2_{(df)} = \sum \frac{(O - E)^2}{E}$$

where O is the observed count, E the expected count, and Σ the sum. We again rely on degrees of freedom (*df*), which in this case is the number of rows − 1 times the number of columns − 1, or (r − 1)(c − 1). *T* represents the total count, or $a + b + c + d$. If we expect the null hypothesis to be true, we would expect the counts in each cell to be the same across the exposed and unexposed groups. Thus, for the first cell, the expected rate would be the proportion of exposed times the number of cases, or $((a + b)/T)(a + c)$; now there's no effect of being exposed. To identify the *P* value associated with the chi-squared statistic, again we look for the value of *df* in a chi-squared table, with larger values of a chi-squared test statistic coming from a larger difference in observed minus expected, and therefore less likely to be due to chance. If sample sizes are small, the chi-square test may have problems. In those cases, we use the Fisher's exact test instead.

OUTCOMES OVER TIME, PART 2—STATISTICAL PROCESS CONTROL (SPC) CHARTS

Statistical process control (SPC) charts extend the capabilities of run charts, discussed above, by helping us see when variation in a process over time is statistically significant (special cause variation) and when it is just noise or routine variation (common cause variation). Originally described by Walter Shewhart in the 1920s, the SPC chart informs the reader about variations in a process. Shewart built SPC charts to understand variations in Bell Labs, to move beyond understanding when the output of a process differed from some standard or control or when the output varied from that control by a test of statistical difference.[13] Instead, the method informs us about the *process* itself in order to move away from measures strictly focused on outputs and instead get to the heart of the processes that produced those outputs to improve and control unnecessary variations.[14]

Let's take as an example a clinical outpatient team that wanted to study how long it took an outpatient team to get a patient from check-in at the front desk back to the exam room (known as *getting roomed*). We have already made a process map of this in Chapter 8; now we can look at some of the data we may have collected when we built that map. As we recall, getting a patient roomed involves multiple steps: (1) greeting a patient; (2) getting the patient's updated insurance information; (3) moving the patient to a cubby to take his or her vital signs; and (4) walking the patient to an available room for the PCP. Figure 14-7 is used to illustrate an SPC for 25 consecutive patients. The *x*-axis represents both patients and time because the patients are consecutive. The control limits are 1, 2, or 3 standard deviations from the mean (in our case, 7.2 minutes). Almost all our patients are put in a room within 10.9 minutes; 1 patient took 25 minutes to get roomed.

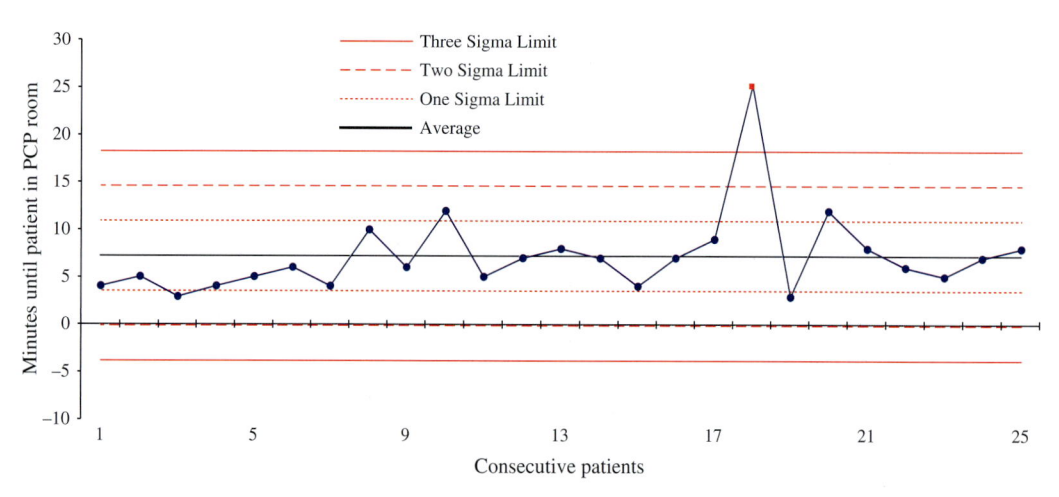

Figure 14-7 • A statistical process control chart, plotting the number of minutes it takes to room each consecutive patient in an outpatient primary care office. (Source: From ASQ.org.)

Similar to the run chart, SPCs provide much of the data in the method by which they are presented: we see the order of the data points, their timing, and their relationship to one another. But SPCs also let us see what variations may be due to chance and what may be due to a reason (termed *special cause variation*).[15] When we see variation that appears to be due to chance (but, as in our case, may exceed what we want for our patients), we have to work on the constraints of the system, which is to say the way in which our system is designed to produce this output.[15] However, when there is special cause variation, we have to study that specific example, understand it, and work to eliminate the cause of that variation.

There are a range of criteria for identifying special cause variations.[15,16] Among the criteria with the greatest agreement are the following:

- A run of seven or eight data points on one side of the mean
- Two of three consecutive points more than 2 standard deviations away from the mean in the same direction
- A run of seven or eight points trending up or down in the same direction[15]
- A point outside the control limit, which is the line indicating a 3-SD variation from the mean

In our example, our first seven data points are on the lower end of the mean. If we study this area of special variation, we may find that because these are the first seven patients who arrived, while all the rooms were available, while later in the morning, PCPs might be running late and their rooms may not be open. We also see a single patient well outside the 3-sigma control limit, which suggests special-cause variation, as well.

As in other aspects of data, the type of data, whether continuous or discrete, determines the type of SPC that is most useful. For continuous data, like our example of how long it takes to get a patient into a PCP's room, we use similar charts to the example given here. Referred to as an individuals chart or *x*-chart, this chart plots the actually observed values with the measure of central tendency as the mean or $\bar{x}$. This is often paired with a chart of the moving ranges, which allows us to see the changes between individual observations. For our graph, the X-*mr*-chart looks like Figure 14-8.

Figure 14-8 highlights exactly how much of an outlier there is for patient 18, who stood out in the last chart, as well. We also see that that there are periods of less variability (at the beginning of the day, and sometime after patient 11), while at other points, there are big differences between patient experiences. This highlights a strength and a weakness of

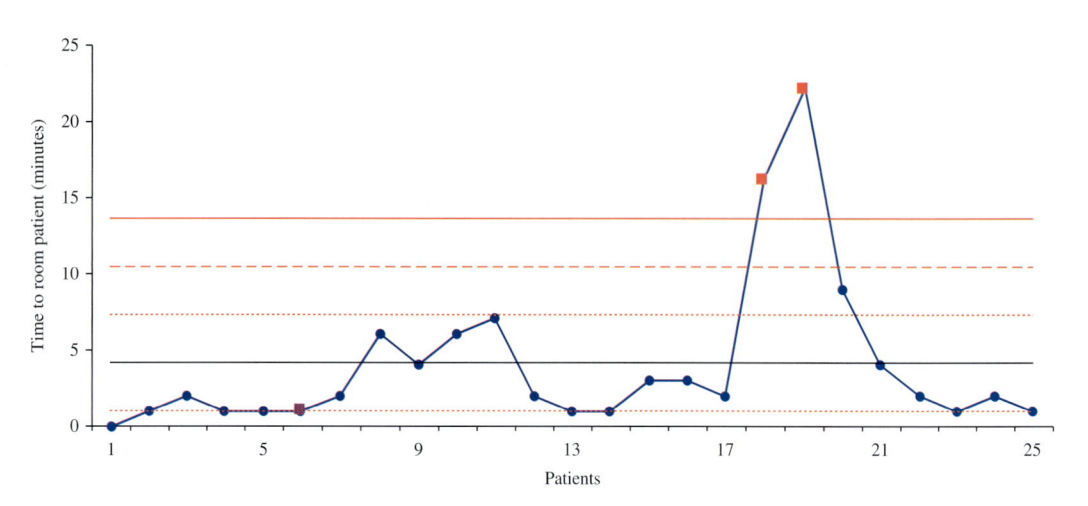

Figure 14-8 • An X-*mr*-chart of the moving ranges between consecutive patients of the time required to room patients in a PCP office.

SPC charts: they are most powerful in the hands of the frontline user, who can best look to understand the drivers of special cause variations and what to understand of the system itself. Imagine a medical assistant who could tell you that once you get beyond 15 patients, you are now frequently into midday, and many people excuse themselves to go to lunch at that time, reducing the number of frontline staff available to room patients. In the absence of this deeper understanding, SPC charts communicate only the most general sense of the process to outside users.

For additional discrete data, such as proportions or counts, we must use different assumptions to calculate the measures of central tendency and to identify control limits that are meaningful to the data. Table 14-3 describes the other candidate SPC charts that accommodate discrete data.

EVERYDAY ANALYTICS

This chapter has provided a range of essential tools that help form the foundation for the subsequent chapters in this book. While these future chapters develop more multivariable techniques or emphasize the power of machine learning, the ability to look at one's raw data and perform straightforward tests of difference on those data will permit you to see where there is signal and where there is noise. We would encourage you to always return to the basics of your data to understand what the information is telling you about healthcare.

Table 14-3 SPC CHARTS BASED ON TYPES OF DATA

Type of Data	Example	Chart Type	Calculation for Central Tendency	Working Example	Upper and Lower Control Limits
Proportions	Mortality among patients admitted with sepsis, by month	p-chart	$\bar{p} = \dfrac{\sum_{i=1}^{n} x_i}{\sum_{i=1}^{n} n_1}$, where x represents an event and n represents patients	$\bar{p} = \dfrac{25\,deaths}{120\,sepsis\,cases} = 0.2$ deaths from sepsis, on average	$\bar{p} = \pm 3\sqrt{\bar{p}(1-\bar{p})/n_i}$
Incidence, or count data with low frequency events or where the underlying population does change	Central-line infections per patient-day	u-chart	$\bar{u} = \dfrac{\sum_{i=1}^{n} u_i}{\sum_{i=1}^{n} n_i}$, where u represents the total events and n represents the total person-time	$\bar{p} = \dfrac{2\,infections}{400\,patient-days} = 0.005$ infections per patient-day, on average	$\bar{u} = \pm 3\sqrt{\bar{u}/n_i}$
Incidence, or count data where the underlying population does not change	Coronary artery bypass graft (CABG) cases admitted from the operating room on Mondays	c-chart	$\bar{c} = \dfrac{\sum_{i=1}^{n} c}{n}$, where c represents the total events and n represents the total time periods	$\bar{c} = \dfrac{24\,admissions}{8\,Mondays} = 3\,admissions$ following CABG every Monday	$\bar{c} = \pm 3\sqrt{\bar{c}}$

KEY POINTS

- Before any analysis takes place, *look* at your data.
- You will need to summarize your data using summary statistics and measures of central tendency. Consider carefully any assumptions that you make when collapsing your raw data into summary statistics, as these assumptions will be compounded in later analyses.
- Understand different types of data (e.g., continuous or discrete) because that will determine how you ask questions about your data.
- Consider the power of simple displays of data over time, such as run charts, to highlight and understand the relationship that time has on your process of interest.
- Beware the common mistakes in data presentation: strange and distracting eye effects, the tempting three-dimensional graph, the overused pie chart, and too many notes and annotations.

Box 14-1   CASE

Maria is the chief medical officer at Arbitrary Regional General Hospital (ARGH). She conducted a staff satisfaction survey and has summarized the results below. The survey asked her staff to rank how satisfied each person was on a scale of 1 to 5, with 5 being the most satisfied and 1 being very unsatisfied. The survey also asked several questions of the respondents. Maria de-identified the survey so people would answer honestly.

** Note that, for the purposes of this worked analysis, we will say that these satisfaction data can be treated as continuous values, which is to say you can take the mean of these values. Chapter 15 on surveys does offer meaningful caution about whether this is an ok practice. But for the purposes of this case, let's throw caution to the wind. **

Respondent	Satisfaction	Month of Survey	Job	Gender	Age	Vacation days taken this month
1	5	8	RN	F	42	4
2	4	8	RN	M	35	7
3	5	8	MD	F	60	5
4	3	1	RN	F	55	0
5	3	1	MD	M	45	0

Respondent	Satisfaction	Month of Survey	Job	Gender	Age	Vacation days taken this month
6	5	1	MD	M	62	1
7	1	3	MD	F	30	0
8	3	3	MD	F	35	0
9	4	3	RN	M	37	5
10	5	8	MD	F	65	7

These data lead Maria to ask several questions:

1. How is ARGH doing in staff satisfaction? Does everyone feel the same way or are there differences of opinion?
2. What are some characteristics or features of the people who are less satisfied?
3. Maria is interested in making sure everyone ranks at least 4 or more on the survey (better than neutral). She wants to introduce a Bring Your Pet to Work day to boost satisfaction. When should she do this and with whom?

Worked solutions

How is ARGH doing in staff satisfaction?

We can start by looking at these data, using the visual techniques we described. We can look at a bar graph of our results:

Summary of staff satisfaction

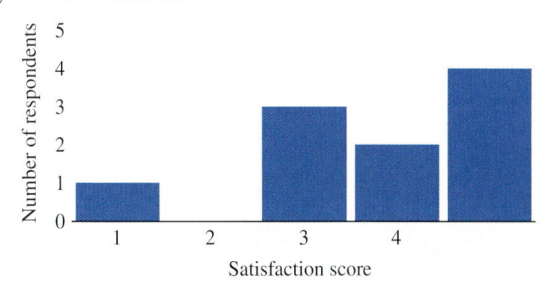

In general, it looks like many people are pretty satisfied. But there is a group at 3 and a single person at 1.

Another way to ask this question is what is the mean of the satisfaction scores. This is calculated as the sum of all of the values (38) divided by the total number in the population (10), for an average of 3.8.

If we are interested in the standard deviation, we have to calculate the difference each value is from the mean, square these answers, sum these squares, divide by $n-1$ for the *variance*, and then take the square root for the standard deviation. All common spreadsheet programs have a function

(continued)

Box 14-1 CASE (continued)

to do these calculations for you, but it is worth doing them once by hand to make sure you understand what's going on. The result looks like this:

Value	Mean	Difference from mean	Square of difference from mean
5	3.8	1.2	1.44
4	3.8	0.2	0.04
5	3.8	1.2	1.44
3	3.8	−0.8	0.64
3	3.8	−0.8	0.64
5	3.8	1.2	1.44
1	3.8	−2.8	7.84
3	3.8	−0.8	0.64
4	3.8	0.2	0.04
5	3.8	1.2	1.44

The sum of the differences from the mean = (1.44 + 0.04 + 1.44 + 0.64 + 0.64 + 1.44 + 7.84 + 0.64 + 0.04 + 1.44) = 15.6.

Divided by n − 1 = 9, this is 15.6/9 = 1.73, the variance.

The standard deviation is the square root of the variance or 1.32.

So, Maria's average score is 3.8 with a standard deviation of 1.32. By comparison, if the one person who rated a score of 1 wasn't in the data set, how would these change? (Answer: new mean: 4.1, new standard deviation 0.93, a small change in mean but also a more narrow standard deviation).

If we are interested in the median, we need to sort our satisfaction scores in ascending or descending order:

1
3
3
3
4
4
5
5
5
5

We see the median, which lies between our 5th and 6th values, is 4.
What are some characteristics or features of the people are less satisfied?
We have a number of variables and ways to compare these respondents. How about women versus men? The mean satisfaction of women is 3.7 as compared with men, which is 4. So perhaps women are less satisfied then men.

It looks like the month might matter. The average satisfaction in August (month 8) is 4.75 while the average satisfaction in the winter months (January and March) is 3.2.

Nurses are also more satisfied on average (4) than doctors (3.7).

And we can see if age has something to do with it. How would you try that?

Maria is interested in making sure everyone ranks at least 4 or more on the survey (better than neutral). She wants to introduce a Bring Your Pet to Work day to boost satisfaction. When should she do this and with whom?

If we take our finding about gender from above, that women are less satisfied than men, we can also stratify by nurses and doctors. Maybe women and men feel differently whether they are nurses or doctors (a term called *effect modification*, which we will come back to Chapter 16). If we look at these means, we would find that:

Doctors (avg satisfaction)		Nurses (avg satisfaction)	
M	F	M	F
4	3.5	4	4

It seems like female physicians may be a good target for Bring Your Pet to Work day.

That said, if we look at a scatter plot of days of vacation and average satisfaction, we might draw a different conclusion:

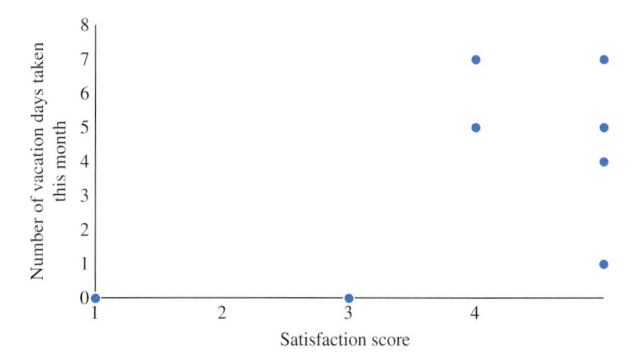

It seems that people who rated 3 or 1 had taken no vacation days this month, while those who rated 4 or 5 all had. Put another way, the average satisfaction score for people who took no vacation days was 2.5, while the average satisfaction score everyone else was 4.7. So maybe instead of pets, a day off might help staff satisfaction!

REFERENCES

1. Strunk W, White EB. *The Elements of Style*. 50th anniversary ed. New York, NY: Pearson Longman; 2009.
2. Tufte ER. *The Visual Display of Quantitative Information*. 2nd ed. Cheshire, CT: Graphics Press; 2001.
3. Perla RJ, Provost LP, Murray SK. The run chart: a simple analytical tool for learning from variation in healthcare processes. *BMJ Qual Saf*. 2011;20(1):46–51.
4. Little JDC, Hauser JR, Urban GL. *From Little's Law to Marketing Science: Essays in Honor of John D.C. Little*. Cambridge, MA/London: MIT Press; 2015.
5. Fisher RA, Bennett JH, Fisher RA, Fisher RA, Fisher RA. *Statistical Methods, Experimental Design, and Scientific Inference*. Oxford, UK/New York: Oxford University Press; 1990.
6. Goodman SN. Toward evidence-based medical statistics. 1: The *P* value fallacy. *Ann Intern Med*. 1999;130(12):995–1004.
7. PIOPED Investigators. Value of the ventilation/perfusion scan in acute pulmonary embolism. Results of the prospective investigation of pulmonary embolism diagnosis (PIOPED). *JAMA*. 1990;263(20):2753–2759.
8. Dressler R, Dryer MM, Coletti C, Mahoney D, Doorey AJ. Altering overuse of cardiac telemetry in non-intensive care unit settings by hardwiring the use of American Heart Association guidelines. *JAMA Intern Med*. 2014;174(11):1852–1854.
9. Law AC, Stevens JP, Hohmann S, Walkey AJ. Patient outcomes after the introduction of statewide ICU nurse staffing regulations. *Crit Care Med*. 2018;46(10):1563–1569.
10. Centers for Disease Control and Prevention. *National Diabetes Statistics Report, 2017*. Accessed May 24, 2019, from https://www.cdc.gov/diabetes/pdfs/data/statistics/national-diabetes-statistics-report.pdf.
11. Cohen SH, Gerding DN, Johnson S, et al. Clinical practice guidelines for Clostridium difficile infection in adults: 2010 update by the Society for Healthcare Epidemiology of America (SHEA) and the Infectious Diseases Society of America (IDSA). *Infect Control Hosp Epidemiol*. 2010;31(5):431–455.
12. Stevens JP, Nyweide DJ, Maresh S, Hatfield LA, Howell MD, Landon BE. Comparison of hospital resource use and outcomes among hospitalists, primary care physicians, and other generalists. *JAMA Intern Med*. 2017;177(12):1781–1787.
13. Shewhart WA. *Economic Control of Quality of Manufactured Product*. New York, NY: D. Van Nostrand Company, Inc.; 1931.
14. Mohammed MA. Using statistical process control to improve the quality of health care. *Qual Saf Health Care*. 2004;13(4):243–245.
15. Mohammed MA, Worthington P, Woodall WH. Plotting basic control charts: tutorial notes for healthcare practitioners. *Qual Saf Health Care*. 2008;17(2):137–145.
16. Lee K, McGreevey C. Using control charts to assess performance measurement data. *Jt Comm J Qual Improv*. 2002;28(2):90–101.

SURVEY-BASED DATA
Pitfalls and Promises 15

INTRODUCTION

Surveys have always been part of medical research. However, over the past two decades, the ease of quickly administering surveys to large numbers of people has markedly increased—first, because of the ability to deliver surveys by email, and more recently because of the widespread availability of web-based, easy-to-use, professional-appearing survey tools.

This ease of use comes with a downside, though. First, it is almost effortless for administrators to overwhelm their clinical staff with the number of surveys administered. Physicians and nurses commonly report being "surveyed to death," and this overuse of surveys leads to a degradation in the quality of all responses. Second, *surveys are deceptively hard to do well.* The purpose of this chapter is to provide an overview of the reasons for surveys, of methodological steps needed to conduct and analyze a good survey, and of a few common pitfalls to avoid.

PERHAPS THE MOST IMPORTANT THING YOU'LL LEARN IN THIS CHAPTER

If there is one thing we want you to leave this chapter with, it's this: surveys are easy to get wrong—and, for the uninitiated, bad surveys look remarkably similar to good surveys. Survey research is a highly specialized methodology. *If you are making critical decisions based on a survey, consider getting specialist help.*

This has been known for a long time. In 1895, Caroline Miles wrote an amazingly prescient passage. We'll address many of her insights and concerns as we work through this chapter, because they still hold true today:

> *To ask questions is easy, but to make the questionnaire an instrument of precision is very far from easy. It has more ways of going wrong than the chronoscope ... To say nothing of the general difficulty of*

Key Point

Surveys can be much trickier than they appear. If you are making critical decisions based on a survey, consider getting specialist help.

selecting truly cardinal points for questioning about, and the special rhetorical difficulty of framing questions that shall be perfectly clear as to the information required without at the same time prejudicing the answers to be received ... What allowance must be made for influences that might unconsciously mold the answers? ... Some of these sources of error can be avoided, some must be recognized and allowed for and some must forbid the use of the method except under uncommon circumstances.[1]

In the 21st century, Jones and colleagues summarized the dilemma facing the modern healthcare delivery scientist:

There is a widespread perception that surveys are easier to conduct than other research methodologies. However, in reality, rigorously designed, implemented and analysed survey research requires substantial planning, time and effort. Conclusions drawn from survey research may be misleading or invalid if the design of the questionnaire is poor, the sample inadequate, or unrepresentative of the target population.[2]

We couldn't agree more.

WHAT ARE SOME OF THE MAIN PURPOSES OF SURVEYS?

Surveys can serve innumerable purposes, and we won't attempt to exhaustively list them here. However, we do think that it is worth knowing a few of the major categories of work that surveys are used for in healthcare. These groups (adapted from Jones[2]) are not formal conceptual structures, but may be useful pragmatically.

Conditions and Concepts for Which the Ground Truth Is Patient-Reported (or Provider-Reported)

Many important outcomes and concepts can only be measured by asking people. Satisfaction with care, assessment of experience, how well dyspnea is controlled, and quantification of physician burnout are all examples of these. Over the past decade, there has been a significant emphasis on patient-reported outcomes (PROs), patient-reported outcome measures (PROMs), and patient-reported experience measures (PREMs).[3] These kinds of outcome measures are increasingly used in research, public reporting, and payment. They may be broad-based measures of health status or quality of life (such as the SF-36),[4] disease- or condition-specific (such as the Seattle Angina Questionnaire,[5] or joint-specific patient-reported outcomes), or focused on patients' experiences of care [such as the Hospital Consumer Assessment of Healthcare Providers and Systems (HCAHPS)].[6]

Epidemiological Surveys

Epidemiological surveys make inferences about population-level health characteristics based on a sampling methodology and questionnaires. Patients, physicians, or other providers can be respondents in these kinds of surveys, which might be focused on disease prevalence, risk factor exposures, practice patterns, or on treatment variation. Administered over time, these surveys can also provide insight into temporal changes in diseases, symptoms, and clinical practice. For example, these surveys have been used to quantify answers to questions as diverse as the prevalence of autism,[7] how much the burden of cutaneous leishmaniasis has increased in Brazil,[8] and what percentage of Americans cannot afford a $400 emergency expense.[9] Many nationally important health data resources are also survey-based, such as the National Health and Nutrition Examination Survey (NHANES), the Medical Expenditure Panel Survey (MEPS), the Health and Retirement Study (HRS), the National Health Interview Survey (NHIS), the Behavioral Risk Factor Surveillance System (BRFSS), and even the U.S. Census.

Attitudes of Patients, Physicians, or Staff Members

Assessing attitudes is an important aspect of survey research, and this type of survey is highly prevalent in healthcare delivery settings. Examples include:

- Questionnaires to assess attitudes toward new technologies, such as electronic health record (EHR) implementation[10]
- Patient safety culture surveys[11]
- Physician and employee engagement surveys[12] or perceptions of one's work environment[13,14]
- Investigations of patients' attitudes toward various physician practice characteristics, such as type of attire[15]
- Quantifying patients' attitudes toward different types of communication, such as preferences between electronic and over-the-phone communication for receiving biopsy results[16]
- Understanding physician attitudes toward techniques for quality improvement[17,18]

Understanding Organizations

Another use of surveys is to understand organizations. For example, surveys have been used to understand ICUs organizational processes,[19-21] an organization's readiness for change,[22,23] and understanding a hospital's work environment and organizational traits—and how they relate to patient and clinician outcomes.[24,25]

Assessing Knowledge

Knowledge assessments are ubiquitous—after all, we've all grown up taking quizzes and tests throughout our education and careers. However, surveys can also be used to measure a population's knowledge of particular diseases, diagnostic criteria, or therapeutic techniques, among other things. The population being surveyed can be patients, providers, or others in the health system—and can be locally specific (e.g., in a single hospital), or broad-based and nationally or internationally representative.

These kinds of studies can sometimes have quite an impact. One example of this type of study that had a major global impact was Iberti et al.'s multicenter study of whether physicians who used pulmonary artery catheters understood what the information from these invasive monitoring devices actually meant. They found that—on average—physicians misinterpreted the pulmonary artery catheter information 33% of the time. A subsequent survey-based study found similar miscomprehension, even when the population being studied was limited to ICU physicians.[26,27] This was one of the pieces of evidence that helped lead to dramatic reductions in the use of this invasive technology in ICUs worldwide.

Another example of this type of survey focused on ventilator-associated pneumonia. At the time, a specific surveillance definition was used for pneumonia by the Centers for Disease Control and Prevention (CDC). This definition was incorporated into several required public reporting programs and was used in several pay-for-performance programs. A nationally representative survey used case vignettes of patients with possible ventilator-associated pneumonia and asked respondents from 43 hospitals to decide whether these patients met the criteria for ventilator-associated pneumonia. Hospitals' classification as pneumonia versus not pneumonia was nearly random (Fleiss κ 0.13, a statistic that measures level of agreement across respondents, with 0–0.2 representing little to no agreement and 0.8–1.0 representing perfect agreement). Some hospitals rated 0% of vignettes as pneumonia; others rated 100% as pneumonia[28] (and they saw the same vignettes!). This was one of several pieces of evidence used to sunset the prior national definition of ventilator-associated pneumonia.

OVERVIEW OF CONDUCTING A SURVEY

This section reviews some of the important steps in planning, designing, administering, and analyzing a survey.[29]

Crisply Defining the Goal of the Survey

One of the most important steps of designing a survey is ensuring that you have clearly defined the goal of the survey. As Coggon et al. wrote: "The first and often the most difficult question is: 'Why am I doing this survey?' Many studies start with a general hope that something interesting will emerge, and they often end in frustration."[30]

What specific question or questions are you trying to answer? Are there any existing surveys that have been validated that you could use to answer your questions? Are you confident that a survey is the best way to answer these questions? Are you confident that the survey will provide the necessary answers, from the intended sample? Who will use the results? How will the answers to these specific questions be used? Is your written statement of objectives unambiguous enough that others can read it and understand what you are trying to do?

> **Key Point**
>
> Crisply define (and write down) the key objective of your survey. This will save substantial difficulty later.

Deciding Whom You Will Survey: Population, Survey Frame, and Sampling Approach

In defining your objective, you will have developed an operational definition of whom you should survey. Physicians in your hospital? Patients of a certain age in your state? A nationally representative sample of nurses who care for patients with stroke?

You should define the overall population from which you wish to sample. If it is a small population (e.g., all physicians in one division in your hospital), then you will simply try to enroll them all. In many cases, though, when you are interested in a large population, you will need to sample from that population. *Sampling* is a way to collect a smaller number of surveys and use them to make inferences about an overall population. The *sampling frame* is your closest approximation to the overall population of interest. For example, you might be interested in all people in Texas, but your sampling frame might be a list of all phone numbers in the state. To be able to make these inferences, the critical part is that your sampling approach needs to create a sample that is representative of the overall population. In many cases, a random selection out of the population is best. In other cases, you will stratify the population and then select

> **Key Point**
>
> Survey samples need to be representative of the overall population in which you are interested. This is usually accomplished by some version of random sampling; a convenience sample is almost always biased.

randomly from within strata. But the key point is that randomness helps to create a representative sample.

This is the point at which you will need to calculate the *sample size* for the survey, which will be driven by your overall question and by the level of precision you need in your survey. In this context, precision is conceptually related to confidence intervals, as discussed in Chapter 14. In general, the larger your sample size, the better the chance that you would get the same estimate if you repeated the survey again in the same population. Put another way, as you increase sample size, precision increases (and confidence intervals become smaller).

There are a couple of points about sampling approaches that are common and warrant mention. First, you may wish to stratify your sampling approach if there are specific characteristics that you want to make sure are present in the sampled population (age, sex, race, and educational level are common stratification variables); in some cases, you may wish to specifically oversample some groups of particular interest, such as those of particular race, age, etc. Second, logistically, you also need to figure out how you will identify the actual people whom you'll contact from the population of interest. How will you get in touch with them? You will need to decide the mode of the survey. Will it be mailed? Done via a web survey? Emailed? Conducted via phone? Conducted in person? If you use multiple modes, you should realize that responses may vary systematically with different modes of survey administration.[31] Further, you will also need to consider how frequent your follow-up will be ahead of time—will you email once a week until you achieve your desired response rate? Or follow-up only once with nonresponders?

Sometimes the logistical approach requires two-stage sampling. In this approach, you contact an organization first (e.g., a hospital), obtain lists of eligible participants (e.g., pharmacists at the hospital), and then sample from within each of these clusters. Stratification, multimodal surveys, and two-stage sampling all require additional steps and calculations, both in planning the survey (for sample size) and analyzing it (to handle correlation within clusters and to reweight the sample so that it reflects the overall population). This is technically intricate, and we recommend working with a statistician or survey methodologist with expertise in these matters if you require a complex sampling approach.

Regardless of these analytical complexities, an important point to keep in mind is that your sampling approach should be driven by the question you're trying to answer—hence the importance of crisply identifying your survey's objectives at the outset.

Caution

Different survey modes (e.g., in-person, telephone, postal, or electronic surveys) may have significantly different responses, even when the same questions are asked.

Designing the Survey Instrument (Questionnaire)

Designing a good questionnaire requires expertise. There are many pitfalls of survey instrument design that can inadvertently cause bias and incorrect conclusions. For this reason, you should use an existing, validated survey instrument for your survey whenever possible. Instruments that have been carefully designed and previously validated are much less likely to suffer from design flaws that lead to biased results than ad hoc questionnaires. What does it mean to use a validated instrument? It means that you use the whole instrument, in the way it was originally worded, and with the order of the original questions preserved. As we'll see later in the chapter, just changing the order of questions (let alone their actual wording) can markedly change how people respond to the survey. That means that the original validation of the instrument may no longer apply.

Language in survey instruments needs to be clear, concise, and appropriate for educational level. Each item should only ask one question—it is surprisingly common to encounter *double-barreled questions* in surveys. An example of this sometimes-unanswerable type of question might be, "How important are patient safety and patient satisfaction?" or "Does your hospital have dedicated programs to recruit women and underrepresented minorities?" (How should you answer if your hospital has a program to recruit women, but not underrepresented minorities?) These would be better broken into individual questions. Questionnaires should be as short as possible to achieve the overall objectives of the survey. The ordering of questions is important—both because question ordering can introduce bias but also because respondents may be less likely to complete questions later in the survey.

You will also have to choose what kind of response is available for each question. Perhaps the most common is a rating scale, commonly called a *Likert-type scale*. (By the way, *Likert* is commonly mispronounced as "LIKE-urt." The correct pronunciation is "LICK-urt." For a fascinating story involving Rensis Likert himself, see Roger Wimmer's discussion.[32]) These are multipoint, ordinal scales. For example: "Strongly disagree—Disagree—Neutral—Agree—Strongly Agree" would be a common scale. The anchors for these types of scales need to be clear and understandable for each respondent, which can be challenging. Each scale entry is sometimes paired with a number (e.g., Strongly disagree = 1, Disagree = 2). Be careful when analyzing these options because it is tempting to treat them as continuous variables, but the distance between 2 and a 3 isn't always than same as the distance between 3 and 4.[32] Variations on these kinds of scales include 10-point scales and visual analog scales, which

Caution

Small changes in survey wording can have large effects on survey results. Therefore, use an existing, validated instrument whenever possible.

Key Point

Language in survey instruments needs to be clear, concise, and appropriate for educational level.

Key Point

Avoid double-barreled questions—question types that combine two questions into one.

Key Point

Questionnaires should be as short as possible (though of course, no shorter!) because this encourages completion of the survey.

offer respondents more granularity in response. Of note, you must also consider whether you want a "neutral" category in a Likert-scale. This may degrade the interpretation of your results (e.g., everyone selects neutral for confusing or challenging questions) but there are some questions or instances in which neutral response may be helpful; this decision is context-specific.

Finally, a free-text response provides the most flexibility for the respondent and can be very useful for helping you understand respondents' thinking. However, free-text responses are difficult to analyze even with modern machine-learning techniques. A common practice is to give an opportunity for respondents to provide a free-text comment on questions or sections of the survey, which may offer the ability for interesting qualitative analyses in addition to the survey's quantitative elements.

More sophisticated surveys may adapt their questions as a respondent answers items on the questionnaire. A simple form of this approach is branching logic. For example, if one question is "Are you a physician?" and the answer is "No," it doesn't make sense to then ask, "What medical school did you attend?" Therefore, you might design the survey so it suppresses this question. More sophisticated adaptive surveys leverage item-response theory to develop models of the questionnaire-taker as the survey progresses. A common type of this is the computer-adaptive test, which attempts to select questions that are appropriately challenging to each test-taker. Similar approaches can be used in health-related surveys to help tailor them to individual respondents in a way that gathers information more efficiently than conventional, nonadaptive surveys.[33] For example, a patient might provide enough information in a few questions to estimate her or his overall rating accurately on a particular dimension of quality of life (say, physical functioning). There is little information to be gained by asking further questions in this domain, and the patient's time can be used more efficiently by moving the questioning to other quality-of-life dimensions.

Cognitive Testing and Revision of the Survey

If you have written your own survey instrument, you need to evaluate it before administering the survey broadly into the population from which you are sampling. *Cognitive testing,* or *cognitive interviewing,* is the process of having a potential respondent take the survey and provide insight into his or her thought process. A common approach is to ask the respondent to think aloud while reading, considering, and answering each question. This lets you see whether they are interpreting the question is the way that's intended, helps you understand whether all the information needed is there, and often identifies quite unexpected problems in the instrument.

Caution

Don't skip pretesting your survey! This is a critical step that helps you find and fix problems. It's tempting, but don't skip this step.

It also can identify issues with survey flow. Another approach is to use specific, scripted probes about survey items or about potential areas of concern with the instrument.[34,35]

As you proceed with cognitive testing, you will very likely find that your survey instrument needs revision. Cognitive testing is helpful in identifying weak spots in your instrument and assumptions that you have made, but that respondents will not make. You may need to revise the instrument several times during this process.

Pilot Testing and Revision of the Survey

Pilot testing is often considered a kind of "dress rehearsal" for the full survey. In a pilot test, you recruit subjects and administer the survey using all the procedures you anticipate using for the full survey—but with a small sample of the overall population. Pilot testing helps you identify problems in the end-to-end survey process and is an important step in administering large surveys. You can test alternative phrasing for questions and also analyze the responses to ensure that you are beginning to see some of the expected results. It is important that respondents who participate in the pilot are not resampled for the final survey because they are likely to answer differently from first-time survey-takers. For this reason, when you are doing surveys of small populations (e.g., all the cardiologists at two hospitals), it may not be feasible to conduct a pilot test because you would contaminate too great a proportion of the overall population of interest.

Administering the Survey and Collecting Responses

A major goal of survey administration is to achieve the highest response rate possible. This is because low response rates decrease the precision of the estimate you're trying to make. How does this work? Remember that a key element of defining confidence intervals (CIs) is *variance*. *Nonresponse* means that you have no information about how that person would have responded, so it effectively increases the sampling variance, meaning that your confidence intervals increase. It can also introduce nonresponse bias into your analysis, which is a problem that cannot be overcome by simply increasing sample size. How much nonresponse bias is created by low response rates is a matter of significant current debate—and likely varies with each survey. But in general, nonresponse bias is a form of selection bias (see Chapter 13), and it can cause the data you collect to tell you one thing, while the truth in the population is actually quite different.

So, what should you do? First, if you are administering surveys in person or via phone, you should train your staff so that survey administration is consistent. Second, there is a prolific body of research on techniques

Key Point

Cognitive testing, or *cognitive interviewing,* is the process of having a potential respondent take the survey and provide insight into their thought process. A *think-aloud* process is an efficient approach identifying problems with the survey, as are more structured approaches.

Key Point

In larger surveys, pilot testing is a critical step that is a small-scale dress rehearsal for the full survey.

> **Key Point**
>
> Incentives for survey participation as well as follow-up contacts, improve survey response rates.

to maximize response rates—enough studies, in fact, that multiple meta-analyses specifically address techniques for improving response rates.[36-39] A Cochrane review[40] amassed studies of 121 strategies to improve response rates in postal and electronic surveys. Table 15-1 highlights some of these findings. The table is not meant to be exhaustive, but rather illustrative of some of the approaches studied for improving response rates. While the relationship between response rates and survey quality may not be as clear as once believed, it remains likely that better response rates lower total survey error.

Table 15-1   SOME APPROACHES TO INCREASING SURVEY RESPONSE RATES

	Technique	Comment
Postal Surveys		
👍	Monetary incentives	Trials showed that monetary incentives nearly doubled response rates. Larger incentives were more effective. Notably, lotteries (rather than unconditional incentives) were generally ineffective.
👍	Nonmonetary incentives	Trials also showed that nonmonetary incentives (e.g., a key ring) increased response rates, though by less than monetary incentives.
👍	Timing of incentives	Incentives given at the time of receiving the questionnaire (rather than on returns of the survey) increased response rates.
👎	Providing the survey results to participants	Offering to provide the survey results to participants (as an incentive) did *not* increase response rates.
👍	Shorter questionnaires	Shorter questionnaires increased response rates by more than 60%.
👍	Personalizing the survey	Personalizing the survey (e.g., with a personal cover letter, sometimes hand-signed) increased response rates.
👍	Single-sided pages	Using single-sided surveys, rather than double-sided, increased response rates by more than 20%.
👍	Using special mailing modes	Response rates increased by about 75% when special delivery modes (such as registered mail) were used.
👍	Using stamps on return envelopes	Using stamps, rather than prepaid envelopes, improved response rates.

	Technique	Comment
👍	Precontacting recipients	Recipients who were precontacted to let them know that a survey was coming were almost 50% more likely to respond.
👍	Follow-up reminders	Follow-up reminders significantly increased response rates, especially when the survey is reincluded in follow-up messages.
👍	Providing an assurance of confidentiality	Providing an assurance of confidentiality increased the odds of responding by one-third.
Electronic Surveys		
👍	Incentives	Nonmonetary incentives nearly doubled response rates; the effect estimate of monetary incentives was imprecise. Larger nonmonetary incentives did not appear to have a larger effect. For healthcare professionals, monetary incentives seemed to have a larger impact than nonmonetary incentives.[54] Notably, lotteries (rather than unconditional incentives) were generally ineffective.
👍	Providing the survey results to participants	Offering to provide the survey results to participants (as an incentive) increased response rates.
👍	Shorter questionnaires	Shorter questionnaires increased response rates by more than 70%.
👍	Personalizing the survey	Personalizing the survey (e.g., using the recipient's name in the salutation) increased response rates by about 25%.
👍	Putting a picture in the email invitation	In two trials, putting a picture in the email invitation *tripled* the odds of a response.
👎	Including the word *survey* in the subject line	Including *survey* in the subject line reduced the response rate by about 20%.
👍	Follow-up reminders	Follow-up reminders significantly increase response rates.[55]

Adapted from Edwards et al[40]

Analyzing the Results

Analyzing survey responses can be simple if you used a straightforward, representative sample and received a high response rate with little item-level nonresponse. However, this is often not the case. The goal of this section is to highlight a few potential pitfalls that commonly arise in survey analysis so that you are familiar with them.

Basic Principles

First, keep your eyes on the prize. Remember your study objective: the main, key question you are trying to answer. As you work through your analyses, *remember the primary reason that you did the survey.* Answer that question first.

Second, as with any study, you should look at your data—the raw responses at the individual level, and then crosstabs. Are there strange patterns or unexpected missingness or item nonresponse? Exploratory analysis can be quite helpful in finding problems in the data themselves, and can identify issues in need of data cleaning.

Accounting for Your Sampling Approach

We should say at the outset that analyzing some surveys will require specialist expertise. For example, if you used a complex survey design (e.g., a stratified sampling design, multimodal surveys, or two-stage sampling), you will need to account for your sampling approach in the analysis. That can be quite complex.

Dealing with *Item Nonresponse*

You will need a strategy for dealing with *item nonresponse,* when a subject fills out part of the questionnaire but skips some questions. This is a type of missing data, a topic more fully reviewed in Chapter 13. Complete case analysis, where you drop all responses with any missing items, is the simplest way to deal with item nonresponse. Unfortunately, it is usually also a poor way to handle the issue because it tends to drop a large number of responses (reducing power), and it will often yield biased results. More sophisticated methods, such as *multiple imputation,* are commonly used to handle item nonresponse. These methods are likely to provide less-biased estimates than complete case analysis or simple imputation methods, but are more complex to implement. (See Chapter 13 for more details.)

Assessing Reliability

All practical research has measurement error. The goal of a survey, and of each item on a survey, is to create a standardized stimulus that elicits a consistent response from subjects, so as to minimize measurement error. *Reliability* refers to the statistical measurement of this property: how reproducible are the surveys' results?[41] (This does not mean that the results are correct, or that they represent the truth: a survey can be systematically biased, but consistently so.) But a survey is unlikely to be useful (or valid) if its results vary widely when given to the same subjects in the same situation. Reliability is commonly measured in three ways:[41]

- *Test-retest reliability.* If you administer a survey and then, later on, give it to the same set of respondents, do you get the same answers? There are two important caveats for this type of reliability assessment. First, some things in fact change over short periods of time (e.g., emotional states); a good instrument would reflect those changes, and so care is required in the application of this criterion. Second, if the time between survey administrations is too short, respondents may simply remember their responses from the prior administration and repeat them. This is called a *practice effect* or *training effect.*
- *Alternate form reliability.* In this reliability assessment, you readminister the survey and repeat an item, but change the wording slightly while examining the same concept. For example, you might simply change the order of responses in the response scale: "Never—Sometimes—Frequently—Always" versus "Always—Frequently—Sometimes—Never." Rewording the question itself can also be done, but it requires great attention to keep from changing the underlying concepts being measured.
- *Internal consistency reliability.* In many surveys, you will include several items that measure the same general concept—for example, physicians' trust of hospital management or patients' self-reported physical functioning. Having multiple questions that measure the same concept can increase the reliability of the overall survey. Survey domains are said to be internally consistent when these theoretically related questions are tightly correlated. This correlation is commonly assessed using *Cronbach's alpha*. In this measure, $\alpha = 0$ means there is no covariance between the survey items, and α approaches 1.0 as items have higher and higher covariance (and the number of items becomes very large). That is, a Cronbach's alpha value that is closer to 1 implies that the survey items in a given domain are more likely to be measuring the same underlying concept because they vary together in similar ways. As a concrete example, Banzett's multidimensional dyspnea profile (MDP) is an instrument that helps quantify a patient's experience

Key Point

The goal of a survey is to create a standardized stimulus that elicits a consistent response from subjects, so that measurement error is minimized. *Reliability* refers to the statistical measurement of this property: How reproducible are the surveys' results?

Key Point

Three approaches to measuring reliability include test-retest, alternative wording, and internal consistency. The latter is often quantified using Cronbach's alpha.

of breathlessness.[42] One domain of questions focuses on sensory qualities of shortness of breath (e.g., chest tightness) and another on the emotional response (e.g., anxiety) to dyspnea. In this study, Cronbach's alpha ranged from 0.82 to 0.95, suggesting high reliability of the domains being measured.

Assessing Validity

Validity is the idea that a survey, or just a question, measures what it intends to measure. An item that intends to measure anxiety should not measure pain, for example. There are numerous aspects of validity; a few that are commonly discussed are the following:[41]

> **Key Point**
>
> Validity is the idea that a survey, or just a question, measures what it intends to measure.

- *Face validity.* Face validity is the idea that each question looks reasonable to someone who knows the field that you are trying to measure. This is essentially a casual review by an expert or experts. It is the weakest type of validity, and some do not consider it a separate aspect of validity.
- *Content validity.* Content validity is similarly subjective, but it generally involves an organized and more systematic review of the instrument. Have you captured the important aspects of what you are trying to measure? Do the scales make sense? Do experts in the field agree that, upon review, the content of the questionnaire seems valid? Content validity could be provided by the cognitive interviewing process described above.
- *Criterion validity.* While face validity and content validity need to be established before fielding a survey, criterion validity is assessed based on responses to the instrument. Types of criterion-related validity include:
  - *Predictive validity*: Do responses on the survey predict future events or behavior? For example, hypertension medication adherence reported on a survey should predict future blood pressure control.[43]
  - *Concurrent validity*: Do responses on the survey agree with a gold-standard criterion measured at the same time? For example, a question that asks hypertensive patients about their average blood pressure might be compared against records from their home blood pressure monitor, or a survey question that asks patients about their cholesterol level might be compared against a lab test in their medical record. For example, an important step in the development of the Family Satisfaction in

> **Key Point**
>
> Face validity, content validity, criterion validity, and construct validity are commonly discussed when assessing survey validity.

the Intensive Care Unit (FS-ICU) instrument was assessing its correlation with other instruments that should measure similar concepts (in this case, the Quality of Dying and Death instrument, as well as nurse-assessed quality indicators).[44]

- *Construct validity*. Construct validity attempts to assess how well an instrument actually measures what it is trying to measure, especially when what it is trying to measure is an abstract concept, such as clinical reasoning, engagement, or burnout. Introduced in 1954,[45] the idea of construct validity remains a subject of active scholarship[46] and debate in the 21st century.[46] Some argue that it is essentially the grand unifying theory of validity, subsuming both content and criterion validity,[46] while others have gone so far as to argue that "construct validity has not proven to be a way to validate psychological constructs that have no clear referent in reality."[47] Regardless, measuring construct validity is difficult, and agreement that construct validity exists may come only after many years, and after many researchers have focused on a topic.[41]

  - *Convergent validity* is one type of construct validity, which asks how well the item or survey correlates with things that it should theoretically correlate with.
  - *Discriminant validity* is another aspect of construct validity, which focuses on whether the item or survey can tell the difference between things that it should theoretically be able to distinguish ... even if those concepts are closely related.

SOME PITFALLS

As easy as they are to administer, there are many pitfalls to surveys. We highlight a few of them here.

1. It's Easy to Write Questions that are Hard (or Impossible) to Answer.

Write simply. Questions need to be understandable to those responding to your survey. Use common words, not methodological and technical jargon. Do you imagine this is impossible to accomplish because your topic is complex? A great book to read is Randall Munroe's *Thing Explainer: Complicated Stuff in Simple Words*, in which he uses only the 1,000[1] most

---

[1] Or, as "thousand" isn't one of the thousand most common words, the "ten hundred" most common words.

common English words to explain airplane cockpit controls, tectonic plates, living cells, and computer data centers.[48]

Avoid *double-barreled questions*[49]—questions that actually ask two questions in one. "Do you agree that patient safety can be compromised by low nurse staffing or having too many patients in the clinic?" is an example. How should you interpret a "No" or "Yes" response to this? It's hard to tell.

2. Writing Response Scales can be Tricky.

There are several potential errors when you are writing Likert-type response scales for questions. A common one is a "forced choice," where you don't give the respondents the ability to say that they don't know the answer to the question. (Adding a "Don't know" category is typically recommended.) Similarly, scales can be unbalanced, or they can have anchors that don't make sense to respondents.

3. Even Subtle Changes in Question Phrasing can Markedly Change Results.

A 1987 Gallup poll asked a question in two subtly different ways—simply changing whether "who" or "which party" came first in a question (Table 15-2). The question was about whether the respondent cared about who won the 1988 U.S. presidential election. Putting "which party" in the first clause

Table 15-2 DRAMATIC EFFECTS OF QUESTION PHRASING ON SURVEY RESPONSES

Question Phrasing	Care a great deal	Don't care very much	Don't know
"Generally speaking, would you say that *you personally* care a good deal **which party** wins the presidential election in 1988 or that you don't care very much **who** wins?"	54%	40%	6%
"Generally speaking, would you say that *you personally* care a good deal **who** wins the presidential election in 1988 or that you don't care very much **which party** wins?"	76%	20%	4%

Note: Highlights are added to show the actual differences between the questions, which are easy to miss on a first reading.
Source: Adapted from Idid,[56] with source data from Ornstein.[57]

of the question *doubled* the rate at which respondents replied that they "Don't care very much."

4. Open-Ended vs. Closed-Ended Questions can also Markedly Change Results, Even when the Question is Identical and Respondents can Volunteer an Answer.

A 2008 Pew Research poll asked, "What one issue mattered most to you in deciding how you voted for president?" In one version of the question, respondents were simply asked the question. In the closed-ended question, they were read five options but could volunteer an option not listed. One of the five options was "the economy." Respondents in the closed-ended version of the question cited the economy as the single most important factor in their presidential vote 58% of the time, compared to 35% in the open-ended version—a relative difference of 69%.[50]

5. The Ordering of Questions Matters.

Even with perfect individual questions, your survey can vary markedly based on which questions come first. For example, a randomized study evaluated question order in a bullying victimization survey among middle schoolers. When students were asked specific bullying questions first, and then a general question, the prevalence of bullying victimization increased by 45%, compared to the opposite question order.[51] Similar magnitudes of effects are seen across very different domains. For example, a 2008 Pew Research poll asked whether Republican leaders should work with President Barack Obama or stand up to him on important issues. They also asked whether Democratic leaders should work with Republican leaders or stand up to them on important issues. When the "What should Republican leaders do" question was asked first, respondents said "Work with Obama" 66% of the time. If that question was asked second, respondents said "Work with Obama" 81% of the time—a 23% relative increase.[50]

6. Convenience Samples are Almost Always Biased.

Convenience samples are convenient, but that's essentially their only advantage. Avoid them for quantitative survey research. Instead, try to get a representative sample of the population you're interested in. That also means that you need to make sure your surveyed population includes people with insight into the question you're most interested in. For example, if you are interested in the effect of poverty on health behaviors, but your sample only includes people with an income of >$100,000 per year, your survey has a problem. Be attentive to your sampling frame and think through whether your sampling approach might introduce bias. Recognize that convenience samples almost always result in a biased population.

7. The Mode of Survey Administration Matters.

Even with exactly the same questions, the mode in which a survey is administered can affect responses quite dramatically.[31] Do not assume that modes are equivalent, or interchangeable, unless you've conducted a specific study to document this. For example, a study of the Hospital Consumer Assessment of Healthcare Providers and Systems (HCAHPS), which is used for public reporting and payment of U.S. hospitals, found that patients who were randomized to telephone/interactive voice response systematically rated hospitals more positively than those who received mailed surveys. In some cases, these effects were equivalent to a startling 30 percentile points in how hospitals would have been ranked.[52]

8. Nonresponse Bias can be Lethal for Your Survey.

You will always have people who don't respond to your survey. As much as you can, try to determine whether they differ systematically from people who responded. You might be able to do that through demographics (perhaps you know age, sex, education, and profession of respondents and nonrespondents), through other data sources, or through recontacting some people who initially declined your survey. Handling nonresponses is methodologically challenging.

9. Be Cautious When Treating Ordinal Scales as Continuous Variables.

In the analysis phase, it is common to code survey responses with numerical values. For example, surveys commonly ask a demographic question about respondents' race. An analyst might then represent responses in the data set as "1 = American Indian or Alaskan Native, 2 = Asian, 3 = Black or African American, 4 = Native Hawaiian or Other Pacific Islander, 5 = White, 6 = Other."[53]

Here, it is obvious that it would not make sense to calculate a mean or a standard deviation (SD), even though that field is represented numerically in the survey data set. However, Likert-type response scales are often associated with a number as well (e.g., 1 = strongly disagree, 2 = disagree, 3 = neutral, 4 = agree, and 5 = strongly agree). This makes it tempting to measure means, SDs, and other summary statistics that we associate with numerical, continuous variables. It is important to remember that these are ordinal, categorical variables, *not* continuous data. Sometimes it can be fine to treat them as continuous (if usually skewed) data, particularly with large sample sizes—but it is important to make sure that the assumptions of any statistical test you are using are met by the pattern of data you've collected, as discussed in Chapter 13.

10. Correlation is Not Causality: Be Cautious When Interpreting Key Drivers.

A common analysis of survey data focuses on the "key drivers" of a response. For example, you might measure physician engagement and wonder which factors drive this engagement. You then run a regression on the other questions you've asked on your survey—perhaps about time away from work, or satisfaction with support staff, or even the quality of coffee in the cafeteria—and you find that some questions are significantly associated with physician engagement. A common interpretation is that these factors **drive** engagement. That may or may not be true. They are certainly correlated with engagement, but the direction that causality flows is often suspect in these kinds of analyses. (Maybe physicians who are really engaged with your health system think coffee tastes better because they are generally happier at work.)

11. Surveys Can be Really Challenging to Design, Administer, and Analyze Correctly—Don't be Afraid to Get Specialist Help.

We'll end with what we started with. If there is one thing we want you to leave this chapter with, it's this: Surveys are easy to get wrong—and, for the uninitiated, bad surveys look remarkably similar to good surveys. Survey research is a highly specialized methodology. If you are making critical decisions based on a survey, consider getting specialist help.

KEY POINTS

- Surveys are attractive and powerful because they can be quick and relatively inexpensive ways to get information about a whole population.
- Surveys can be much trickier than they appear. If you are making critical decisions based on a survey, consider getting specialist help.

- Survey samples need to be representative of the overall population in which you are interested. This is usually accomplished by some version of random sampling because a convenience sample is almost always biased.
- Use existing survey instruments whenever possible. If you have to write a new instrument, don't skip the pretesting step.
- Numerous pitfalls exist in creating and analyzing surveys. Something as simple as changing the order of identically worded questions can change your results significantly.

REFERENCES

1. Miles C. A study of individual psychology. *Am J Psychol.* 1895;6(4):534–558.
2. Jones D, Story D, Clavisi O, Jones R, Peyton P. An introductory guide to survey research in anaesthesia. *Anaesth Intensive Care.* 2006;34(2):245–253.
3. Weldring T, Smith SM. Patient-reported outcomes (PROs) and patient-reported outcome measures (PROMs). *Health Serv Insights.* 2013;6:61–68.
4. Ware JEJr, Sherbourne CD. The MOS 36-item short-form health survey (SF-36): I. Conceptual framework and item selection. *Med Care.* 1992:473–483.
5. Spertus JA, Winder JA, Dewhurst TA, et al. Development and evaluation of the Seattle Angina Questionnaire: a new functional status measure for coronary artery disease. *J Am Coll Cardiol.* 1995;25(2):333–341.
6. Jha AK, Orav EJ, Zheng J, Epstein AM. Patients' perception of hospital care in the United States. *N Engl J Med.* 2008;359(18):1921–1931.
7. Fombonne E. Epidemiological surveys of autism and other pervasive developmental disorders: an update. *J Autism Dev Disord.* 2003;33(4):365–382.
8. Brandão-Filho SP, Campbell-Lendrum D, Brito ME, Shaw JJ, Davies CR. Epidemiological surveys confirm an increasing burden of cutaneous leishmaniasis in north-east Brazil. *Trans R Soc Trop Med Hyg.* 1999;93(5):488–494.
9. Board of Governors of the Federal Reserve Board. *Report on the Economic Well-Being of U.S. Households in 2016.* 2017. Accessed November 30, 2018, from https://www.federalreserve.gov/publications/2017-economic-well-being-of-us-households-in-2016-economic-preparedness.htm.
10. Morton ME, Wiedenbeck S. A framework for predicting EHR adoption attitudes: a physician survey. *Perspect Health Inf Manag.* 2009;6:1a.
11. DiCuccio MH. The relationship between patient safety culture and patient outcomes: A systematic review. *J Patient Saf.* 2015;11(3):135–142.
12. Macey WH, Schneider B. The meaning of employee engagement. *Industrial and Organizational Psychology.* 2008;1(1):3–30.
13. Lake ET. Development of the practice environment scale of the Nursing Work Index. *Res Nurs Health.* 2002;25(3):176–188.
14. Lake ET, Sanders J, Duan R, Riman KA, Schoenauer KM, Chen Y. A meta-analysis of the associations between the nurse work environment in hospitals and 4 sets of outcomes. *Med Care.* 2019;57(5):353–361.

15. Fox JD, Prado G, Baquerizo Nole KL, et al. Patient preference in dermatologist attire in the medical, surgical, and wound care settings. *JAMA Dermatol.* 2016;152(8):913–919.
16. Choudhry A, Hong J, Chong K, et al. Patients' preferences for biopsy result notification in an era of electronic messaging methods. *JAMA Dermatol.* 2015;151(5):513–521.
17. Linsky A, Meterko M, Stolzmann K, Simon SR. Supporting medication discontinuation: provider preferences for interventions to facilitate deprescribing. *BMC Health Serv Res.* 2017;17(1):447.
18. Scales K, Zimmerman S, Reed D, et al. Nurse and medical provider perspectives on antibiotic stewardship in nursing homes. *J Am Geriatr Soc.* 2017;65(1):165–171.
19. Kohn R, Madden V, Kahn JM, et al. Diffusion of evidence-based intensive care unit organizational practices. A state-wide analysis. *Ann Am Thorac Soc.* 2017;14(2):254–261.
20. Costa DK, Wallace DJ, Kahn JM. The association between daytime intensivist physician staffing and mortality in the context of other ICU organizational practices: a multicenter cohort study. *Crit Care Med.* 2015;43(11):2275–2282.
21. Costa DK, Kuza CC, Kahn JM. Differences between nurse- and physician-assessed ICU characteristics using a standardized survey. *Int J Qual Health Care.* 2015;27(5):344–348.
22. Weiner BJ. A theory of organizational readiness for change. *Implement Sci.* 2009;4:67.
23. Weiner BJ, Amick H, Lee SY. Conceptualization and measurement of organizational readiness for change: a review of the literature in health services research and other fields. *Med Care Res Rev.* 2008;65(4):379–436.
24. Aiken LH, Clarke SP, Sloane DM, International Hospital Outcomes Research C. Hospital staffing, organization, and quality of care: cross-national findings. *Int J Qual Health Care.* 2002;14(1):5–13.
25. Aiken LH, Patrician PA. Measuring organizational traits of hospitals: the Revised Nursing Work Index. *Nurs Res.* 2000;49(3):146–153.
26. Gnaegi A, Feihl F, Perret C. Intensive care physicians' insufficient knowledge of right-heart catheterization at the bedside: time to act? *Crit Care Med.* 1997;25(2):213–220.
27. Iberti TJ, Fischer EP, Leibowitz AB, Panacek EA, Silverstein JH, Albertson TE. A multicenter study of physicians' knowledge of the pulmonary artery catheter. Pulmonary Artery Catheter Study Group. *JAMA.* 1990;264(22):2928–2932.
28. Stevens JP, Kachniarz B, Wright SB, et al. When policy gets it right: variability in U.S. hospitals' diagnosis of ventilator-associated pneumonia. *Crit Care Med.* 2014;42(3):497–503.
29. Statistics Canada. *Survey Methods and Practices (Catalogue No. 12-587-X).* 2003. Accessed April 26, 2019, from https://www150.statcan.gc.ca/n1/en/pub/12-587-x/12-587-x2003001-eng.pdf?st=Qzmqiu9q.
30. Coggon D, Barker D, Rose G. *Epidemiology for the Uninitiated.* 2009. Accessed April 26, 2019, from https://www.bmj.com/about-bmj/resources-readers/publications/epidemiology-uninitiated/.

31. Bowling A. Mode of questionnaire administration can have serious effects on data quality. *J Public Health (Oxf)*. 2005;27(3):281–291.
32. Wimmer R. *Likert Scale—Dr. Rensis Likert Pronunciation*. 2012. Accessed December 13, 2018, from https://www.allaccess.com/forum/viewtopic.php?t=24251.
33. Revicki D, Cella D. Health status assessment for the twenty-first century: item response theory, item banking, and computer adaptive testing. *Quality of Life Research*. 1997;6(6):595–600.
34. Presser S, Couper MP, Lessler JT, et al. Methods for testing and evaluating survey questions. *Public Opinion Quarterly*. 2004;68(1):109–130.
35. Collins D. Pretesting survey instruments: an overview of cognitive methods. *Qual Life Res*. 2003;12(3):229–238.
36. Pit SW, Vo T, Pyakurel S. The effectiveness of recruitment strategies on general practitioner's survey response rates—a systematic review. *BMC Med Res Methodol*. 2014;14:76.
37. VanGeest J, Johnson TP. Surveying nurses: identifying strategies to improve participation. *Eval Health Prof*. 2011;34(4):487–511.
38. VanGeest JB, Johnson TP, Welch VL. Methodologies for improving response rates in surveys of physicians: a systematic review. *Eval Health Prof*. 2007;30(4):303–321.
39. Edwards P, Roberts I, Clarke M, et al. Increasing response rates to postal questionnaires: systematic review. *BMJ*. 2002;324(7347):1183.
40. Edwards PJ, Roberts I, Clarke MJ, et al. Methods to increase response to postal and electronic questionnaires. *Cochrane Database Syst Rev*. 2009;(3):MR000008.
41. Litwin MS, Fink A. *How to Measure Survey Reliability and Validity*. Vol. 7: Thousand Oaks, CA: SAGE; 1995.
42. Meek PM, Banzett R, Parsall MB, Gracely RH, Schwartzstein RM, Lansing R. Reliability and validity of the multidimensional dyspnea profile. *Chest*. 2012;141(6):1546–1553.
43. Morisky DE, Green LW, Levine DM. Concurrent and predictive validity of a self-reported measure of medication adherence. *Med Care*. 1986;24(1):67–74.
44. Wall RJ, Engelberg RA, Downey L, Heyland DK, Curtis JR. Refinement, scoring, and validation of the Family Satisfaction in the Intensive Care Unit (FS-ICU) survey. *Crit Care Med*. 2007;35(1):271–279.
45. TECHNICAL recommendations for psychological tests and diagnostic techniques. *Psychol Bull*. 1954;51(2:2):1–38.
46. Strauss ME, Smith GT. Construct validity: advances in theory and methodology. *Annu Rev Clin Psychol*. 2009;5:1–25.
47. Colliver JA, Conlee MJ, Verhulst SJ. From test validity to construct validity ... and back? *Med Educ*. 2012;46(4):366–371.
48. Munroe R. *Thing Explainer: Complicated Stuff in Simple Words*. Hachette UK; 2015.
49. Choi BC, Pak AW. A catalog of biases in questionnaires. *Prev Chronic Dis*. 2005;2(1):A13.
50. Pew Research Center. U.S. Survey Research: Questionnaire Design. n.d. Accessed December 18, 2018, from http://www.pewresearch.org/methods/u-s-survey-research/questionnaire-design/.

51. Huang FL, Cornell DG. Question order affects the measurement of bullying victimization among middle school students. *Educ Psychol Meas*. 2016;76(5):724–740.
52. Elliott MN, Zaslavsky AM, Goldstein E, et al. Effects of survey mode, patient mix, and nonresponse on CAHPS hospital survey scores. *Health Serv Res*. 2009;44(2 Pt 1):501–518.
53. US Census Bureau. *Race*. 2018. Accessed April 25, 2019, from https://www.census.gov/topics/population/race/about.html.
54. Cho YI, Johnson TP, Vangeest JB. Enhancing surveys of health care professionals: a meta-analysis of techniques to improve response. *Eval Health Prof*. 2013;36(3):382–407.
55. McPeake J, Bateson M, O'Neill A. Electronic surveys: how to maximise success. *Nurse Researcher (2014+)*. 2014;21(3):24.
56. Idid SA. Electoral studies: understanding some research problems. *e-Bangi*. 2017;(1).
57. Ornstein NJ, Kohut A, McCarthy L. *The People, the Press & Politics: The Times Mirror Study of the American Electorate*. Reading, MA: Addison-Wesley Publishing Company; 1988.

16 PREDICTIVE MODELING 1.0 AND 2.0

If we could see the future, could we improve our patients' care? For example, what if we could predict which patients may be at risk of a clinical decline in the next 6 hours?[1-3] What if we knew which patients in a primary care practice were going to skip an essential outpatient appointment?[4-6] And if we implemented an intervention—say, a reminder by phone—could we measure whether our intervention meaningfully improved adherence (or some other outcome)?

Predictive modeling in healthcare delivery science uses the models of biostatistics in healthcare delivery. A key aspect of these more advanced models—compared to those we've looked at earlier in the book—is that we can now begin to look at the role of multiple exposures in achieving the outcome of interest.

WHAT TO EXPECT IN THIS CHAPTER

One of the principles of predictive modeling—like all statistical analyses—is that you must understand the assumptions of your models. In this chapter, we will start with the basic building block of regression analysis. Three types of regression (linear, logistic, and proportional hazards) are workhorses for a tremendous amount of healthcare delivery science, and in fact for all the biological sciences. These regression models make two key assumptions: (1) each observation (or patient) is independent of each other observation; and (2) we understand the mathematical relationship of all the variables well enough that we can describe them accurately with specific functions that have a few parameters (i.e., these regression models are *parametric methods*). Sometimes this second assumption doesn't hold. In those cases, we can turn to *nonparametric methods*, and we'll do that in this chapter—exploring Classification and Regression Tree (CART) analysis. We will also have a section to help you avoid problems, in which we will discuss many of the common pitfalls and land mines inherent with each of these models. We call all of this *Predictive Modeling 1.0.*

Next, we will explore what to do when that first assumption—that each observation is independent of each other observation—doesn't hold. In those cases, one value predicts another value in the dataset. Ordinary linear and logistic regression simply can't deal with these problems. This is tricky to handle, and we'll call it *Predictive Modeling 2.0* to reflect that complexity. We will conclude the chapter with exploring additional methods that handle these issues, but that trade simplicity for complexity. These models better reflect the actual environment in which we deliver healthcare, but they may be harder to describe to other people. For example, we should have the methodologic flexibility to model the hierarchical nature of data (e.g., multiple patients cared for by a single attending physician, or multiple patients housed on a single medical floor in a hospital). The trade-off, though, is that complex models and their results are harder to explain.

PREDICTIVE MODELING 1.0

We have already discussed several univariable techniques in Chapters 13 and 14. These techniques allow us to test, one at a time, whether independent variables are associated with the outcome. When we begin to move toward predictive modeling, we move toward multivariable analysis. At its most fundamental, multivariable analyses are used to see if the independent variable most of interest continues to be important, while removing the effect of all other variables. However, we will find that many of these methods are useful for determining predictive strategies, such as developing scoring systems. We will start with parametric tools and then move to nonparametric tools.

Parametric Tools

Parametric models are models where we assume that we can describe all information about the data within the identified parameters. This typically uses a family of probability distributions and then allows us to create a mathematical model that best fits the data we have. Already, given the nature of our clinical environments of healthcare delivery, we can see that almost any model that we imagine is already almost laughably oversimplified. However, as we move to multivariable models, we can start to ask questions like, "Removing the effect of all other variables, what is the effect of our exposure (or independent) variable on our outcome (or dependent) variable?"

The most common models that appear in most of the medical literature are the models described here. We will spend additional time on many of them later in this chapter as well.

- **Multiple linear regression**—The outcome variable is a continuous value. Independent variables (exposures) can be either continuous or categorical. The result can be interpreted as follows: "For every 1 unit of change in the exposure variable, the outcome will change by the beta-coefficient." For example, you could use multiple linear regression to answer the question, "Given age, sex, blood pressure, and weight, can we predict someone's cholesterol level?" Thus, given these factors, the model would give you a number that is a patient's predicted cholesterol level. We will give worked examples later in this chapter.
- **Multiple logistic regression**—The outcome is a binary variable. Independent variables (exposures) can be continuous or categorical. The result, when transformed into an odds ratio, can be interpreted as "For every 1 unit of change in the exposure variable, the odds of our outcome will change by $e^{\text{beta-coefficient}}$." For example, you could use multiple logistic regression to answer the question, "Given age, sex, blood pressure, and weight, can we predict the likelihood that a patient has a diagnosis of diabetes?" Given those factors, the model would give an estimate of the probability that a patient has a diagnosis of diabetes (technically, it gives an estimate of the natural logarithm of the odds that someone has diabetes, but it is straightforward to convert that to a predicted probability).
- **Proportional hazards regression or Cox regression**—The outcome is the duration of time until the occurrence of an event, such as death or transfer out of the hospital, or the hazard rate. The result can be transformed into a ratio of the two hazards. Presuming the hazard ratio to be 2, the result can be interpreted as, "For every 1 unit of increase in the exposure variable, the relative hazard of our outcome will change by a factor of 2." For example, you could use proportional hazards regression to answer the question, "Given age, sex, blood pressure, and weight, what is the relative hazard that a patient will visit the emergency department for cardiac issues during the next year?"

Correlation and Multiple Linear Regression

Correlation is the strength of any relationship between two continuous variables, X and Y, denoted by the Greek letter ρ (pronounced *rho*).

The parametric value of linear correlation, termed the *Pearson correlation coefficient*, is designated with lowercase r. The value of r has no units and is scaled between −1 and 1. If two continuous variables have no linear correlation, then r = 0. A perfectly positive linear relationship (for an increase of 1 unit in X, there is exactly 1 unit increase in Y) has r = 1. A negative relationship (for 1 unit of increase in X, there is exactly 1 unit of decrease in Y) has an r = −1. Figure 16-1A–C illustrates these three examples.

The correlation coefficient tells us about the strength of the linear association between X and Y but does not tell us anything about cause and effect. As an example, consider two measurements of height and weight of a series of outpatients, with r = 0.6. This tells us that while the variables are related (taller people have greater weights), the value tells us nothing about a causal relationship between the two.

In linear regression, we are able to ask whether the change in one variable (termed the *independent*, the *explanatory*, or the *exposure variable*)

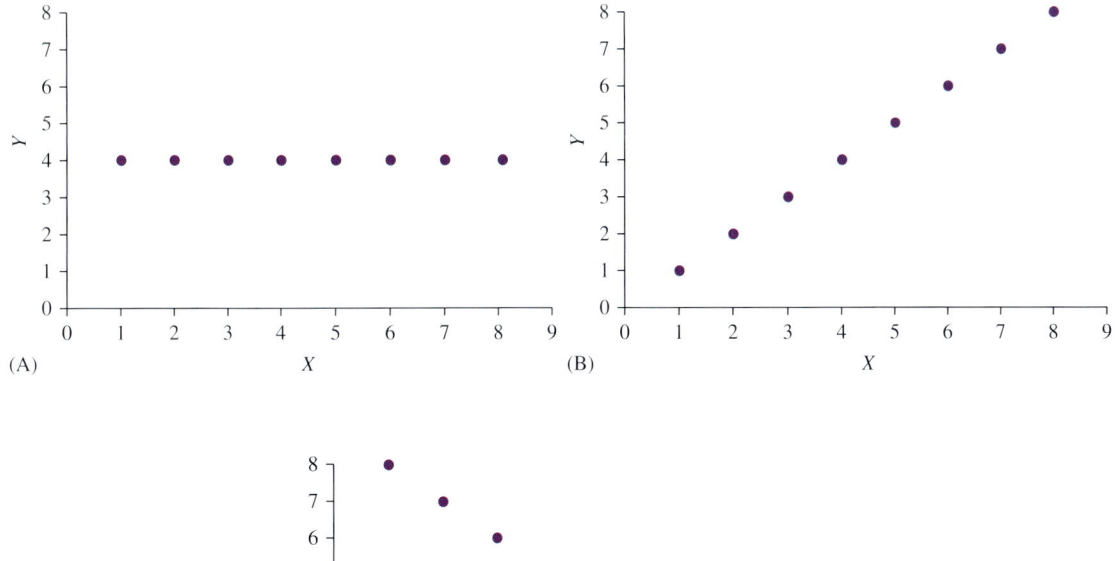

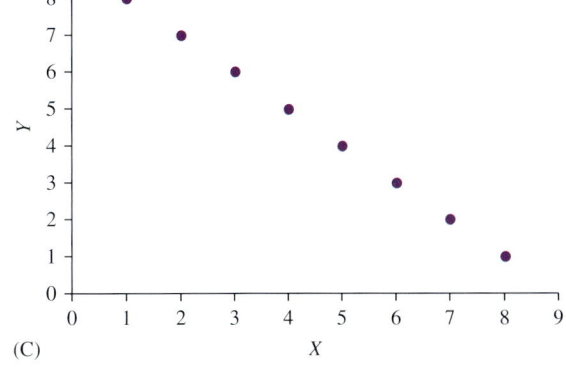

Figure 16-1 • **A.** X and Y have a Pearson correlation coefficient of r = 0. **B.** X and Y have a Pearson correlation coefficient of r = 1. **C.** X and Y have a Pearson correlation coefficient of r = −1.

corresponds to the change in our outcome of interest (or dependent variable). Is admission from a nursing home associated with longer lengths of stay on average for hospitalized patients? What is the relationship between each hour of the afternoon in a primary care practice and the average time waiting to be seen by the physician?

Fundamentally, linear regression graphs the dependent variable on the y-axis and the independent variable on the x-axis, and then generates the line of best fit for the data. Let's look at the example of hours since the primary care practice office opened (at 8 a.m.) versus the number of minutes patients are waiting to see a particular physician. The resulting graph would look something like Figure 16-2. We can fit a line to the graph in Figure 16-2, illustrated in Figure 16-3, which we can then express as an equation:

$$\mu_{y|x} = \alpha + \beta x,$$

where α is the y-intercept of the graph, β is the slope of the line, and where $\mu_{y|x}$ is the average number of minutes that a patient waits x hours from the start of the clinic day. The y-intercept is the mean value of the response y when x is 0 (i.e., at time 0, or when the clinic starts). If β is positive, then as x increases, y increases. In Figure 16-3, the equation is $y = 2.6x - 3.1$.

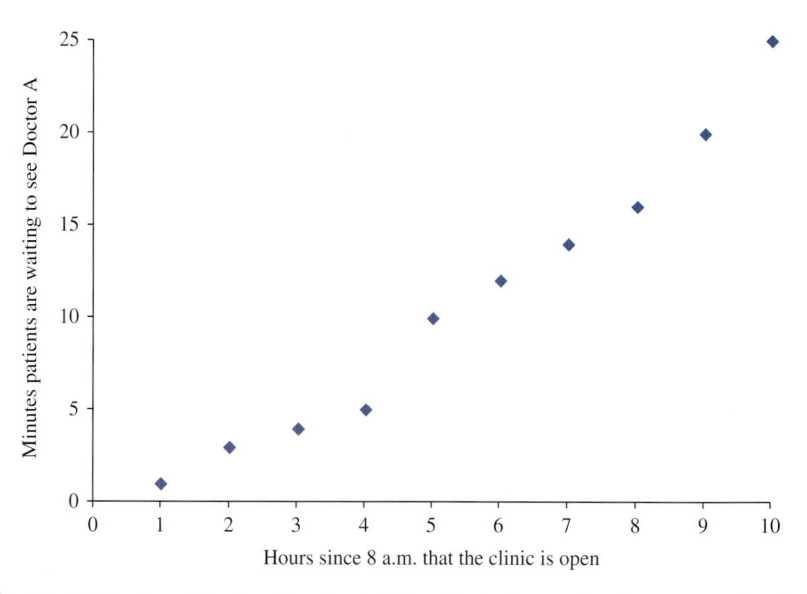

Figure 16-2 • A graph showing the relationship between the hours an outpatient clinic is open (the dependent variable) and the number of minutes that patients must wait to see Doctor A (the independent variable).

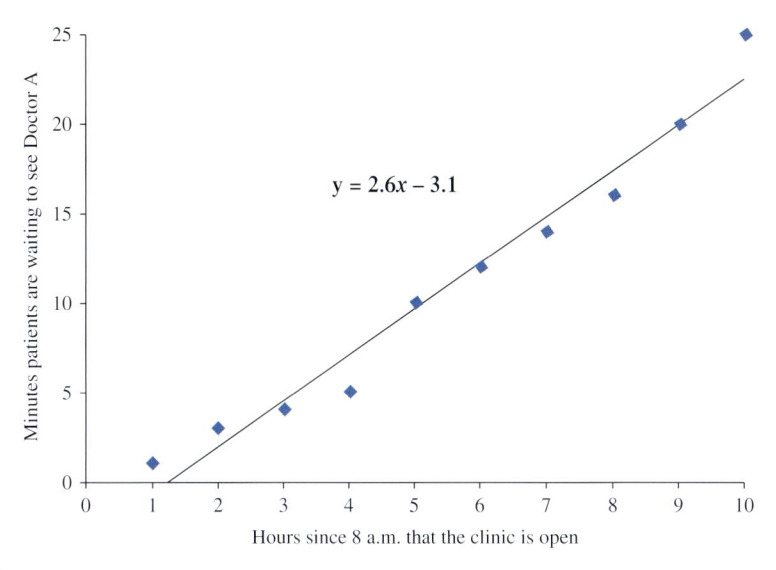

Figure 16-3 • A line fit to the data in Figure 16-2.

To translate our equation into words, we would say that
- At 8 a.m. (the *y*-intercept), the physician starts 3.1 minutes ahead of schedule.
- For every hour after 8 a.m., a patient waits an additional 2.5 minutes on average.
- If a patient arrives at 4 p.m., or 8 hours since the start of the clinic day, our model would predict that, on average, a patient would wait 17.7 minutes for his or her appointment.

In reality, on the day these data were collected, that patient waited 16 minutes for the physician. The true line that we actually fit is

$$y = \alpha + \beta x + \varepsilon,$$

where ε is the error term. When ε is positive, the observed outcome variable falls above the line, and when ε is negative, it falls below the line. The difference between the predicted value and the true value, ε, is termed the *residual*, which is a useful tool to evaluate whether the assumptions necessary to use a linear regression are met. For example, we've plotted the residuals from Figure 16-3 in Figure 16-5, which we will come back to shortly. You can see that there's no particular pattern to the residuals, which is helpful in thinking about the assumptions of linear regression, described later in this section.

Let's start with evaluating how good our predictive model actually is. One method is to consider R^2, or the *coefficient of determination*, which is equivalent to the square of a Pearson correlation coefficient of the same line. This value can be expressed as the fraction of the variability of the observed values of *y* that is explained by our model, or the linear regression

Key Point

The *residual* is defined as the difference between the predicted value and the true value. You should evaluate the residuals of your model to see how your model performed (i.e., did your model predict reasonably well?) and to see if your model meets the assumptions of linear regression.

of y on x. In our case of the model here, R^2 is 0.97, meaning that 97% of the variability in the amount of time that a patient spends waiting for the physician is explained by the variation in the hour of the day.

Next, let's make sure that the assumptions for linear regression actually can be applied to our data. These assumptions are the following:

1. The observations are independent of one another.
2. For any value of x, the distribution of y values is normal, with a mean $\mu_{y|x}$ and a standard deviation of $\sigma_{y|x}$.
3. The relationship between $\mu_{y|x}$ and x is a straight line.
4. For any value of x, the standard deviation of the outcome $\sigma_{y|x}$ does not change. That means that when x is a small number, the standard deviation of the outcome is the same as when it is a large number. This is termed *homoscedasticity*.

Key Point

Take note of the fundamental assumptions of linear regression. Many people don't do this.

There may be a problem here for our prediction model. For example, if we are interested in modeling length of stay versus age for hospitalized patients, we might see that the relationship between age and length of stay is not linear, as we fail to meet our linearity assumption (Figure 16-4). If we graph our residuals, we will see that the residuals at higher values of age are greater than those at lower values of age. If this is the case, unfortunately, our candidate linear model does not meet our assumptions.

We should note, however, this is not an unsolvable problem. To use linear regression for these variables, we can transform one or both variables to a different scale (e.g., squaring a variable or log-transforming it), so as to return to a linear function. But only by transforming our variables can we actually use linear regression in this case, something that we could diagnose only by both knowing the assumptions of the model and looking at our diagnostics.

Let's look at the residuals (or errors) to evaluate how well our line fits the data from our patient wait time model, and see if we can assume homoscedasticity (Figure 16-5). Fortunately, our residuals appear not to violate assumption 3 because they are evenly dispersed on both sides of 0. Put another way, our standard deviation of our predicted outcome ($\sigma_{y|x}$), the distribution of where we would expect to find the values of our outcome based on our predicted mean ($\mu_{y|x}$), should remain constant over all values of x. However, if we graph our errors and see that the residuals exhibit any kind of pattern, as shown in Figure 16-4, we have not met our assumption of homoscedasticity. In Figure 16-4, the residuals get larger as patients get older. In other situations, we might see that residuals swing from positive to negative as the value on the x axis gets larger (or vice versa). If this was the case, the assumptions of linear regression would not be met.

Caution

Make sure that you run diagnostics on your model. There could be something lurking in it that violates the model's fundamental assumptions. It is better to take the time to run diagnostics than to draw the wrong conclusion from an errant model.

But there is still one major problem with our model. It seems unlikely that our variables (duration of wait and time of day) are actually

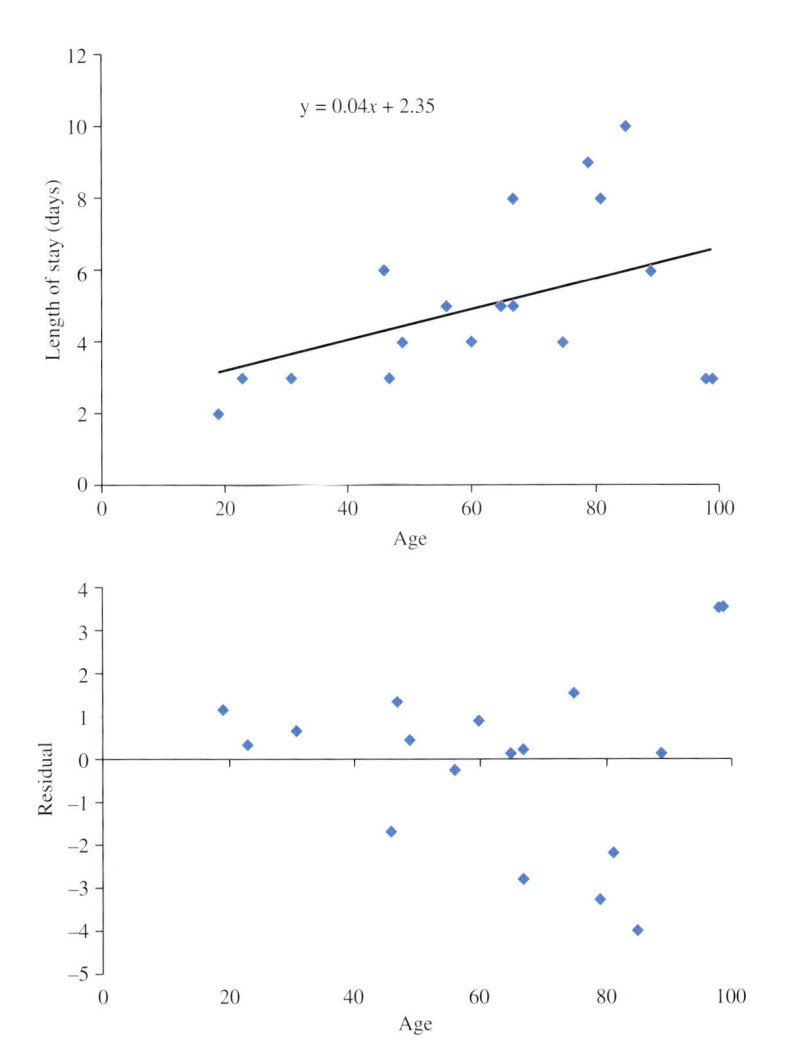

Figure 16-4 • A new model that asks whether length of stay is associated with the age of the patient. In the first graph, we have length of stay and age in the model, with a proposed linear model. The second graph shows the residuals of the model (the observed length of stay − the predicted length of stay, for each individual in the model). However, as patients get older in our population, the residuals get larger. This means that we can't apply a linear regression model to these data in their current form.

independent of one another. As an example, whether a patient has to wait 5 minutes or 30 minutes at 4 p.m. is likely not independent of how long a patient has to wait at 3 or 3:30 p.m. Further, if we measured it for two physicians, the values for y may vary by physician or cluster within each physician. We will consider ways to solve these challenges in the section entitled "Predictive Modeling 2.0," later in the chapter. Other methods, such as queuing theory and discrete event simulations, might be other

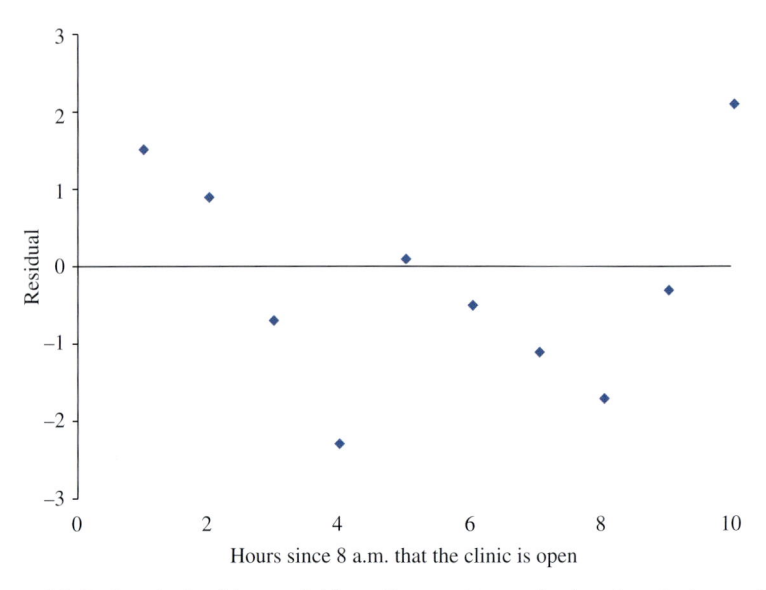

Figure 16-5 • Residuals of the model from Figure 16-3 graphed against the hours since 8 a.m. that our clinic is open.

ways to solve this problem, which will come up in Chapter 19. But for the sake of argument, let's pretend that each patient is completely independent of every other patient.

We're now ready to add more to our model and use multiple linear regression. The same assumptions will still apply (with all the necessary caveats mentioned previously). We can write our new model this way:

$$y = \alpha + \beta_1 x_1 + \beta_2 x_2 + \beta_3 x_3 + \ldots + \beta_q x_q + \varepsilon,$$

where α remains the y-intercept but now we have more than one explanatory variable, x_1 all the way through to x_q, each with its own coefficient. The x-variables can be either continuous or discrete. If we return to our original project, predicting the time that a patient will wait based on the hours since the office opened, we can now ask new questions of our data:

- What are all the factors influencing the patients' wait time?
- What is the relationship between the time since the office opened and the patients' wait time, if all other variables are held constant?

Perhaps we want to include whether the person checking in the patient has been hired in the last 4 weeks or not (β_1 is the coefficient for new hire, where NewHire = 1 if the person were hired in the last 4 weeks, and 0 if not) or whether there is a lunch conference (β_2 is the coefficient for lunch conference, where LunchConference = 1 if there is a lunch conference, and 0 if not). Then we will have a new predictive model that will allow us to predict the patient's wait time based on all three factors (whether the employee behind the desk is new, whether there is a lunch conference, and the number of hours since 8 a.m.). Our new model might look something like this:

$$\text{minutes waiting} = \alpha + \beta_1 \times \text{Newhire} + \beta_2 \times \text{LunchConference} + \beta_3 \times \text{HoursSinceOpening} + \varepsilon.$$

To put our results into words, we could say, "When controlling for new hires and whether there's a lunch conference that day, for each additional hour since the clinic opened, patients will wait Y minutes to see Doctor A." We would also ask, "On days with lunch conferences, how much longer do patients wait, on average, after controlling for new hires and how many hours have passed since the clinic opened?"

How do we know which model is the right one? That is to say, how do we know if we should include new hires and lunch conferences in the model? There is a trade-off to including all the variables we can get our hands on. Imagine that every time we add variables, we slice all our data into smaller and smaller buckets. In this model, we have three variables, each of which has several levels: new hires versus old hires; lunch conference versus no lunch conference; and 10 hours of data. That amounts to $2 \times 2 \times 10$, or 40 different buckets of data. The number of patients in each of those 40 buckets gets smaller and smaller, which makes us less able to draw a statistical conclusion about the exposures (i.e., we lose the power to detect a difference). If we add another two-level variable, such as the sex of the patient, we now have 2×40, or 80 different subsets of data. The cost of each additional variable, particularly for smaller studies, can be considerable (see the section entitled "When Good Models Go Bad," later in this chapter).

So, how do we choose which variables to include? One method is to include all the variables in the model that we think are important. The most important variables should be *confounders*, variables with their own relationship with both the exposure and the outcome (refer back to Chapter 13 for more on this concept). Maybe we think that new hires won't matter because there shouldn't be a relationship between hours since the clinic opened and when staff was hired. A second method is to conduct a series of univariable tests of association and only include variables that meet a statistical threshold for a relationship with both outcome and exposure (e.g., $p < 0.10$ or $p < 0.05$). A third method is to rely on your statistical software. Most statistical packages will make available at least two methods: forward selection and backward selection. These two methods help us select a model with the best fit (i.e., select the model with the highest R^2, which is to say the model that explains most of the variation in the data) while keeping the model as simple as possible. In forward selection, the program adds variables one at a time until one sees the greatest R^2. Backward selection works in reverse, adding in all the variables in the model and then removing them one at a time. There are many other approaches to variable selection in regression, each with its advantages and disadvantages.

Multiple Logistic Regression

Many outcomes in healthcare delivery science that we're interested in are not continuous but rather dichotomous, such as alive or dead, discharged home or to a facility, satisfied or not, infected or not. Our work so far in multiple linear regression falls apart when the y-axis now becomes a 1 or a 0. Instead, we become interested in predicting $p = P(Y=1)$ or the proportion of times our outcome is 1. And because we need to limit p to a value between 0 and 1 that is always positive while still attempting to fit a line, we use the odds of an outcome, which for any probability p is equivalent to $\frac{p}{p-1}$. Now our model becomes

$$\ln\left[\frac{p}{1-p}\right] = \alpha + \beta x,$$

and the method we are using is logistic regression. And we can use this model to predict the likelihood that our event of interest (e.g., death, discharge home, total satisfaction) will happen based on our exposure variables (e.g., severity of illness, exposure to early cardiac catheterization, age over 65).

The interpretation of our β coefficients is different than with linear regression, particularly with indicator (i.e., categorical) variables. We will use as an invented example a hypothetical study of whether patients admitted between 7 p.m. and 7 a.m. (the night shift) are more likely to die in the hospital than patients admitted during the day shift to the medicine floors of our hospital. Our exposure variable is an indicator variable where $\beta_{night\ shift} = 1$ if the patient is admitted at night and 0 if admitted during the day. Our outcome, y, is also a categorical variable, dead or alive. Our resulting logistic regression is the following:

$$\ln\left[\frac{p}{1-p}\right] = \alpha + \beta x,$$

where $\beta_{\text{night shift}} = 0.049$. In this case, the antilogarithm, or $e^{\beta_{\text{night shift}}}$ is the estimated odds ratio (OR) of the response for the two levels of the indicator variable. Said another way, $e^{\beta_{\text{night shift}}} = 1.05$, or the odds of death in the hospital is 5% greater when admitted at night compared to during the day. Multivariable logistic regression works similarly to multivariable linear regression, in that each estimate becomes the OR if all other variables are held constant. In our example, if we also added in the severity of illness of the patient, we would have a new ratio of the odds of death if admitted at night, controlling for severity of illness.

Logistic regression relaxes many of the assumptions that are required under linear regression, including the requirement that we have a linear relationship between the independent and dependent variable, that the residuals be normally distributed, and any requirement for homoscedasticity. But never fear—there are still rules to follow. The assumptions are:

1. The independent variable must be binary (or, in ordinal logistic regression, the independent variable must be ordinal and categorical).
2. Every observation must be independent.
3. Each predictor variable must be linearly related to the log of the odds of the outcome.

> **Key Point**
> Take note of the fundamental assumptions of logistic regression. Many people don't do this.

Assumptions 2 and 3 should be carefully considered as we use multiple logistic regression to understand and predict in healthcare. For example, if multiple patients return to visit the primary care office multiple times per month, we are violating the second assumption of independence if we conduct our analysis with the unit of analysis as office visits—because a single patient appears more than once in the data. Similarly, many common independent variables in healthcare, like length of stay and age, fail rule number 3. For example, it is unlikely that every decade of life is linearly related to the natural log of the odds of death as the decade before. Patients who are between 70 and 79 may be twice as likely to die compared with those between 60 and 69, but patients who are between 80 and 89 may be ten times as likely to die than patients in their 70s. If this is true, the relationship between decade and log odds of death isn't a straight line. However, if we include decade of life blindly in our model without testing this assumption, we risk underestimating the strength of the relationship with the dependent variable.

Creating a Scoring System or Prediction Rule

Multiple logistic regression can also be used to build a predictive score for an event. This can be accomplished in the following way:

1. Build a logistic regression model with all relevant variables included in the model.
2. Use the β or the odds ratios from each variable, rounded to integers, to assign points for each variable (e.g., if the β for a given variable is 2.1, that variable receives 2 points if positive, 0 points if negative).
3. Add up the points for each patient to identify a score.
4. Identify a threshold for when subjects are likely to have an event.
5. Build a 2 × 2 table to see how the cutoff performs with the actual data and calculate the specificity and sensitivity of the rule.
6. Validate the results. This can be done in several ways, including generating the original score in a *derivation data set* (e.g., 80% of the original data set) and then testing with the remaining data (the *validation data set*). Alternatively, one can bootstrap a smaller data set. *Bootstrapping* the data means generating a series of data from samples from the original data set and then testing the prediction rule with all these new data sets. Even better, test it in entirely new data from a different site. Some methods of evaluating prediction rules are presented in Chapter 18.

To make a score usable, make sure to use integers rather than multiple significant digits from the estimate, keep all points positive, and turn continuous variables into categories in the model. For example, rather than include age in the model as a continuous variable, create a categorical variable that equals 1 if the patient is older than 65, and 0 otherwise. In doing these steps, you are trading some model accuracy for simplicity and usability. We have included a case from the literature below to help you walk through these steps..

Once you have a candidate score, you will need to weigh the risk of false positives as opposed to false negatives. If we are developing a score to identify sick patients in the emergency department (ED), a false negative (reassuring us that the patient is well when he or she is not) may be more dangerous. However, if we have limited resources in our ED and we are concerned about alarm fatigue, a false positive may be more of an issue.

Multiple straightforward and more complex scores[7–12] have been created in the literature and are potentially useful for creating healthcare delivery strategies that can be calculated at the bedside for rapid clinical assessments, or with the aid of decision support tools. Box 16-1 walks through a case of building a predictive rule for patients with clinically suspected infection in the emergency department, based on work by Shapiro and colleagues.

Box 16-1 HOW TO BUILD A PREDICTION RULE

In this case, we will walk through how to build a prediction rule using logistic regression. We will use the work from Shapiro and colleagues[13] to estimate a way to predict mortality in a population of ED patients. We would recommend you review this reference to see how the authors derived this prediction rule.

Questions
Here are two example patients.

Patient 1: An 85-year-old otherwise healthy woman presents to the ED from home with a pneumonia on chest x-ray. She is breathing quickly (tachypnea) but is not confused, nor does she have any lab abnormalities.

Patient 2: An 85-year-old woman presents to the ED from a nursing home with a pneumonia on chest x-ray. She has 20% bandemia, low platelets, and is actively hypoxic and confused. She is in septic shock.

Using the Shapiro et al. paper, identify how the authors built their prediction rule and apply it to these patients. What are the scores for Patient 1 and Patient 2? What does the score estimate their mortality to be? And how sure are you of that estimate?

Responses
Identify Table 3 in the Shapiro et al. paper, which we have replicated here. First, the authors derived a set of independent predictors of mortality. Then, using the odds ratios for their point system, they rounded each odds ratio to an integer. You could also do this using their beta-coefficients.

Variable	Beta-coefficient	Odds Ratios	Points
Intercept	−5.45		
Terminal illness	1.8	6.1	6
Tachypnea or hypoxia	0.98	2.7	3
Septic shock	0.98	2.7	3
Low platlets	0.93	2.5	3
Bandemia	0.82	2.3	3
Age >65	0.77	2.2	3
Lower respiratory tract infection	0.66	1.9	2
From a nursing home	0.62	1.9	2
Confusion	0.5	1.6	2

(continued)

Box 16-1 HOW TO BUILD A PREDICTION RULE (continued)

How would you use this score? Let's illustrate how to use such scores in our given scenarios.

Variable	Score	Patient 1	Patient 2
Terminal illness	6	0	0
Tachypnea or hypoxia	3	3	3
Septic shock	3	0	3
Low platelets	3	0	3
Bandemia	3	0	3
Age >65	3	3	3
Lower respiratory tract infection	2	2	2
From a nursing home	2	0	2
Confusion	2	0	2

Patient 1 has a score of 8. Patient 2 has a score of 21.

Now, how do we use this in our prediction model?

In Figure 2 in the paper, Shapiro et al. present the results from their derivation and validation steps. We've replicated the output here, with the risk of death score for first the derivation group, and then the validation group.

Score	0–4	5–7	8–12	12–15	> 15
Derivation	2%	2%	8%	20%	50%
Validation	1%	4%	9%	16%	39%

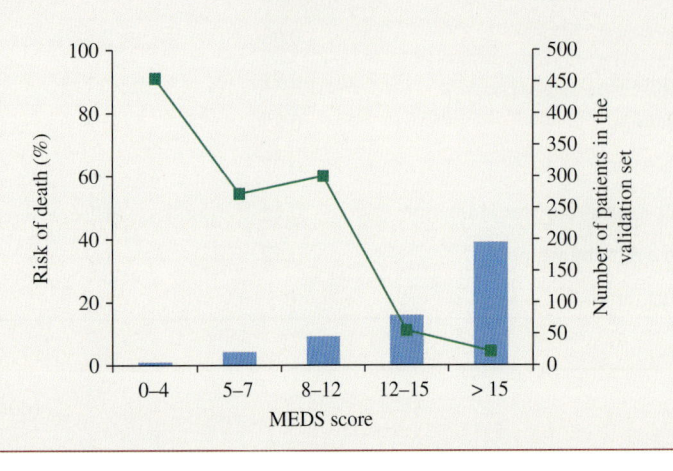

> Based on the validation cohort, these two patients have very different risks of death. Patient 1 has a risk of death of 9% (still pretty high!). Patient 2 has a risk of death of 39% (very high!).
>
> But how certain are we about Patient 2's risk of death? Her score is very high. However, if we look at how many patients were in the validation set with high scores, that was very few. That said, clinically, she seems at risk of mortality!

When Good Models Go Bad

Prediction models are filled with challenges. But there are major risks to us getting things wrong. In healthcare delivery, we are often building prediction models to focus limited resources in clinical settings. If we build a model to alert the intensive care unit (ICU) to sick patients on the floor, we want to get it right. Here are several land mines to watch out for.

Inaccurate and Models

It probably goes without saying that, to be useful, a predictive model needs to have some level of accuracy that is useful. If the model can't predict anything, it's not helpful. The most common measure of overall discrimination for models that predict binary outcomes is the area under the receiver operating characteristic curve (AUROC), and the most common measure of discrimination is the Hosmer-Lemeshow test. These are reviewed in Chapter 18's sections "Discrimination" and "Calibration," respectively. These are useful tests to get a handle on whether your model has reasonable predictive accuracy.

Additionally, the density of data available in the electronic health record (EHR) makes it tempting to include all possible independent variables in the model. This leads to three important consequences: the increased likelihood of a type I error (thinking that something is true when it is not, or a *false positive*), a type II error (obscuring something that is true from being seen, or a *false negative*), and a type III error (thinking that something has one effect when it has the opposite effect). A standard solution has been that, for every 10 or 20 events or outcomes, only 1 variable should be included.[14,15] As an example, if a study has 1,000 participants but 50 deaths, we should include between only 2 and 5 variables in our model. Unfortunately, we can't try to get around this problem by noting that there are 950 survivors and trying to include 95 variables; mathematically, we'll run into the same problem.

Caution

Unstable models come from the siren song of too many variables.

Overfitting and Underfitting

An *overfit model* is one that follows the data too closely. Overfitting creates a model that is both ungeneralizable and draws spurious conclusions—a bad combination! Overfitting comes from incorporating too many parameters, or variables, into the model. *Underfitting,* which happens either when we left out necessary parameters from our model or we chose the wrong model structure (e.g., a linear model for nonlinear data), is also a concern, as it risks drawing the wrong conclusion about the relationship between the variables and the outcome. We can run into both underfitting or overfitting when we have too few outcomes.

> **Caution**
> Overfitting and underfitting can make a prediction model useless.

Let's walk through two examples to illustrate this. First, consider the risk of the rare outcome. Let's say our analytic team wants to create a model to predict something that should never happen, like surgery that is performed on the wrong side of a patient. The investigators find out that this is an exceedingly rare event. There have been two wrong side surgeries in the past 10 years. Our analytic team puts together a model that includes surgeon experience, time of day, number of surgeries performed by the surgeon in the last week, and urgency of the procedure. We already know that we have a problem with this model because it will be overfit to our rare outcome—too many variables are included. As a result, if our model tells us there is an association seen between physician experience and the risk of wrong-side surgery, we can't know if that association is real. Similarly, if the analytic team picked even fewer variables for the model, the chance that they somehow managed to pick the correct variables out of all possible variables in the universe also would be low. We would need to change our methods (i.e., seek additional institutions to collaborate with to increase the number of outcomes or consider an alternative method of investigation, such as root cause analysis) to explore the drivers of wrong-side surgery.

In a second example, Nate Silver points out the risks of overfitting a model too closely to the data. In his compelling and easily digestible book about modeling and prediction, *The Signal and the Noise*, Silver describes the Japanese earthquake analytics that led the country to build the Fukushima reactor to withstand an 8.6 earthquake on the Richter scale. Based on data collected between January 1964 and March 2011, their model predicted that an earthquake of 9.0 magnitude would occur once every 13,000 years. The model that they built tightly fit a model of all modern data. Unfortunately, the earthquake later that year exceeded 9.0 and destroyed the Fukushima reactor. Had they drawn a more conservative model—a line less tightly fit to the data—they would have learned that the chance of a 9.0 magnitude earthquake occurring was closer to 1 in 300 years.[16]

Consider the Interaction

Not every variable is as straightforward as we might first suspect. Sometimes the effect of one independent variable on the outcome depends on another independent variable. Let's take another hypothetical example: Imagine that we are interested in whether there are differences between whether men or women are referred to specialist care. We have built a logistic regression model with the outcome of referral to a specialist. Our independent variables are patient sex (male and female) and patient age (under 65 years old and over 65 years old). When we include our variables in this way, we assume that the relationship between the variables is additive: There is an effect of sex; there is an effect of age; and the effect of the two together is the sum of these two coefficients. But what if young men are referred the least often, followed by younger women, then by older women, and finally, older men are referred the most? Now we know that older age reduces a woman's chance of seeing a specialist, but younger age increases her chances. This relationship between two variables is termed an *interaction*, or *effect modification*. Mathematically, the model goes from looking like this:

$$\text{seeing a specialist} = \alpha + \beta_1 \times \text{Female} + \beta_2 \times \text{Age}_{>65} + \varepsilon$$

to looking like this:

$$\text{seeing a specialist} = \alpha + \beta_1 \times \text{Female} + \beta_2 \times \text{Age}_{>65} + \beta_3(\text{Female} \times \text{Age}_{>65}) + \varepsilon.$$

By adding a new variable, the interaction between Female and age >65, we can estimate the coefficient β_3, which quantifies the additional effect of being a woman over the age of 65. Only by including and testing an interaction would this relationship between sex and age be visible. Interaction terms are not generally included by default in statistical packages—you have to include them yourself.

Caution

Effect modification or interaction is an opportunity to better understand your data and create a model closer to reality.

Consider Collinearity

Collinearity is defined as the state in which two variables are so similar as to include essentially the same (or at least very similar) information to explain the outcome. An extreme example is the variables *age in years* and *age in days,* which are perfectly collinear. One can see a variable is collinear with another when the standard error of the first variable in the model

> **Caution**
>
> *Collinearity* is a wasted variable that leads to estimates that are confusing to interpret.

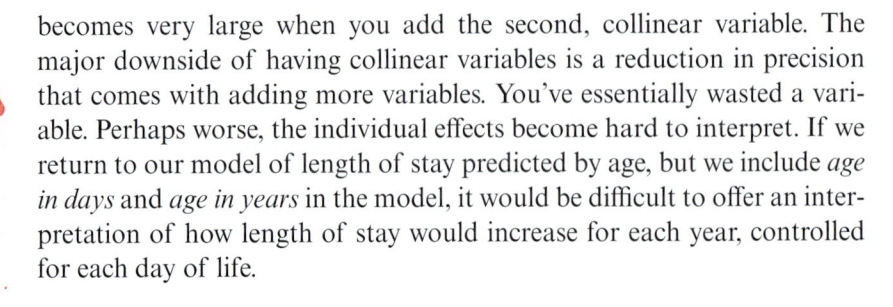

becomes very large when you add the second, collinear variable. The major downside of having collinear variables is a reduction in precision that comes with adding more variables. You've essentially wasted a variable. Perhaps worse, the individual effects become hard to interpret. If we return to our model of length of stay predicted by age, but we include *age in days* and *age in years* in the model, it would be difficult to offer an interpretation of how length of stay would increase for each year, controlled for each day of life.

The Strong Effect of Outliers

Occasionally, a single value for an observation may be grossly different from all other values and may have a strong effect on both the mean and the variance. Outliers require careful attention to one's data. Occasionally, an outlier may represent a true value (like a patient who stayed in the hospital for 400 days), which may lead the analyst to either delete this value or transform the variable to create less of an effect of such a large value. In other circumstances, a variable may have an incorrect value (like a length of stay of 4,000 days instead of 40 days) that was simply miscoded or miscalculated. These represent data that require cleaning. In either circumstance, however, without careful attention to outliers, the resulting model may be substantially miscalibrated.

> **Caution**
>
> Outliers can distort results and may sometimes result from errors in data recording that have gone unnoticed.

Nonparametric Tools

Nonparametric tools are particularly useful when no rational order seems inherent in the data we are examining. For example, when the variable in nature does not assume any obvious distribution, reverting to a nonparametric solution may be more appropriate. In this case, methods that use ranks, like the Wilcoxon Signed Rank Test, inherently do not require assumptions about distributions to make univariable comparisons.

In the setting of predictive modeling, Classification and Regression Tree (CART) analysis is a handy nonparametric strategy that allows the user to include multiple variables with neither prespecified interactions nor model statements. We will discuss CART models next, but also return to them in Chapter 17, because these become useful in understanding other tree-based models.

Classification and Regression Tree (CART)

The purpose of CART is to build a decision rule or prediction model without a prespecified hypothesis to guide the model. The design itself is resistant to many of the problems that we have identified in this discussion, including outliers and large numbers of variables. A CART splits our data into smaller and smaller piles so that the data in each pile are increasingly similar to each other and increasingly different from the other piles. The result is a tree-based model with each small pile of data as one of the leaves. At the starting point, or the *root,* all the observations are sequentially split into the best class (for categorical data) or regression model (for continuous data). Each branch, or *node,* is a subset of the observations and can either split further into *daughter nodes* or be a *terminal node.* The split is often binary on the value of a specific variable and whether a condition is met or not (e.g., age is >65 or <65). When an observation arrives at a terminal node, it gets assigned to a class.

The splitting strategy is designed to make each daughter node purer than the parent nodes. Put another way, the daughter nodes reduce the number of cases that are misclassified at each subsequent branch. At each stage, every possible way of splitting the observations is considered. The tree can grow and grow until none of the nodes can be split further; an extreme would be if the observations are split until only one observation lives in each leaf. However, this version of the tree would create an unwieldy structure that is overfit to the data and is poorly generalizable to other data sets and circumstances. To counteract this problem, one can restrict the growth of the tree by limiting the size of each node to a specific, predetermined number of observations.

To test a tree's predictive ability and judge its misclassification rate, much of what we've already discussed still applies. First, the tree can be generated on a derivation or test set of data. Second, the tree is then applied to a second set of data, the validation set. As more than one tree can be created from any set of observations, the tree with the minimum misclassification rate can then be selected.

A simplified example is illustrated in Figure 16-6. We have modeled the likelihood that a patient will be discharged from the hospital to an extended care facility. Each node is categorical, for simplicity. Under each node is the number of admissions. Nodes that go to the right are "No," while nodes to the left are "Yes." Beneath each terminal node is the probability of discharge to an extended care facility and number of admissions that remain. The first clear split is whether a patient is admitted from an extended care facility, followed by age, followed by length of stay. Reading backward, a patient who has been hospitalized for 10 or more days, is over 65 years old, but was not admitted from an extended care facility has a 65% chance of admission to an extended care facility upon discharge.

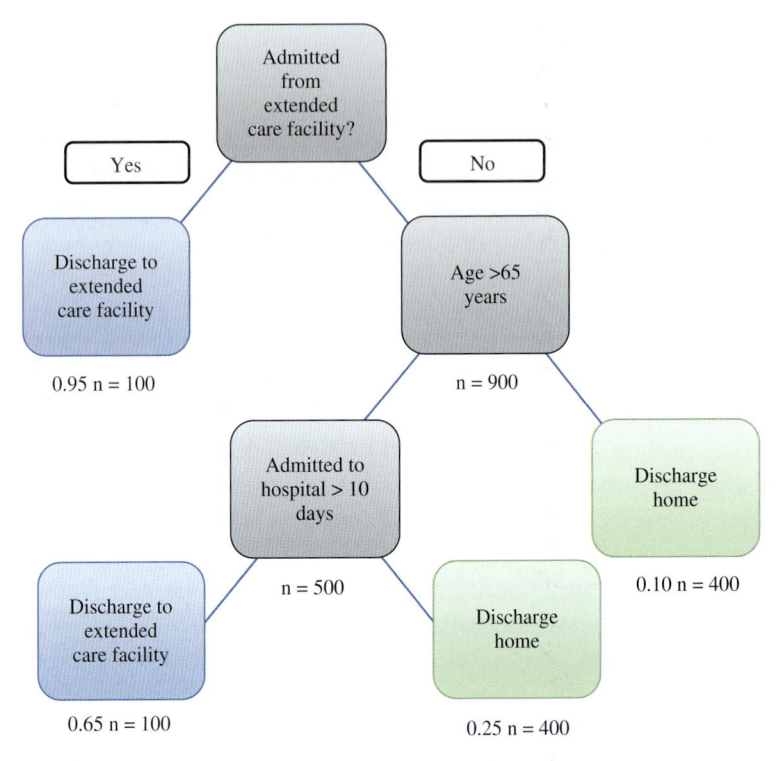

Figure 16-6 • A CART model designed to predict whether a patient will be discharged home from the hospital or to an extended care facility. The probability of discharge to an extended care facility is included at each terminal node.

Unlike other nonparametric modeling strategies or predictive methodologies, CART is relatively interpretable. In the example given here, outliers with excessively long lengths of stay do not change the outcome of our model. We also do not need to transform any part of our model, like length of stay, which often has a decidedly nonnormal distribution. So, what are the downsides? For one, CART trees quickly overfit the data, particularly if the branches are not pruned back or the tree is not validated. For another, we don't have a good way of quantifying how our tree performs. This type of modeling does not permit any confidence interval or ability to measure how much this has changed our pretest probability of an event happening. CART remains one tool among others when we consider the right approach for prediction. CART and its extension, random forest, are covered in more detail in the next chapter.

PREDICTIVE MODELING 2.0

Up to now, we have based all of our predictive modeling and design on the assumption that all our observations are independent of one another. For example, we have assumed that all hospital admissions are independent events. We have ignored that, in the real world, data cluster together and have multiple layers. Clinical values can be clustered within a patient, such as multiple vital signs or lab values over time. Patients can be clustered within a care unit or clinic. Alternatively, patients can all be cared for (i.e., clustered within) the same physician. And physicians may all work at (i.e., be clustered within) the same hospital.

Why is clustering important? We can imagine that these relationships should matter to our model. Patients will have some baseline heart rate or blood pressure; each measurement of that one person's heart rate or blood pressure is much more likely to be close to the baseline than a random, independent number. Hospital systems behave the same way. Patients in a given hospital are almost always more like each other than they are like patients in another hospital—and many of these factors aren't captured in a patient's EHR. For example, the culture of a specific hospital may mean that few or many lab tests are ordered, or specialists are called upon rarely or routinely.[17] The use of hospital resources in general appears to be clustered by geographical region.[18]

As an example, let's say that we were interested in predicting the likelihood of ICU admissions from the ED of 18 hospitals in a state. Critical to our planning for ICU beds, we include in our model patient characteristics (e.g., age, smoking history, and comorbidities), risk factors on admission (e.g., severity of illness, need for vasopressors, and need for mechanical ventilation), number of patients in the waiting area of the ED, and available ICU beds at time of admission. What type of clustering may exist in our data that may be relevant to this study? Perhaps some EDs have a lower threshold for admitting patients to the ICU than others, such that there is a defining culture of the ED about ICU admissions, and our model should cluster at the level of the ED. Maybe there isn't a dominant culture, but the ED physician and his or her management largely determines the likelihood of admission, so in that case, our model should cluster at the level of the physician. Finally, maybe the likelihood of admission changes by time of year, with influenza season changing the likelihood of admission. In this last case, we would need to cluster by month or season. Each of these could be tested and refined to see the predictive capabilities of our model and to best accommodate the realities of healthcare delivery with the appropriate mathematical approximation of

Key Point

Data in healthcare exist in hierarchies and clusters. Consider whether a model that accommodates clustered data is most appropriate for your question.

reality. Now, we can ask questions about between-subject variation (e.g., how different are physicians from each other) and within-subject variation (e.g., how do physician behaviors change over time).*

Perhaps most important, when we use models that accommodate the clustering of data, we make sure that we don't overstate the precision of our estimate and describe a statistically significant difference when none exists. Earlier in the chapter, we noted that if we have more observations, we increase our ability to detect a statistical difference. Further, 1,000 observations are better than 100 for making sure we're seeing the truth in the data. But if those 1,000 observations came from only 10 people (e.g., 10 patients with 100 repeated measures of heart rates each), we don't actually have 1,000 independent observations at all.

In the remainder of this chapter, we will discuss two types of models: linear mixed effects models (both random and fixed effects) and generalized estimating equations, which accommodate clustered data (i.e., they make sure that we include all 1,000 observations, but stipulate that the data come from only 10 patients). Keep in mind that both of these models are crucial not only for expanding your predictive analytics, but also for thinking ahead to how best to model and understand common risk adjustment strategies. We will delve into the latter in more detail in Chapter 19. Also, keep in mind that we are now becoming increasingly complicated statistically, so we would recommend seeking statistical assistance when putting these models into practice.

Linear Mixed Effects Models

We will start with linear mixed effects models and two simplifications of these models, random effects and fixed effects. And if we want to extend our model to include nonnormal data, we can use *generalized linear mixed effects models*, which we won't discuss here. Linear mixed effects models allow each cluster of data (e.g., each ED, each hospital, each state) to have its own separate, mathematical identity. In our example of EDs and their admissions to ICUs, we can imagine that each ED has a hospital-specific culture. We can measure that culture in some ways and with some variables

---

*The careful observer will recognize that we're predicting a risk of a binary event with this example. Patients are either admitted to the ICU or not, and so we're predicting the probability of that event. This is common throughout healthcare delivery science, and we found that it might be easier to think through the concepts of clustered data and mixed effects models than a model with a continuous outcome. But in reality, we couldn't use models relying on a Gaussian distribution (linear models). Instead, we would need models based on a binomial distribution with a logit link (derived from logistic regression). Alternatively, we could estimate the count of ICU admissions, which is a model that we haven't discussed, called the *Poisson model*.

(or parameters), but not others. We can capture the trajectory of each of these EDs (i.e., its "ED-ness") as a so-called random effect, which encompasses all the unmeasurable and site-specific features of the individual EDs (or patients with repeated measures over time, or hospitals, or however we have clustered our data). We now divide our parameters for our model into *random effects*, unique to the particular clustered variable (ED, in our case), and *fixed effects*, population characteristics shared by all admissions (e.g., patient variables like gender and age). All the local character of each individual ED gets captured in the random effects for each ED. Let's quickly also return to our model from earlier in the chapter, which predicted patient wait times based on the hour of the day. Here, we might want to study all the doctors in the practice and then use a random effect for each doctor, to capture the individual "doctor-ness" of each person.

When we get an answer from our mixed effects model, that result is termed a *marginal average response*. In our case about ICU admissions from the ED, our model will predict the average likelihood of ICU admission from the ED, *averaged over all the individual contributions of each ED*. Put another way, our results tell us what the average effect is of our population-averaged exposure (e.g., the gender of a patient) on our outcome (admission to the ICU from the ED).

These models allow us to ask questions of both between-ED and within-ED variations. This is the power of a linear mixed effects model. We can ask how much of the variation in likelihood of ICU admission is due to each individual ED and how much is explained by, for example, the marginal contribution of the gender of patients in all the EDs. These models also tolerate unbalanced data between clusters (or EDs, in this case) or over time, which is to say that these models can accommodate if one ED has many more observations (i.e., patients) than another. And because of the specificity of each model, we can take the model we build and apply it to any specific ED, rather than simply generate output for all EDs, everywhere.

The most simplified version of a linear mixed effect model is a *random intercept model* (we can also have just a fixed effects model, too, which we'll discuss next). In this model, the difference between the marginal average treatment effect and the subject-specific treatment effect is a subject effect b, in addition to the within-subject error. So, put another way, each ED in our example gets its own y-intercept and error term. But in a random intercept model, we assume that the slope of each ED's line is the same as all the other EDs. Put another way, in a random intercept model, we account for baseline differences in EDs but assume that the effect of the fixed effects is identical across all the EDs. If we think this last point may not be true and we want to make this more complicated, we can give each ED its own slope, called a *random slope* model.

> **Caution**
>
> A linear mixed effects model requires assumptions about the hierarchy of the model and the relationship of measures within each level of the hierarchy (the covariance structure).

One of the biggest challenges of a linear mixed effects model is the requirement that we have to make even more assumptions about how the data are related to each other. We have to propose a *covariance structure* for the model, or how we think the data within clusters are related to each other, before we can calculate our model. There are multiple covariance structures available. Let's use the example of heart rate and repeated measures of heart rate in a single patient over time. We have to make a few assumptions to identify the right covariance structure to use in our analysis. First, we could assume that the measures of heart rate are independent even if they come from the same person (a *simple* covariance matrix). Second, we could assume that the *covariance* (or the relationship between heart rates) decreases over time (an *autoregressive* covariance matrix), which is to say heart rates measured now are more related to each other than heart rates measured later. Third, we could assume that the relationship between heart rates is always the same (an *exchangeable* covariance structure). Whatever we decide, our covariance structure is yet another assumption that we build into our model. Models like generalized estimating equations, discussed next, take this particular choice away from us.

Another type of model that we can use is a model limited only to fixed effects. In contrast to random effects, a *linear fixed effects model* allows us to remove the effects of variables that don't change over time (time-invariant confounders).

Why would we want to do that? As a type of model derived from econometrics, it was designed to address the concern from earlier in the chapter that any regression model can account only for the confounders that can be identified and measured. Instead, a fixed effects model says that we can include specific group designations that capture the unchanging (i.e., time-invariant) characteristics of our study population, both unmeasured and measured, which then can be included as parameters in our model. These are our fixed effects, unchanging group parameters. By adding in these group-designation variables, we allow our model to control for all the heterogeneity encompassed in the fixed effects. But, importantly, these can't be the variables we're interested in. We will be controlling for these fixed effects, not exploring them further. Instead, the variable we're interested in studying needs to have at least two or more repeated measures because subjects will serve as their own controls. In a fixed effects model (and this is important), we now ignore the between-subject (or group) variation and ask questions only of the within-subject (or group) variation.

Let's return to our example of our efforts to model the likelihood of ICU admission from the EDs at various hospitals and identify how we could use a fixed effects model. Say that we are interested in whether a full ED waiting room (presented as a binary variable, full or less than full) affects the likelihood of ICU admission. Now we're no longer going to spend any time comparing ED to ED, like we did in the random-intercept model. We're only focused on the full waiting room issue. So we are going to make the EDs their own fixed effects in our model and remove all of the uniqueness of each ED (i.e., the measured and unmeasured confounders associated with each ED). And, to make our model even more complicated, we also want to remove the measured and unmeasured confounders associated with the reason for ICU admission, so we will include diagnosis as another, separate fixed effect in our model. And now, when we have a result about the relationship between a full waiting room and ICU admission, we can interpret this information as the marginal effect of a full waiting room versus a not-full waiting room on ICU admission within each ED within each diagnosis. In essence, in a fixed effects model, each ED is compared to itself at different times, but not compared to each other.

So why not always use fixed effects models? First, we may actually be interested in time-varying covariates alongside time-invariant covariates. When we limit our analyses only to fixed effects, we cannot ask questions of the time-invariant covariates. Second, our fixed effects model is less efficient than a mixed effects model. Often, the between-subject variation is much greater than the within-subject variation, and much of the true difference (and, therefore, statistical ability to answer our question) may be lost.

Generalized Estimating Equation (GEE) Models

Linear mixed effects models are really useful. They allow us to ask questions about how groups vary between each other (e.g., how much do EDs vary, one from another), or how to try to remove the effects of clustering altogether. But one of the greatest challenges we have with these models is whether we have some sense of how the individuals are related to each other (the covariance structure)—as a result, fitting the right model can be hard. The next model we'll discuss, the *generalized estimating equation* (GEE) model, is a flexible alternative when you have both correlated (clustered) data and either binary or continuous outcomes. And, so long as the population is large enough, the model does not require us to make any assumptions about the covariance structure, as mixed effects models do. The model is used when we are interested in questions that span the whole population and lets us make population-wide statements.

In GEE models, we are interested in either a categorical or a continuous response variable Y and a set of explanatory X variables that can be either categorical, continuous, or a combination. As in mixed effects models, we no longer have to abide by the independence assumption of the models described in the section entitled "Predictive Modeling 1.0," earlier in this chapter. We can assume that the responses Y are not independent, but rather are correlated or clustered. Similarly, we assume that the errors are correlated. Because of how the GEE model is fit (i.e., using estimates rather than a likelihood function, making GEE models semiparametric), we can't rely on the same type of model-fitting tools. For these reasons, GEE models typically need large numbers in order for the standard errors to come closer to estimating the true ones.[19]

Returning to our question about EDs and ICU admission, how could we use a GEE? We want to ask again about whether a full waiting room (versus a less-than-full waiting room) changes the odds of ICU admission. Let's imagine that there are multiple patients who visit EDs more than once, and that admission to the ICU from one visit to the ED to the next are not independent. A GEE model is useful here. We want our unit of analysis to be "ED visit," and we want to cluster visits within patients. Thinking about how to build the right covariance matrix for this is somewhat hard. We'll let the GEE do it for us. But first, we would need to assure ourselves that we had sufficient numbers of patients in this study that we could use the modeling process used in GEE.

How many is enough? We now need to make sure that we have enough observations and enough clusters or groups. There are several recommendations about how many groups (in our case, how many patients), and how many members of the group are needed (in our case, visits to the ED). Some authors have suggested that more than 50 groups are needed, with more than 20 members per group, while others have reduced the number of groups to 10 and the members per group to 5.[20] If we have enough patients in our analysis and enough repeat visits among many of them, we can create a model in which we ask what patient and provider characteristics affect admission to the ICU, given that the tabulation of patients visiting the ED more than once is not an independent observation.

GEE models allow us to ask questions population-wide. So if we want to ask whether full waiting rooms change the odds of ICU admission, we could design our model to cluster visits within patients (GEE models are frequently designed with one level of clustering, but can accommodate more).[21] Then we would include a number of other potential confounders measured on each patient, physician, and ED. Finally, we could look at the relationship between a full waiting room and the odds of ICU admission.

TAKING PREDICTIONS TO THE NEXT LEVEL

We have covered several predictive strategies in this chapter: linear models, multivariable models, accommodating various types of outcome data, understanding clustered data, an initial look at the models that can accommodate clustered data, and some nonparametric strategies that can help us understand and predict outcomes. In the next chapter of this book, we will move to discussing other methods that do not require upfront hypotheses about how variables should relate to each other, but instead take advantage of the underlying data structures themselves.

KEY POINTS

- Figure out the type of data you have (binary? continuous?) and then decide which model makes sense.
- Consider carefully the assumptions that are required for each type of model. Linear regression models have the most rigid assumptions.
- Prediction rules are often derived from multivariable logistic regression models. Use the simple steps included in this chapter to build one—but remember to validate your new rule!
- CART is a straightforward way of using nonparametric methods, while still being able to explain the resulting model. Consider using this method when you are uncertain of which variables are important and how they relate to one another.
- Healthcare data is inherently clustered data. If you ignore a hierarchy, you risk estimating your standard error incorrectly and making your P values look smaller than they should be.

REFERENCES

1. Kipnis P, Turk BJ, Wulf DA, et al. Development and validation of an electronic medical record-based alert score for detection of inpatient deterioration outside the ICU. *J Biomed Inform*. 2016;64:10–19.
2. Churpek MM, Adhikari R, Edelson DP. The value of vital sign trends for detecting clinical deterioration on the wards. *Resuscitation*. 2016;102:1–5.
3. Howell MD, Ngo L, Folcarelli P, et al. Sustained effectiveness of a primary-team-based rapid response system. *Crit Care Med*. 2012;40(9):2562–2568.
4. Goldman L, Freidin R, Cook EF, Eigner J, Grich P. A multivariate approach to the prediction of no-show behavior in a primary care center. *Arch Intern Med*. 1982;142(3):563–567.
5. Alaeddini A, Yang K, Reddy C, Yu S. A probabilistic model for predicting the probability of no-show in hospital appointments. *Health Care Manag Sci*. 2011;14(2):146–157.
6. Goffman RM, Harris SL, May JH, et al. Modeling patient no-show history and predicting future outpatient appointment behavior in the Veterans Health Administration. *Mil Med*. 2017;182(5):e1708–e1714.
7. Wells PS, Anderson DR, Rodger M, et al. Excluding pulmonary embolism at the bedside without diagnostic imaging: management of patients with suspected

pulmonary embolism presenting to the emergency department by using a simple clinical model and d-dimer. *Ann Intern Med.* 2001;135(2):98–107.
8. Cohen ME, Liu Y, Ko CY, Hall BL. An examination of American College of Surgeons NSQIP Surgical Risk Calculator accuracy. *J Am Coll Surg.* 2017;224(5):787–795, e781.
9. Escobar GJ, Greene JD, Scheirer P, Gardner MN, Draper D, Kipnis P. Risk-adjusting hospital inpatient mortality using automated inpatient, outpatient, and laboratory databases. *Med Care.* 2008;46(3):232–239.
10. Churpek MM, Yuen TC, Winslow C, Meltzer DO, Kattan MW, Edelson DP. Multicenter comparison of machine learning methods and conventional regression for predicting clinical deterioration on the wards. *Crit Care Med.* 2016;44(2):368–374.
11. Churpek MM, Snyder A, Han X, et al. Quick sepsis-related organ failure assessment, systemic inflammatory response syndrome, and early warning scores for detecting clinical deterioration in infected patients outside the intensive care unit. *Am J Respir Crit Care Med.* 2017;195(7):906–911.
12. Seymour CW, Liu VX, Iwashyna TJ, et al. Assessment of clinical criteria for sepsis: for the Third International Consensus Definitions for Sepsis and Septic Shock (Sepsis-3). *JAMA.* 2016;315(8):762–774.
13. Shapiro N, Wolfe RE, Moore RB, Smith E, Burdick E, Bates DW. Mortality in emergency department sepsis (MEDS) score: a prospectively derived and validated clinical prediction rule. *Critical Care Med.* 2003;31(3):670–675.
14. Peduzzi P, Concato J, Kemper E, Holford TR, Feinstein AR. A simulation study of the number of events per variable in logistic regression analysis. *J Clin Epidemiol.* 1996;49(12):1373–1379.
15. Harrell FEJr, Lee KL, Matchar DB, Reichert TA. Regression models for prognostic prediction: advantages, problems, and suggested solutions. *Cancer Treat Rep.* 1985;69(10):1071–1077.
16. Silver N. *The Signal and the Noise: Why So Many Predictions Fail—But Some Don't.* New York: Penguin Press; 2012.
17. Stevens JP, Nyweide D, Maresh S, et al. Variation in inpatient consultation among older adults in the United States. *J Gen Intern Med.* 2015;30(7):992–999.
18. Wennberg JE, Fisher ES, Stukel TA, Sharp SM. Use of Medicare claims data to monitor provider-specific performance among patients with severe chronic illness. *Health Aff (Millwood).* 2004;Suppl Variation:VAR5–VAR18.
19. Zeger SL, Liang KY. Longitudinal data analysis for discrete and continuous outcomes. *Biometrics.* 1986;42(1):121–130.
20. Hox JJ, Moerbeek M, van de Schoot R. *Multilevel Analysis: Techniques and Applications.* 3rd ed. New York: Routledge; 2017.
21. Shuts J, Ratcliffe SJ. Analysis of multi-level correlated data in the framework of generalized edstimating equations via xtmultcorr procedures in Stata and qls functions in Matlab. *Stat Interface.* 2009 2:187–196.

PREDICTIVE MODELING 3.0: MACHINE LEARNING

17

Machine learning and artificial intelligence (AI) are very trendy right now, with coverage in the popular press, accompanied by more than 45,000 articles on PubMed, and more every day. Part of this popularity is certainly because of some major advances in machine learning's capabilities: recent studies have achieved results that simply weren't possible just a decade ago. But this popularity also runs the risk of overpromising what machine learning can actually deliver in healthcare, at least in the short and medium term.

How should a health system leader engage with machine learning? The goal of this chapter is to give you an understanding of some of the key points of machine learning. Specifically, we are hoping to help you develop an intuition for how machine learning works and what it can do ... but we are specifically *not* trying to teach you how to implement machine learning algorithms. We assume that you've read the chapters that come before this one, focused on data in healthcare and traditional epidemiological modeling techniques—and we'll build on that knowledge to help you better understand machine learning, AI, and what they can do in healthcare.

DEFINITIONS: WHAT IS ARTIFICIAL INTELLIGENCE? MACHINE LEARNING?

General Versus Specific Artificial Intelligence (AI)

An important distinction separates general from specific AI. Artificial general intelligence (AGI) is the stuff of science fiction—a computerized intelligence that can learn, handle any task that a human intelligence can take on, and become self-improving. AGI would be able to handle the same range of problems that a human could (or more) and do them as well as (or better than) a human. This is also sometimes called *strong AI*, and, importantly, it does not exist today. However, AGI is an active area of research for many groups around the world.

Key Point

Artificial general intelligence (AGI)—a computerized intelligence that can learn, handle any task that a human intelligence can take on, and become self-improving—does not exist today, though it is an area of active research.

On the other hand, specific AI (also called *narrow AI* and *weak AI*) focuses on one specific, narrow task (hence the name) and gets really good at doing that one task. For example, you can now search through your home photos to find all the pictures of cats (or flowers, meals, or family members) without ever having tagged your photos with information about what's in them. Similarly, a research team trained an algorithm to identify diabetic retinopathy from photos.[1] That algorithm was then shown to be better than U.S. board-certified ophthalmologists, but just at that one, narrow problem.[2] Ask the algorithm to fill out a form, have a conversation, or go grocery shopping, and the difference between general and specific AI becomes immediately apparent.

Specific, narrow AI seems likely to materially affect healthcare in the coming years—and in fact, we are already beginning to see its impact. AGI seems likely to be quite a long way off—though with the caution that any exponential technology acceleration may seem very far off until suddenly it's here.

> **Key Point**
> Specific (or narrow) AI focuses on one particular task. It may have outstanding (and even superhuman) performance on that one task, but its skills cannot generalize to other problems. This kind of AI exists and is in use today.

Machine Learning and *Artificial Intelligence* (AI)

The terms *machine learning* and *artificial intelligence* are often used interchangeably, though they are different. John McCarthy, one of the pioneers of AI, defined it as "the science and engineering of making intelligent machines."[3] Another way of thinking of AI is that it is the discipline involved with creating machines that *appear* intelligent, whether that apparent intelligence is visual perception and classification, language processing, or AGI. Machine learning is usually regarded as being one of many possible techniques to achieve AI (Figure 17-1). The canonical definition of *machine learning*—"the ability to learn without being explicitly programmed"—is often attributed to Arthur Samuel. Another important characteristic is that machine-learned algorithms should perform well on data they've never seen before. Showing remarkable foresight, Samuel noted: "Programming computers to learn from experience should eventually eliminate the need for much of this detailed programming effort," a statement that has clearly been borne out with today's advances in deep learning.[4] What that means is that machine learning systems learn from examples rather than being programmed with large numbers of IF-THEN statements.

Many early AI systems did not actually use machine learning, but instead were programmed by experts in the field working with computer scientists. For example, IBM's Deep Blue was a computer program that in 1997 defeated Garry Kasparov, the world champion in chess. This was a remarkable achievement because it is estimated that there are at least 10^{120} possible ways that a game of chess can play out (the so-called *Shannon*

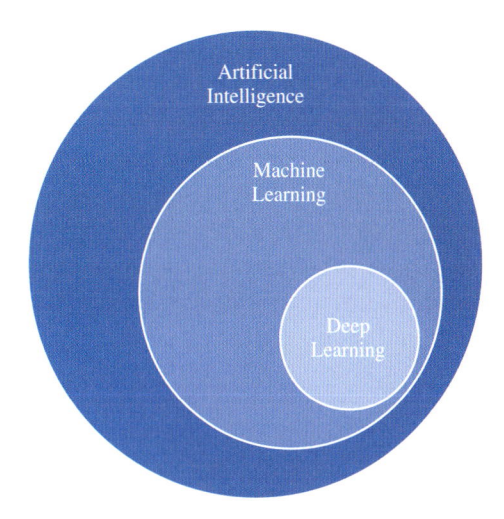

Figure 17-1 • The relationships between AI, machine learning, and deep learning.

number). Deep Blue was a type of AI known as *symbolic AI* (sometimes called *good-old-fashioned AI*) that was created specifically to play world-class chess. It used very efficient algorithms to search through hundreds of millions of decision trees for any given move to sort through how to respond to a particular situation in a chess game.[5] Even today, many AI systems have a blend of machine-learned and handcrafted components.

A different approach was taken by DeepMind, whose AlphaGo defeated professional players of Go (an ancient two-player game of strategy, played on a 19 × 19 grid), and then the world champion at the game in 2016. This was also a remarkable accomplishment, one that most had predicted would require at least another decade of development to achieve because the number of legal positions in a Go game is about 2×10^{170}. (This is an almost unimaginably large number—the number of atoms in the observed universe is estimated to be about 10^{80}.) AlphaGo was never programmed to respond to particular situations in Go. Instead, it was told what the rules of the game were and what "winning the game" meant. It then used a data set of 30 million positions from games of Go and *learned* how expert humans played. Using this as a starting point, it then played itself many, many times using a technique called *reinforcement learning*—in the process, learning about tactics and strategies that were associated with winning.[6] A subsequent version of AlphaGo learned only by playing against itself, without human knowledge, and quickly exceeded the performance of previous versions.[7] Both Deep Blue and AlphaGo appear intelligent—playing chess and playing Go are both complex, hard things to do—but they used quite different approaches to achieve their goals.

Key Point

Machine learning is the discipline of designing systems that can learn without being explicitly programmed. The key insight is that it is now often easier to program a computer to learn from examples than to hard-code it with specific instructions.

A BRIEF HISTORY OF ARTIFICIAL INTELLIGENCE

Origin, Springtimes, and AI Winters

The modern conception of AI seems to have begun in the 1950s. At the start of the decade, Alan Turing published a paper called "Computing Machinery and Intelligence."[8] This paper begins with the startling question: "I propose to consider the question, 'Can machines think?'." John McCarthy introduced the term *artificial intelligence (AI)* in the proposal for a 1956 conference on the subject.[9]

Over the intervening decades, AI has gone through several cycles of enthusiasm and hype ... followed by retrenchment, reduced research funding, and pessimism. The negative periods are often called *AI Winters*. After the first bout of enthusiasm in the 1950s and 1960s, the first AI Winter began in the mid-1970s, following a series of negative studies culminating in the United Kingdom's Lighthill report, which found that AI had profoundly failed to live up to its inflated expectations. A resurgence occurred in the late 1970s and early 1980s, followed by a second AI Winter that lasted well into the 1990s, and perhaps 2000s. Thawing began in the late 1990s. Important discoveries (like Hinton's, LeCun's, and others' work on backpropagation of errors in the mid-1980s) were accompanied by popular successes, such as IBM Deep Blue's defeat of the world champion in chess in 1997. This thawing accelerated in the late 2000s.[10–14]

Why Is Now Different?

There are at least three reasons why many feel that we are now in an AI springtime that is meaningfully different from past decades. This seems particularly true in healthcare.

Better Algorithms

We can see the impact of the development and implementation of new algorithms in dramatic improvements in computer vision performance. A common problem in AI is classifying images: Is this a cat? A dog? A person? A sandwich? The ImageNet Large-Scale Visual Recognition Challenge is an annual event that has been held since 2010. In 2011, a high-performing algorithm had about a 25% error rate. In 2012, there was a marked, sudden improvement compared with prior years—this improvement (and every subsequent winner of the challenge) has used a type of algorithm called *deep learning* (Figure 17-2). The technical improvements in these algorithms are among the major changes that make today's machine learning and AI different from what came before.

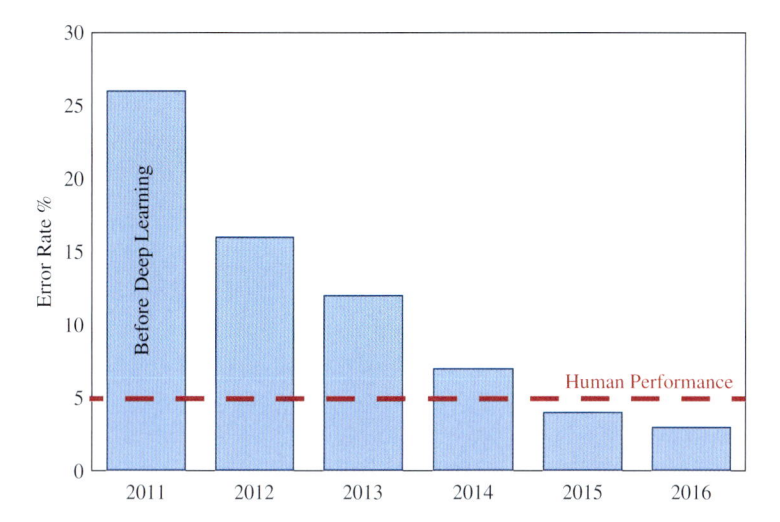

CHAPTER 17 | PREDICTIVE MODELING 3.0: MACHINE LEARNING

Figure 17-2 • Improvement in image recognition with deep learning. The ImageNet Large Scale Visual Recognition Challenge is an annual challenge that has been running since 2010. In 2012, a type of deep learning network (a CNN) resulted in marked improvements in machines' ability to classify and identify images.

The 2012 ImageNet results heralded the rise of deep learning. Other technical advances (such as pretraining and other data augmentation techniques) also created capabilities that hadn't existed before.[15]

More Computing Power

Training machine learning algorithms can be extremely computationally intensive. Historically, statistical computation was done by central processing units (CPUs). A key insight in the 2000s was that graphics processing units (GPUs) significantly reduced the training time for neural network algorithms. GPUs were developed largely to enable low-latency video games; but why would they help with machine learning, and in particular deep learning? It turns out that a particular computationally intensive part of training the networks is repeated multiple *matrix multiplication*. It turns out that GPUs are very good at doing many calculations all at once because they have large numbers of cores and threads—with the tradeoff that each of these cores is much simpler than a CPU core. This characteristic, which originally was developed to allow very rapid graphics processing, turns out to be very good at doing very fast matrix multiplication ... thus speeding up deep learning training. Today, there are systems and processors that have been specifically created to speed up deep learning applications.

How much of an increase in computation applied to machine learning does this represent? An analysis in 2018 showed that, since 2012, the amount of computation used in the largest reported AI training studies has increased by a startling 300,000 times. The amount of computation doubled every 3.5 months (compared to an 18-month doubling period according to Moore's Law.)[16]

More Data

Availability of data is key to machine learning, especially in healthcare. Over the past decade, the U.S. health system has rapidly digitized. In 2008, only 1.5% of U.S. hospitals had a comprehensive electronic health record (EHR).[17] By 2015, this number was 90%, and it has continued to rise since then. One report estimated that the amount of healthcare data in 2013 was 153 exabytes and would grow to 2.314 zettabytes by 2020.[18] This is an almost incomprehensible amount of data. Table 17-1 gives an intuitive sense of the scale of these numbers.

Table 17-1 HOW MUCH DATA IS AN EXABYTE?

A kilosecond ago …	was less than 20 minutes ago.
A megasecond ago …	was about 12 days ago.
A gigasecond ago …	Ronald Reagan was president.
A terasecond ago …	was before recorded history.
2 petaseconds ago …	the dinosaurs went extinct.
An exasecond ago …	was before the Big Bang.

Note: Today's healthcare data is now measured in petabytes and exabytes. It can be almost impossible to get a realistic conception of the scale of these numbers. This table uses an analogy of time to help provide some sense of scale.

TRANSLATING EPIDEMIOLOGY TO MACHINE LEARNING

One of the challenges in understanding machine learning is that this field uses very different terms to refer to common terms from epidemiology and biostatistics—same meaning, but different terms. This sounds trivial, but it is actually a significant barrier to learning. Table 17-2 reviews common, analogous terms between the fields.

Table 17-2 TRANSLATING EPIDEMIOLOGY TO MACHINE LEARNING

Epidemiology Term	Machine-Learning Term
Outcomes (Dependent variables)	Labels
Potential predictor variables (Independent variables)	Features
Positive predictive value	Precision
Sensitivity	Recall
Model coefficients (e.g., β coefficients)	Weights
Model intercepts	Bias terms
R × C table (e.g., a 2 × 2 table)	Confusion matrix
Derivation set	Training data
Multinomial logistic regression	Softmax classifier
Randomized trial	A/B testing
Outcome measurement error	Noisy labels
Fitting (a model)	Training
Bootstrap aggregation	Bagging
LASSO	L1 regularization
Ridge regression	L2 regularization

Note: Many terms in machine learning have analogous concepts and terms in epidemiology and biostatistics.

CATEGORIES OF MACHINE LEARNING USED IN HEALTHCARE

There is no crisp, bright line between traditional epidemiological/statistical models and machine learning. Instead, the lines are blurry. The Framingham Risk Score, designed to gauge an individual's cardiovascular risk, is a good example of this, as Beam and Kohane elucidated.[19] This score predicts a 10-year risk of cardiac adverse events by assigning various points to risk factors like age. This doesn't sound like machine learning, but the risk points were entirely learned from data using a proportional hazards model. When we ask a traditional statistical program to do forward-, stepwise-, or backward-selection of variables in a logistic regression, the program is making decisions about which variables belong in a model based on statistical factors.

Beam and Kohane argue that we can look at these kinds of analytical frameworks as a progression from fully/mostly human supervised to increasingly more decision-making by the machine—with a progression from clinical wisdom to regression methods to random forests to neural networks.[19] Here, we will follow that approach, with particular attention to some approaches that have documented successes in healthcare. Because more traditional statistical and epidemiological models (like logistic and linear regression and hierarchical models) have been covered in previous chapters, the rest of this chapter will focus on models that are usually called *machine learning models*.

What Is the Machine-Learning Algorithm Trying to Optimize? The Importance of the Loss (or Cost, or Objective) Function

> **Key Point**
>
> Machine-learning algorithms have a numerical function that they seek to minimize or maximize. This is often called a *loss function (or cost function, or objective function)*. For example, the sum of the square of errors is a common loss function, just as in many traditional modeling techniques.

Even though this chapter is not focused on implementation details of machine learning, it is important to realize that each machine learning algorithm has something that it is trying to optimize. The goal of the algorithm is usually to maximize or minimize something: for example, the goal might be to minimize some measurement of the amount of prediction error (e.g., the sum of the squares of the error in a prediction*). This goal has various names—the *objective function, cost function,* or *loss function*. Here's the key point: Each algorithm starts with various configurations (e.g., parameters) under its control and then tweaks them, with the goal of minimizing or maximizing this particular function. Many advances in machine learning have had to do with ways to minimize the loss function in computationally efficient ways.[20]

Supervised and Unsupervised Learning

For the rest of this discussion, we will focus mostly on *supervised learning*—the kind of machine learning where you give the algorithm labeled examples of what you want to predict or classify (e.g., a data set in which you know how long a patient's length of stay was, or whether she or he was readmitted, or the rating of the healthcare experience), and then the algorithm learns the best way to classify or predict the label. *Unsupervised learning* means that the data set does not have labels for what you want to

---

* Why use the sum of the square of errors instead of just the sum of errors (or the sum of the absolute value of the errors)? Because you would usually prefer several small errors in prediction than a few big errors. If your algorithm misses by 1, $1^2 = 1$. If it misses by 2, $2^2 = 4$. But if it misses by 5, $5^2 = 25$ (and $10^2 = 100$, and so on).

classify or predict. Unsupervised machine learning algorithms are commonly used for cluster analysis (finding similar groups). For example, Vanfleteren et al. used unsupervised learning and identified that patients with chronic obstructive pulmonary disease (COPD) have five types of comorbidity clusters. Similarly, Seymour et al. used unsupervised clustering methods to identify phenotypes in sepsis. Today, however, most practical applications of machine learning in healthcare result from supervised methods.[21,22] The rest of this chapter will focus on supervised learning.

Tree-Based Models

Tree-based models are statistical approaches to classification that mirror decision trees or clinical pathways: You start with the most important factors and follow the branch points until you reach a prediction. This has the advantage of being clinically intuitive. For example, if you were interested in predicting whether someone has a high-enough risk for a heart attack in the next ten years that you should prescribe statins, you might first ask, "Does this person have diabetes?" Anyone who said "Yes" would be high-risk. Among people who said "No," you might then ask, "Do they smoke?" People who said "Yes" would be high-risk. Among people who said "No," you might then ask about their blood pressure or cholesterol, and so on until you had classified people into risk categories.

Classification and Regression Tree (CART) Analysis

Classification and Regression Tree (CART) analysis is one of the more common tree-based methods and is well established in the healthcare literature. We covered this concept briefly in Chapter 16, but we will now reframe it in terms of machine learning, and as a component of more sophisticated methods. While classification and regression are different (classification models give a categorical outcome, and regression models a continuous outcome), the concepts are the same. The method is based on recursive partitioning and, because it does not require parametric assumptions, it can inherently handle skewed continuous data and multicategory predictors. Each value of a potential predictor is evaluated based on how well it splits the sample into what you're trying to predict. Good predictors split the population into unequal populations: one group with a high percentage of the outcome of interest and another with a low percentage of the outcome. How does it do this? It minimizes the loss function (usually based on either the sum of squared errors for continuous predictors, or the Gini index for categorical predictors). The algorithm then continues partitioning the data set until you reach a stopping criterion, which is typically a certain number of patients in one of the child nodes. Extending the tree metaphor, there is also a *pruning* technique, in which less-informative branch points (known as *leaves*) can be excised, making a more parsimonious tree.

A good example of CART in practice is a *JAMA* study looking at the risk of a patient with acute decompensated heart failure dying in the hospital.[23] This study used ADHERE, a large heart failure registry, and included 33,046 patients in the derivation cohort and 32,229 patients in the validation cohort, with an overall mortality rate of 4.1%. The CART approach found that the most important single factor was blood urea nitrogen (BUN) ≥43 md/dL (Figure 17-3). Patients who had that factor had a mortality rate of 8.98%; those who didn't had a mortality rate of 2.68%—more than a threefold difference in risk. The next most important factor was systolic blood pressure (<115 mmHg or ≥115 mmHg), followed by creatinine levels.

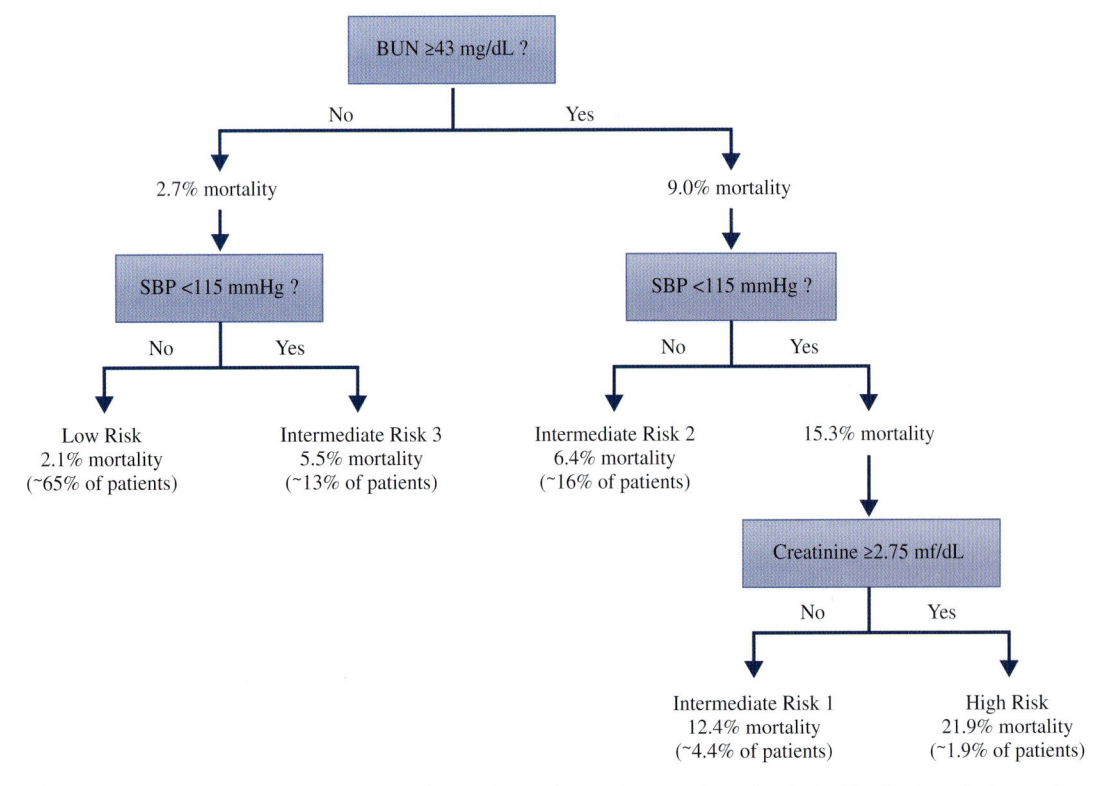

Figure 17-3 • Example of CART analysis, focused on risk-stratifying patients by their risk of in-hospital mortality among patients with acute decompensated heart failure. (*Adapted from Fonarow et al.*[23])

Random Forests

The CART approach has the advantage of being easily interpretable to clinicians, but at the cost of being generally less accurate in risk stratification than more complex models. Decision-tree approaches are also often fragile because they turn out to be particularly at risk of varying a lot in reaction to small changes in training data (that is, they often overfit to the data). Random forests are an extension of decision trees that mitigate some of these shortcomings (at the cost of increased computation and somewhat decreased clinical interpretability).

How do random forests work? (In other words, how does a random forest grow?) First, you create many data sets that vary a bit from your original data set. *Bootstrapping* means generating a series of data from samples from the original data set, and then testing the prediction rule in all these new data sets. This computational approach creates many data sets, which are sampled out of the data set that you actually have at hand. It does this by random resampling with replacement, which means that some observations will usually get sampled more than once (by chance alone), so each bootstrapped data set will vary somewhat from the original. This is useful in helping to avoid overfitting, and bootstrapping is used in many traditional and machine learning techniques.

Bootstrapping is common enough, in both traditional models and machine learning, that it is worthwhile having some intuition for how it actually works. Figure 17-4 shows an example of bootstrapping for a hypothetical data set showing 10 observations of age and favorite color. The leftmost part of the figure is the original data set. The other three data sets were actually created by the bootstrapping procedure. If we focus on Bootstrap 1, we first randomly selected an observation from the original data set. In this

> **Key Point**
>
> Random forests are a machine-learning extension of decision-tree analysis methods like Classification and Regression Tree (CART) analysis. They generate the forest of decision trees by bootstrapping.

Original Data Set			Bootstrap 1			Bootstrap 2			Bootstrap 3	
	Age	Favorite Color		Age	Favorite Color		Age	Favorite Color		Age	Favorite Color
1	23	Red	1	70	Green	1	45	Yellow	1	73	Orange
2	24	Blue	2	73	Orange	2	29	Red	2	43	Orange
3	27	Indigo	3	34	Violet	3	24	Blue	3	23	Red
4	29	Red	4	43	Orange	4	27	Indigo	4	27	Indigo
5	30	Green	5	73	Orange	5	34	Violet	5	45	Yellow
6	34	Violet	6	24	Blue	6	24	Blue	6	34	Violet
7	43	Orange	7	30	Green	7	23	Red	7	30	Green
8	45	Yellow	8	30	Green	8	73	Orange	8	30	Green
9	70	Green	9	70	Green	9	45	Yellow	9	24	Blue
10	73	Orange	10	30	Green	10	43	Orange	10	23	Red

Figure 17-4 • Bootstrapping; observations that are highlighted are duplicated by the bootstrapping procedure.

case, row 9 (age = 70, favorite color = green) got selected, and it became observation 1 in the new data set. Then, we selected another random observation (row 10, age = 73, color = orange), which became observation 2. And the process continues until we get to the fifth time, when something interesting happens. Here, we randomly choose again—but this time, we get the same observation as one of the previous ones (i.e., row 10, age = 73, color = orange). In this way, Bootstrap 1 varies somewhat from the original data set, as do Bootstrap 2 and Bootstrap 3. (It can be shown that bootstrapping leaves out about one-third[†] of the original observations for each new data set.) In Figure 17-4, the colored highlights show duplications from the original data set that make each data set vary from the original. In practice, you usually make many copies of these bootstrapped data sets (e.g., hundreds or more). You can then run your model over many data sets that vary slightly from each other, which helps to detect (and prevent) overfitting.

Now that we have many data sets that vary somewhat from each other, we could just run CART over each data set and then average the result (or, for a classification task, use a majority-vote approach). This would indeed be an improvement over a single decision tree and has in fact been used (the procedure is called *bagging*, which turns out to be a contraction of *bootstrap* and *aggregating*). This approach is a type of *ensemble* model—a model that combines numerous other models' estimates into a single one. However, this approach has an important residual problem—namely, that the decision trees tend to be correlated with each other. This makes intuitive sense: if something is a very strong predictor, it will tend to stay at the top of the decision tree because you are just randomly resampling, and most of the data are the same.

Random forests reduce the correlation between bagged decision trees using a clever mechanism. At each node in the decision tree, you randomly select a subset of the possible predictor values, and the algorithm can consider *only* these variables at that node. A common approach is to let the algorithm have access to approximately the square root of the total number of predictors at any node. This restriction helps reduce overfitting and improve the overall accuracy of the technique.[24] An example of the use of random forests in healthcare is Hsich et al.'s study of predictive factors for survival in chronic systolic heart failure.[25] (They used an extension of random forests called *random survival forests*.). They enrolled 2,231 patients with systolic heart failure who had a cardiopulmonary stress test. They followed these patients for 5 years; 33% of the patients died over this period. They had access to 39 potential predictor variables, and at each branch, they allowed the model to have access to the square root

---

[†] Or, about $1/e$ as you get to larger number of bootstraps ... but $1/e \approx 0.37$; hence, the approximation of "about a third."

CHAPTER 17 | PREDICTIVE MODELING 3.0: MACHINE LEARNING

of the total number of variables. They created a total of 2,000 random trees for their forest. This allowed the identification of peak VO_2, serum BUN, and exercise time as the most important variables in a clinically understandable way, with overall model performance similar to that of a Cox proportional hazards model. For those interested in random forests, this paper is a clear example of the application of these approaches to healthcare data.

Other Tree-Based Approaches

Numerous other tree-based machine learning approaches exist. These are largely extensions of the concepts described here, with various techniques to improve model accuracy, computational efficiency, or both. For example, Adaptive Boosting (AdaBoost) uses the idea that hard-to-classify observations can be weighted more heavily for future learning. Generalized to the term *gradient boosting*, this conceptual approach is now commonly implemented using the open source XGBoost tool.

Support Vector Machines

Support vector machines (SVMs) begin to move out of realms that are familiar to epidemiologists and into areas that use words like *hyperplane* and, yes, *support vectors*. There is a straightforward conceptual approach to understanding SVMs, though. At their core, they are classifiers: Given a set of features (what we might call *potential predictor variables*), is a particular observation more likely to be A or B? Is the patient more likely to be readmitted or not? To have influenza? To achieve functional recovery after surgery?

To start with, imagine that you could describe a patient based on a number of features (potential predictor variables): age, systolic blood pressure, low-density lipoprotein (LDL) cholesterol, and so on. Now, imagine that you could plot where a patient is in some multidimensional space. A patient who is 56 years old, with a systolic blood pressure of 145 and an LDL of 158 would be at (56, 145, 158) in this space. Another patient might be at 42, 130, 86.

In Figure 17-5, using made-up data, we've shown an example. This is simplified into two dimensions because it is much easier to understand—but the actual space can be 3, 50, or 200+ dimensions. (It's just hard to hold those in your head!) In this example, we are interested in predicting a patient's overall emotional state: happy or sad? We have only two features: the patient's age and overall rating on a standard functional quality-of-life assessment (something like the SF-36). For our training data, we know every patient's true state (happy versus sad), their age, and their quality-of-life score.

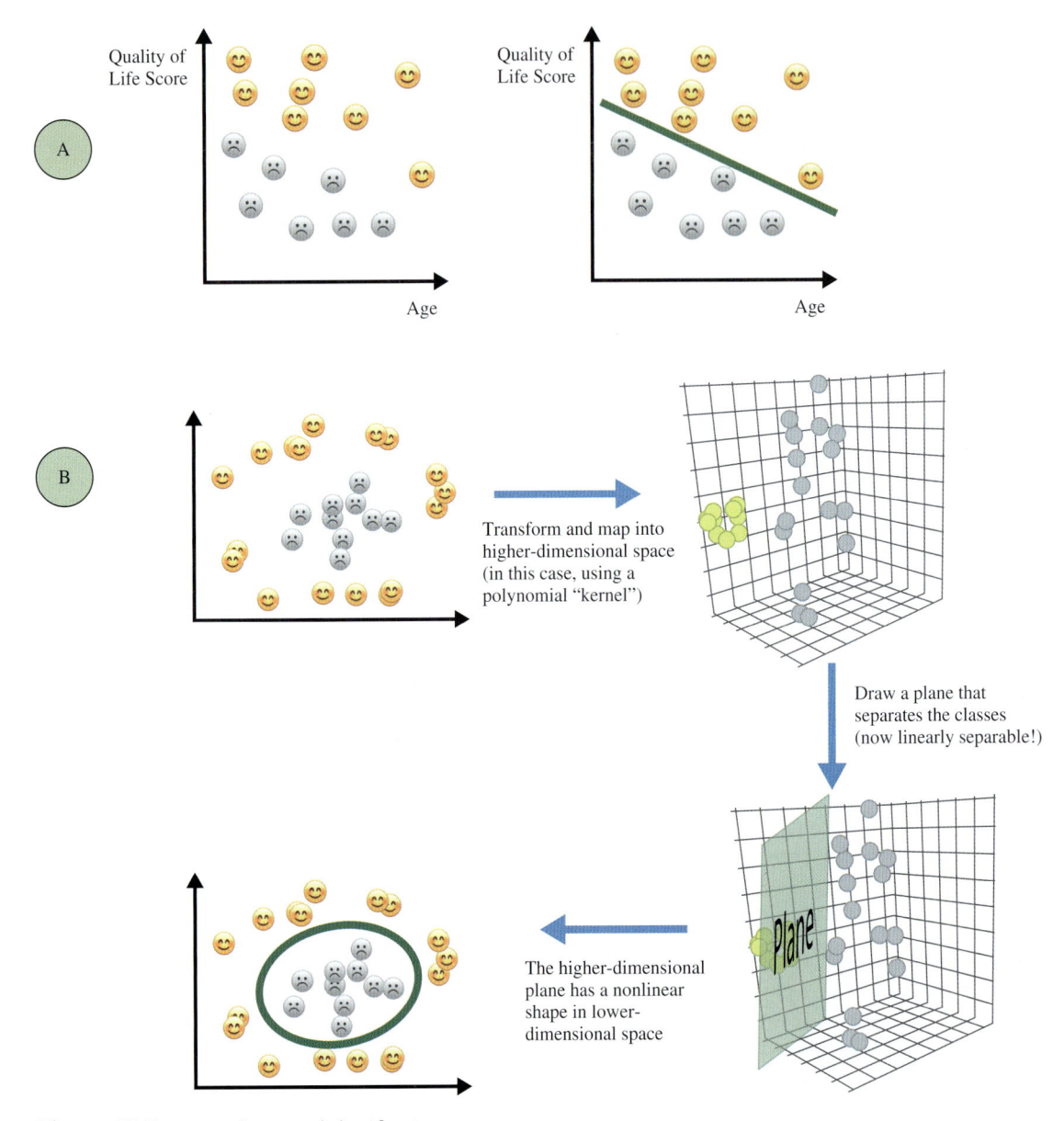

Figure 17-5 • Hyperplanes and classification.

For the data shown in Figure 17-5A, it is obvious that we can draw a line that cleanly separates "happy" from "sad." *This is exactly what an SVM does.* It draws the best line it can find to separate the classes that we are interested in predicting or classifying (here, "happy" versus "sad"). This line is called a *hyperplane* because SVMs usually operate in a large number of dimensions (not just two), and a line in many dimensions is given this name. You can think of the hyperplane (the line in Figure 17-5) as a *decision surface*. If the SVM has done its job, on one side of the decision surface, patients are much more likely to be happy than sad.

How does an SVM draw this hyperplane? It is a *maximum-margin* classifier: it tries to maximize the perpendicular distance between the plane and the nearest observations on either side of the hyperplane. The vectors of the closest examples are called *support vectors*, which is actually how this approach got its name. That makes good intuitive sense if you think of it in two dimensions: You want the line to do the best possible job separating the classes (in this case, "happy" and "sad"). The support vectors are actually examples from your training sets, and the most difficult ones to separate. When using an SVM, removing the other examples (the ones that are farther from the hyperplane than your support vectors are) or moving them around a bit usually will not significantly change the classifier.

But, in real life, data are never as simple as those shown in Figure 17-5A, where the data are linearly separable. Where does an SVM draw a hyperplane if it's impossible to separate the classes linearly? First, you can choose to accept some errors—for example, by minimizing the distance to the misclassified examples that are on the wrong side of the hyperplane. It's worth noting that when the data aren't linearly separable and there is some misclassification, a linear classifier can still be quite useful—even though there are many choices to make that represent tradeoffs between elements such as accuracy in the training data and size of the margin.

In Figure 17-5B, the relationships are more complex. It's quickly obvious to the eye that the classes are quite separate, and no straight line can fully separate "happy" from "sad" in this data set. If an SVM only makes lines or planes, how can it do nonlinear separation and classification? The SVM uses something called a *kernel*, or a *kernel trick*. This is not the same kernel as your computer's operating system (nor of your popcorn!). Rather, a kernel transforms the data in a way that makes separation more possible. One way to think about it is that a *kernel* is a function that adds dimensions to your data set and transforms its contents in a way that lets the SVM find a hyperplane. Put another way, by adding derived variables and increasing the dimensions, you can achieve more expressiveness. The key to an SVM is measuring distances from the data points (calculated using the inner product), and kernels let you define different ways to compute the inner product, like those that we had transformed to a higher dimension, but without the complexity cost involved in that transformation.

Key Point

Support vector machines are classifiers: Given a set of features (what we might call *potential predictor variables*), is a particular observation more likely to be A or B? They do this by drawing lines (or planes, or hyperplanes) that maximize the margin between these decision surfaces and different groups of data.

Figure 17-5B gives an example of this. It uses a polynomial function to remap two-dimensional data into three dimensions in a way that separates them. In this case, X becomes X^2, Y becomes Y^2, and ($\sqrt{2} \times X \times Y$) becomes Z. When you plot this transformed data (the middle plot in panel B), you find that now you can draw a plane that cleanly separates "happy" from "sad." A two-dimensional projection of this plane also separates the points.

When thinking through this example, it is important to remember that an SVM usually operates in many more dimensions than two. One of the advantages of the kernel approach is that there are some computational efficiencies that mean that all these points don't actually have to get mapped back and forth between dimensions. The choice of kernel clearly becomes very important in the overall performance of the algorithm, and there are ways to let the algorithm learn the best kernel when needed.

Deep Learning Models

> **Key Point**
>
> Deep learning is the modern incarnation of artificial neural networks and is responsible for many of the most impressive feats of machine learning and AI.

Deep learning represents the modern incarnation of artificial neural networks, the core ideas of which have been around for many decades. The structure of these networks takes its inspiration (at least vaguely) from biological neural architecture—with the key insight that deep and wide connections among many simple processing units can lead to complex and surprising functions. Each neuron in our brain, after all, is in some ways not very complex: It takes a certain number of inputs (from its dendrites), combines them, and "decides" whether to activate and thus fire a signal forward down its axon. In this section, we will walk through three important types of deep learning: convolutional neural networks (CNNs), recurrent neural networks (RNNs), and deep reinforcement learning. While these are by no means the only types of deep learning, they have each found current uses in healthcare in significant ways.

Perceptrons: The Basic Building Block

> **Key Point**
>
> A *perceptron* is the basic building block of neural networks. Understanding how perceptrons work is helpful for fostering intuition about more complicated networks.

You can think of a perceptron as an artificial neuron, the basic building block of more complex neural networks. A *perceptron* is a single-layer, single-node neural network that—like a neuron—takes numerous inputs, combines them, and then "decides" whether to activate or not.

Understanding a perceptron is helpful for developing an intuition of what more complicated neural networks are doing (Figure 17-6)—in particular, for understanding what exactly is being learned. Imagine that we wanted to build a classifier for whether a patient has diabetes or not. The perceptron would take several inputs—age, sex, body weight, height, and other characteristics. Every input gets a weight—an actual number that is multiplied by the input. Then, all those products are summed: (factor A *

CHAPTER 17 | PREDICTIVE MODELING 3.0: MACHINE LEARNING

[Figure 17-6 diagram: Factors A–E (etc.) feed into a perceptron with Weights A–E (etc.), a Weighted sum + Bias term, then an activation function check ("Is this greater than the threshold of the perceptron's activation function?"), producing Output.

Annotations:
- "Activation functions are usually nonlinear, which lets the perpceptron handle many nonliear relationships."
- "All of the weights, and also the bias term, are under the algorithm's control – they are what gets adjusted and learned."]

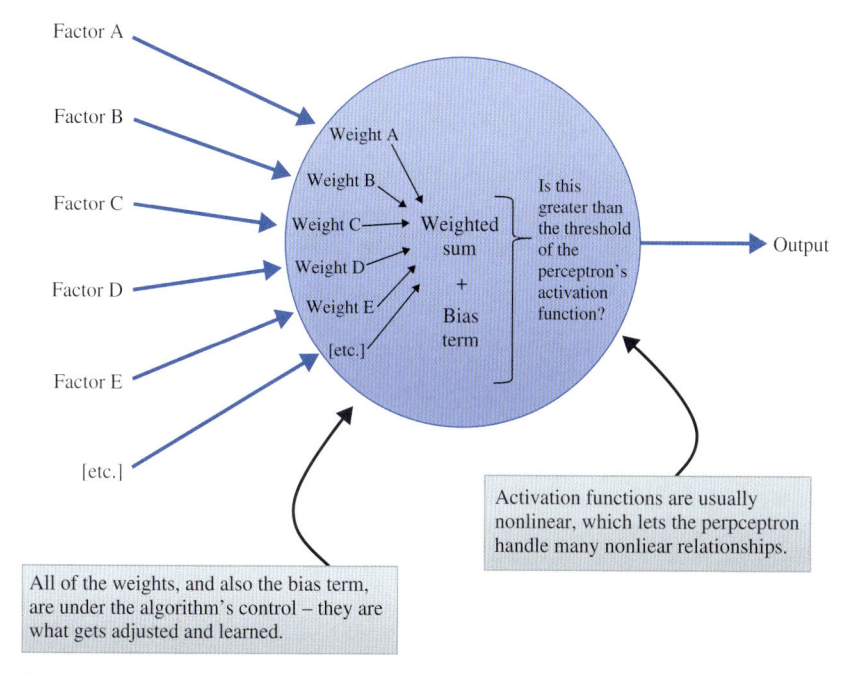

Figure 17-6 • Perceptrons: the basic building block.

weight A) + (factor B * weight B) + (factor C * weight C), and so on. To that number is then added a *bias*, which is just another number (somewhat like the intercept in logistic regression, or the b in the classic equation for a line, $y = mx + b$). That number is then given to an activation function. Originally, the activation function was a step function: If the number that came forward was <0, it returned 0. If it was ≥0, it returned 1. This is called the *Heaviside function*. Other functions are now commonly used, such as the logistic/sigmoid, rectified linear unit (ReLU), and others. (The nonlinearity of these functions becomes important when stacking perceptrons into the many layers of a neural network; this is because stacking linear functions causes the output of the whole network to just be a linear transformation of the first layer's output.)

What is under the perceptron's control? Just the weights and the bias term. Given training examples, the algorithm starts with random weights and a random bias and then varies them based on how much they differ from the correct answer. The function of the weights is obvious: It lets the algorithm treat some factors with more importance than others.

What about the bias term? Imagine that we want to build a classifier for "eligible for traditional Medicare, or not" (and that, as a simplification, age ≥65 means that a person is eligible for Medicare). Our data

Key Point

Like neurons, perceptrons take inputs, sum them up in a weighted fashion, and then have a nonlinear function that decides whether the perceptron activates or not.

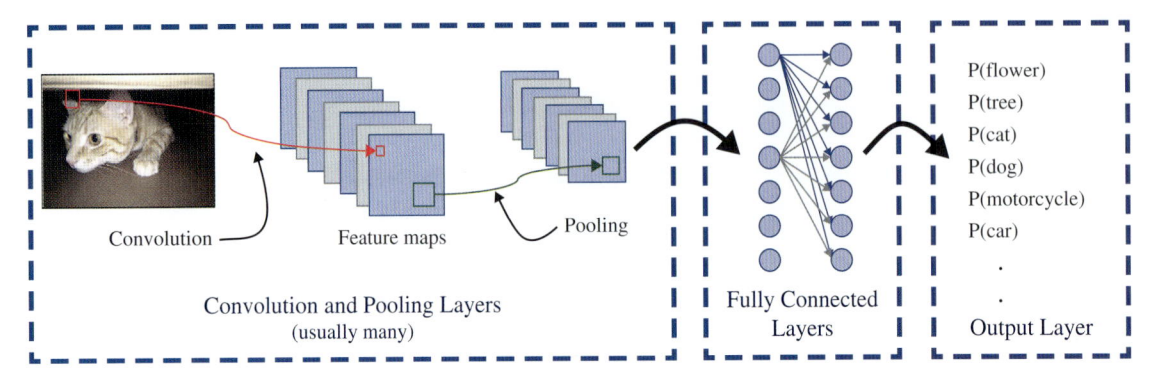

Figure 17-7 • A convolutional neural network (CNN).

> **Key Point**
>
> What do perceptrons actually learn? Only the weights and the bias term—this is all that they can adjust in response to training examples.

set includes inputs of age (in years), height (in meters), and eye color (1 = brown, 2 = blue, 3 = green, 4 = other). We've chosen the Heaviside function as the activation function—the one that returns 1 if the value it receives is ≥ 0, and 0 otherwise. Our perceptron will learn a weight of 0.0 for height and eye color because they are unrelated to Medicare eligibility, and a weight of 1.0 for age. Now, let's imagine that we have a person with an age of 64, a height of 1.7 meters, and green eyes. Given these weights, the number that will be fed to the activation function is 64. We don't want the activation function to fire for people who are 64—only those who are 65 or older. This is where the bias term comes in, which sets the threshold for the activation function, shifting it to the left or to the right. In this case, the perceptron would set the bias term to –65. Combined with weights of 1.0 for age and 0.0 for the other factors, we now have a perfect classifier! The important part about this is what the perceptron learns (the weights and the bias term) and what is set by the investigator (i.e., the data available to the perceptron, the type of activation function, and so on).

Combining perceptrons and their extensions into multiple, connected layers leads to the performance of modern neural networks. Deep neural networks have an input layer, then several hidden layers, and finally an output layer. Each layer of the neural network takes the input of the layer before it and feeds its own output forward to the next layer. This results in a tremendous number of connections (and weights!) among all the neurons in the network.

Convolutional Neural Networks (CNNs)

A common and important task for machine learning—and for healthcare—is image analysis. Perhaps you want to look at a chest x-ray to see if a patient has pneumonia, or at the back of the eye to determine whether a patient has diabetic retinopathy.

CHAPTER 17 | PREDICTIVE MODELING 3.0: MACHINE LEARNING

At first glance, it might seem that you could just give an image to a fully connected neural network. However, there are two important problems with this approach. First, images inherently have spatial structure: If you are looking at a picture of a cat, the eyes are in one place, the paws in another, and the tail in a third. The eyes aren't scattered randomly across the photo. Put another way, pixels at the top left have more to do with each other than pixels at the bottom right. A network to recognize images should deal with this fact. (Many types of data have inherent spatial structures, but we'll stick with images for the rest of this section because they are common and important, and the principles apply generally.) Second, the computational expense of a fully connected approach is very high because the number of connections required for this approach is very large. Imagine a comparatively low resolution image of 1,000 × 1,000—that's 1 million pixels (to put that in context as "low-resolution," every photo your phone takes probably has more than 10 times this number of pixels.). Each pixel is an input into the network. Now, if you fully connected them in a second layer of the network, suddenly you have a trillion connections (1M * 1M)—and even more when you remember that images usually have multiple channels [e.g., red, green, and blue (RGB)].

How do convolutional neural networks (CNNs) deal with these problems? They use mathematical tricks called *convolution* (hence the name) and *pooling*. The particular insight of CNN structures is that they can take into account which pixels in an image are near one another and do it in a way that reduces the computational complexity of the problem by having a network that is only partially connected.

How do they do this? Their first layer is a layer of filters, sometimes called *kernels* or *neurons*. Each filter is a matrix of numbers that is much smaller than the original image. For example, a filter might be 5 × 5 or 3 × 3. You can also think of an image as being a matrix of pixels (height * width). Each pixel might be a number indicating intensity of grayscale, or there might be an additional dimension with different channels (e.g., RGB). The first step of a CNN is to slide this filter around the image, multiply all the numbers, and create a new matrix. It multiplies these numbers using a tool from matrix algebra called the *dot product*. The way this works is shown in Figure 17-8A. With a dot product, you just multiply each cell by its corresponding cell and then add up all the results. Because the filter is smaller than the image, you also have to move the filter around the image. How much you move the filter with each step is called the *stride*. How this all works is shown in Figure 17-8A.[‡]

Key Point

Convolutional neural networks (CNNs) are optimized for image recognition and processing because their architecture takes into account spatial positioning and adjacency.

Key Point

The convolution in a CNN refers to a numerical filter that is applied to detect specific features in an image (or other matrix of data). The weights of these filters are what the network learns and adjusts.

[‡] As you look at Figure 17-8A, you'll notice that the size of the matrix gets a bit smaller when the filter is introduced. Although we haven't done it for this example, it is common to add zeroes at the edges of the image in order to preserve the size of the original image and to capture information at the edge of the image. This approach is called *padding*.

The specifics of how all the multiplication works aren't the important part here. Rather, the critical thing to understand is that (1) different filters can detect different features of an image, (2) each filter has a small field of view, which means that relationships among adjacent parts of the image are important, and (3) a filter is composed of numbers, whose weights are learned by the CNN. Each filter (and there are usually many) creates a new feature map that gets passed forward in the network. Figure 17-8B shows a toy example of this, with an input of a 10 × 10 smiley face, and with three filters that detect different features of the image. The output of each filter is then typically passed to a nonlinear activation function (just as in the perceptron).

There is then a process called *pooling*. How does pooling work? A common approach to pooling is *max pooling*. Here, you might have a 2 × 2 matrix that you wanted to reduce from 4 numbers to just 1. You would simply take the largest number (e.g., "2, 8, 1, 4" would become just "8") and slide the pooling filter around the matrix. Pooling reduces the size of the matrix that gets passed forward, but it also helps prevent mistakes caused by shifting a few pixels left or right (or up or down). This

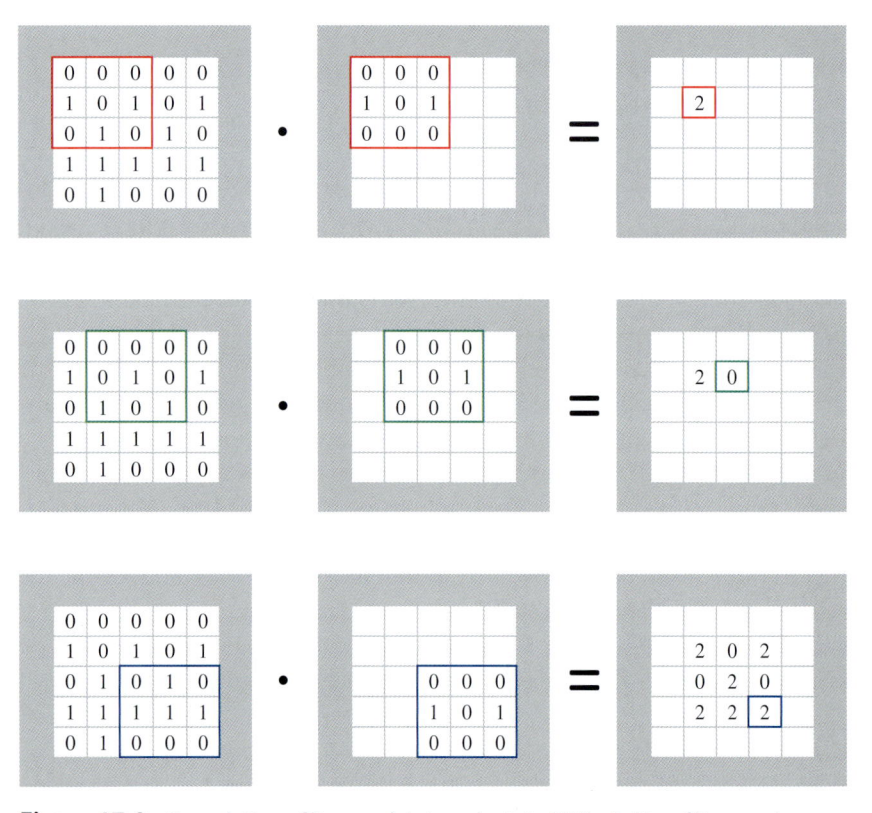

Figure 17-8 • Convolutions, filters, and dot products in CNNs. **A.** How filters work.

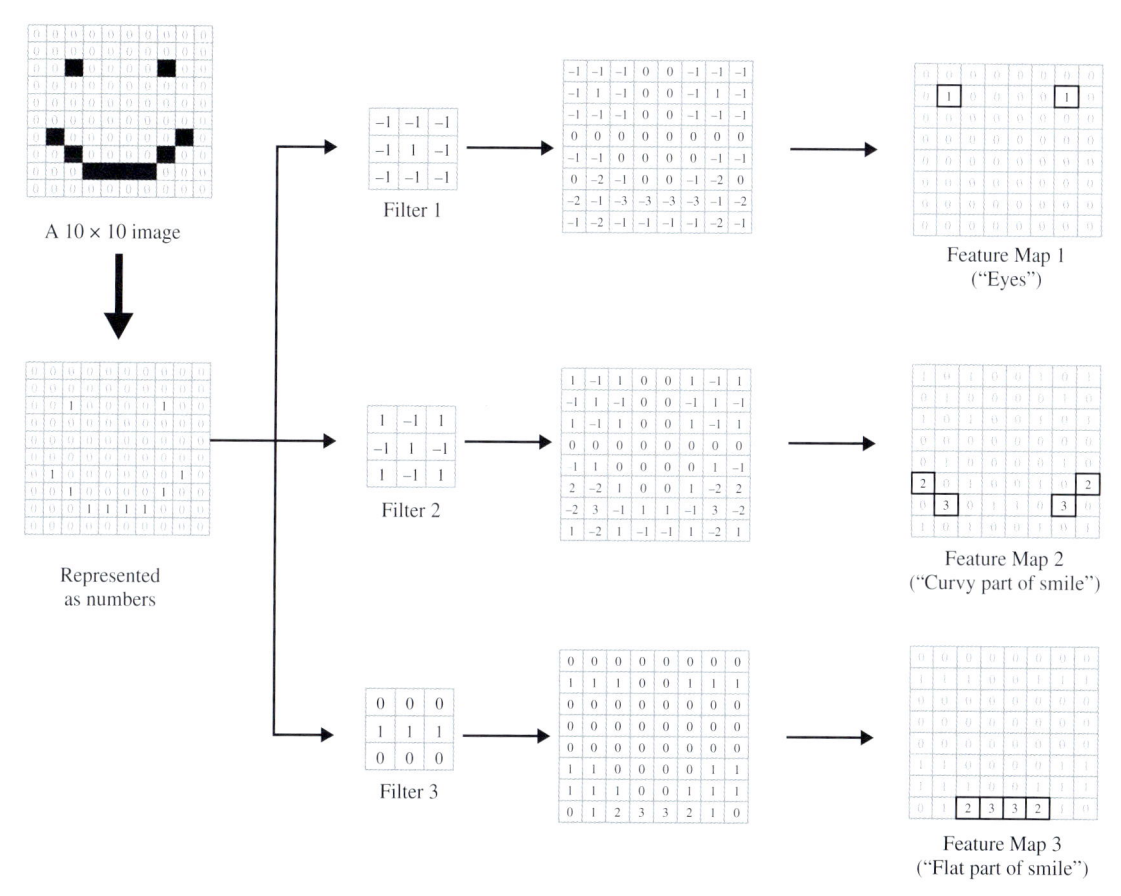

Figure 17-8 • B. How filters detect features. By choosing different weights for each part of a filter, you can detect different features in an image. In the first step, you multiply the filter against the original image to get a new matrix. Here, we have a 3 × 3 filter applied with a stride of 1. In the second step, there is an activation function that introduces nonlinearity into the process. (This example uses the ReLU function, which returns a 0 if the number is <0, and the same number otherwise.) The outcome is that it further highlights the features the filter picked up. In this example, three filters with different weights highlight different parts of the original image. In a CNN, the weights of these filters are learned, not handcrafted.

whole process is repeated a number of times, with the output of each layer of the network serving as inputs for the next.

Eventually, the results are passed to a fully connected layer. This layer has access to all the features and can make connections between them from different parts of the image (unlike previous layers, where features were detected based on adjacency). The output layer then makes a classification or prediction of what the image actually represents. That can be a binary prediction ("Is this a cat?") or, more commonly, it will be a multicategory prediction based on the labels of the training data ("Housecat 0.81, Lion 0.05, Tiger 0.02, Dog 0.01 …").[§]

It is worth emphasizing that—just like the perceptron—the algorithm manipulates weights to minimize the amount of error the CNN has when classifying images. That means that each filter's numbers and patterns are learned, not programmed, as are the weights in the fully connected layer. How does a CNN learn these weights and bias terms? By attempting to minimize the number of errors that it makes on its training data (e.g., categorizing a picture as a cat when in fact it is a dog). This should sound exactly like the loss function described earlier in this chapter. Minimizing a loss function across a many-layered network is a complicated, difficult task. Some of the major advances in deep learning have had to with exactly how this optimization is accomplished.[¶]

Examples of CNNs in Healthcare

There are numerous examples of CNNs in healthcare, ranging from radiology[26] to dermatology[27] to pathology.[28] However, perhaps the most mature example is in ophthalmology, and specifically in the detection of diabetic retinopathy. In December 2016, a *JAMA* publication found that a CNN had a performance in detecting diabetic retinopathy that was equivalent to that of ophthalmologists.[1] The researchers used 118,419 retinal photographs for training and had them graded for the severity of diabetic retinopathy by three to seven ophthalmologists. They then trained a CNN whose architecture was specifically optimized for image classification (called "Inception v3"). They validated the algorithm's performance on a set of 11,711 additional pictures of retinas. For referable diabetic retinopathy, compared to ophthalmologists, the algorithm had an area under the receiver operating curve of 0.99. Subsequent work that used retinal subspecialists as the reference standard (instead of general ophthalmologists) resulted in further improved performance.[2]

Recurrent Neural Networks (RNNs)

As humans, we understand future events in the context of what has already happened. Many important tasks for computer science require understanding sequences of data: Speech recognition, translation, and sentence

---

[§] You will frequently hear computer scientists talk about "softmax" regression. This is a function used to make multicategory predictions, and in epidemiology is usually called multinomial or multiclass logistic regression.

[¶] While the specifics are beyond the scope of this chapter, it is perhaps worth knowing that *gradient descent* and *backpropagation of errors* are critical concepts that have to do with exactly how a neural network chooses these weights.

CHAPTER 17 | PREDICTIVE MODELING 3.0: MACHINE LEARNING

completion are some examples. These are important kinds of problems in healthcare, too, where the order of events matters greatly for predicting what comes next. For example, a patient who receives ciprofloxacin and metronidazole together may have diverticulitis. A patient who receives ciprofloxacin, and then 2 weeks later receives metronidazole, probably had a urinary tract infection followed by *Clostridium difficile* infection (a complication of the original antibiotic). Similarly, a patient who receives insulin and D50 at the same time probably has hyperkalemia, while a patient who receives insulin and then 2 hours later gets D50 probably has hypoglycemia (as a complication of the insulin). The key issue here is that you need to remember what came before—that is, that preceding events change your interpretation of current events.

Recurrent neural networks (RNNs) are an architecture that can remember what happened before. They can take their own prior state into account when handling new features, which means they are useful for tasks where context is important. How do they do this? They have loops. This means that one node has two outputs: first, a regular output, and second, an output that serves as an input for another cycle of the node. Figure 17-9 shows this graphically, in comparison to a non-RNN. This looping lets the network deal with sequences of varying length: for example, a sentence might be 5 words long, or 30. You can also think of an RNN in its unfolded pattern, also demonstrated in Figure 17-9.

How does this work? Imagine a predict-the-next-word task, where the sentence is "In 1986, the president of the United States was Reagan," and

> **Key Point**
>
> A recurrent neural network (RNN) is effective at dealing with sequences of data, as in language or in a medical record.

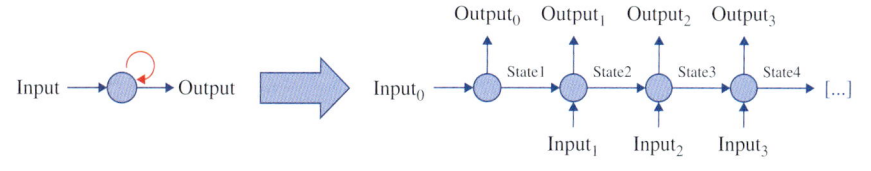

Figure 17-9 • Unfolding a recurrent neural network (RNN).

> **Key Point**
>
> A node in an RNN can "remember" its immediately previous state, because there are loops in the network's architecture (this is the "recurrence" in an RNN).

> **Key Point**
>
> Like perceptrons and CNNs, RNNs learn weights. These weights define how much importance they ascribe to new inputs and to the node's prior state.

> **Key Point**
>
> A Long Short-Term Memory (LSTM) network is an important, specific type of RNN that helps it deal with long-term dependencies in the data.

we give information by word rather than by character. The network's first input will be "In," and it will have no information about its prior state because it is just getting started. For the fourth cycle, it will have information about its state during the third cycle through, and it will get the new input "president." At each step, it will make a prediction about what the next word will be.

In an RNN, each node (or cell, or neuron) has a set of weights that is applied to the new input, and another that is applied to information about the node's previous state. As in perceptrons and CNNs, these weights are what the algorithm actually learns during training.

Given all this, it seems intuitive that an RNN might be good at taking into account the step immediately preceding the current input. That is, RNNs would have good (very) short-term memory. However, if we think about trying to predict "Reagan" in the sentence "In 1986, the year of *The Oprah Winfrey Show*'s national debut, the president of the United States was Reagan," a critical input (1986) comes right at the very beginning of the sentence. The need to deal with this issue of long-term dependencies (along with other problems like the excitingly named *vanishing* and *exploding gradients*[29]) led to the development[30] and refinement of a special kind of RNN architecture, called the *Long Short-Term Memory (LSTM) network*. LSTM networks are an important advance in deep learning, specifically designed to remember things for a long time. The nodes in an LSTM are called *memory cells,* and they have three internal functions (gates) that make them different from vanilla RNNs. These gates control the updating of, and output from, the cell's internal state. The *forget gate* specifically removes information from the cell's current state. For example, if the gender of a sentence's subject changes, it may be useful for the cell to forget the prior subject's gender ("Bob went to the store, so Mary answered the phone when it rang. _____ said 'Hello.'." The correct missing word is *She,* not *He.*). The *input gate* determines what parts of the new information being fed into the cell should update the cell's internal state. For example, we would prefer to ignore new information that is redundant or unimportant. The *output gate* helps select which information from the cell's internal state should be selected to be output at a given time. Together, these gates help the LSTM take long-term dependencies in sequences into account.

Examples of RNNs in Healthcare

RNNs and their variations like LSTMs are increasingly finding use in healthcare, particularly on EHR data and free-text notes. For example, Liu and colleagues found that LSTMs did well at identifying specific medical concepts, even in the absence of hand-engineered features[31];

Mirshekarian used LSTMs to learn about some of the complex dynamics of blood glucose levels;[32] Tsiouris used them to predict seizures from electroencephalograms (EEGs);[33] and Jiang used them to deidentify free-text medical notes.[34] In 2018, Rajkomar and colleagues used LSTMs and some more advanced variants to use full-fidelity EHR data to predict a wide variety of things, including readmission, inpatient mortality, length of stay, and discharge diagnoses, with an accuracy significantly exceeding standard clinical predictive models.[35]

Deep Reinforcement Learning

So far, the machine learning methods we've looked at in this chapter have focused on classification, regression, and prediction. A different category of problem is what we should *do*, given a particular state of the world. Humans learn through feedback from the environment, which reinforces some behaviors and extinguishes others. An example that is often used is how we learn about fire when we are infants: We come in from a cold day and notice that when we move closer to the fire, we get warmer. This is a reward and encourages the behavior. Eventually, though, we get too close to the fire, or even try to touch it, and get burned. This is a powerful negative stimulus, and we learn to not touch the fire.

Reinforcement learning is a computational approach to this kind of learning—learning by trial and error, exploring the environment, and assessing the reward that these actions bring. How do we link situations to actions? Given a situation, what is the best action to take to maximize a reward function? An additional complexity is that some rewards are immediate and others are delayed—and that our actions increase the chance of some rewards but foreclose the possibility of others.

Reinforcement learning has been startlingly effective in situations where the environment can be fully simulated, as when playing games. For example, a deep reinforcement learning algorithm developed human-level control of a number of classic Atari 2600 games—an accomplishment worthy of a *Nature* paper.[36] Similarly, these approaches led to world-champion performance in chess and Go.[6,7] Reinforcement learning is also a natural fit for robotic control,[37] where actions can be tested both in simulation and (often) in the real world with a low risk of major adverse events during training. For healthcare, the ability to learn which treatments are best from observational data is a very important—and very difficult—problem. We are introducing reinforcement learning here because recent research has focused on using this technique to try to discover optimal treatments from observational data. We anticipate that this will become more common over time.

Key Point

Reinforcement learning is a computational approach that in some ways attempts to mimic how humans learn—by trial and error, exploring the environment, and assessing the reward that these actions bring.

Key Point

Reinforcement learning is the machine-learning technique that has led to AI performance that exceeds human performance in games like Atari 2600 video games, chess, and Go.

Reinforcement learning starts with the idea of an *agent,* which learns through trial and error. At a given point in time, the agent finds itself in an environment, and that environment is in a particular state (which may change over time). The agent can then choose one of several actions—and in doing so, it finds a greater or lesser future reward. A key aspect of reinforcement learning is that the desired action can be reduced to a numerical reward function and that the agent will learn to optimize its choice of actions to maximize the reward function. This process is depicted graphically in Figure 17-10.

How does the agent make decisions about actions? This is really a Markov decision process. Markov models are familiar to biostatisticians and epidemiologists from decision analysis, multiple imputation for missing data,

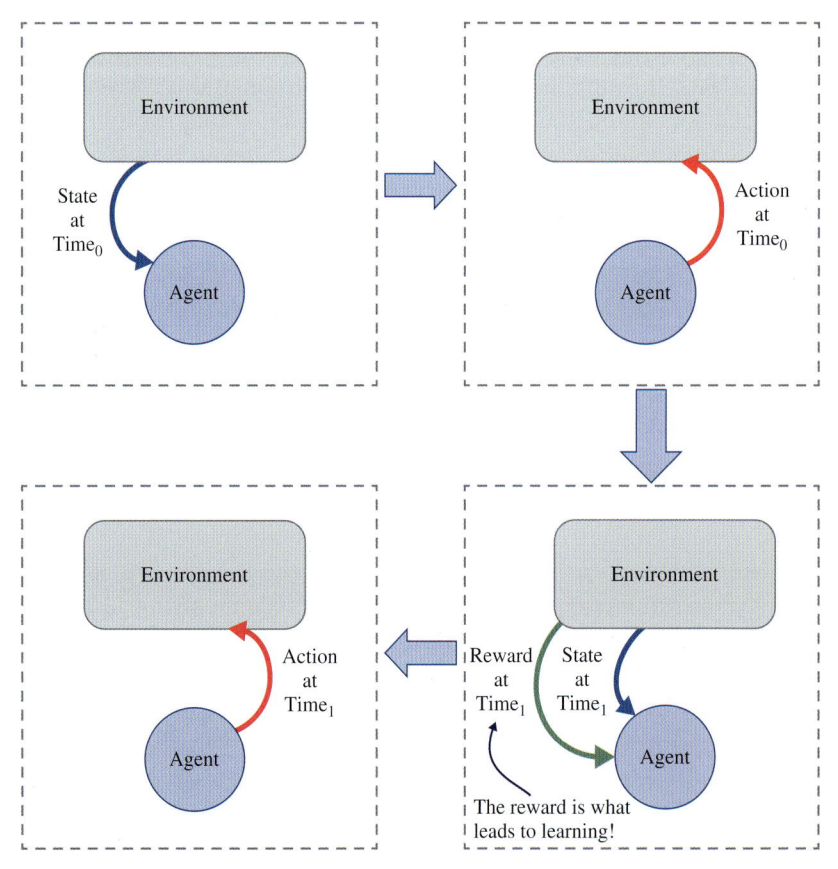

Figure 17-10 • Reinforcement learning. This diagram progresses through four steps, starting at $Time_0$, when the agent perceives the environment. The agent then acts on (or in) the environment, and the clock then advances to $Time_1$. Now, the agent perceives the state at $Time_1$, but it also receives a reward from the combination of its action and the environment. That prompts the agent to take another action. This reward is what encourages learning over time, via trial and error.

and other applications, but it perhaps worth restating that the Markov property is that "the future is independent of the past given the present"[38]—that is, that the current state encapsulates what you need to know to understand the future. (It is worth noting that the complete state of the environment is usually not visible to the agent, and that it improves its map of the environment by exploration—so this is really a partially observable Markov process.)

The agent then optimizes the total value of expected future rewards for a specific action, given a current state. It learns a policy for what to do, typically by evaluating the quality of a specific action, given its current knowledge of the environment's state. You will often hear reinforcement learning called *Q-Learning* because the quality of a given action is calculated in terms of the total expected rewards, using something called the *Bellman equation;* and the agent makes decisions to optimize this numerical (Q)uality. (This is like optimizing the loss function in other methods discussed previously, except that here, we want to maximize the reward.)

There are a couple of subtleties here that are important. First, future rewards aren't usually as good as immediate rewards because (1) they are less certain to occur, and (2) they are in the future rather than the present. Therefore, future rewards are mathematically discounted—but how much they are discounted is in the hands of the modeler, not the algorithm. Second, there is often a tradeoff between what the agent knows in order to provide rewards/to be safe and investigating the environment to capture potentially greater rewards (but with greater risk too).

Figure 17-11 shows a simple game that demonstrates this. In this example, the agent is a mouse. It experiences positive rewards when it ends up in the same square as cheese (yum!), but negative rewards when it ends up in the same square as a T-Rex (yikes!). In the first turn of the game, the mouse knows nothing about its environment, so it moves in a random direction. If it moves up or to the left, 20% of the time it will be startled by the T-Rex (encountering a –10 negative reward). If it moves to the right, and then to the right again, it finds some cheese and receives a reward (+1 reward). It is easy to see how an agent could end up just on the right side of the board and stay there with a reliable (but small) piece of cheese. (This is the real-life equivalent of a category of choice that we face all the time—go to a restaurant we know we like, or try something new.) This is called the *exploration versus exploitation dilemma*. The mouse could just stay on the right side of the board (maybe the best decision, given its information), or it could explore the board (gathering more information about the environment—and finding that a huge piece of cheese might be available). This represents an important parameter that the modeler can set in reinforcement learning agents: Some percentage of the time, the agent can make a random decision, thus gaining more information about the environment.

Over many iterations of playing a game, the agent learns which actions result in the greatest reward and which lead to negative rewards. For a toy game like the one depicted in Figure 17-11, you can imagine directly and exactly calculating the expected reward for every possible action in every square. This approach is practical, and used for small games—it is called a Q-Table (again, for the quality of an action or state, as measured by the expected value of the reward.). However, as games get larger, it becomes impractical and impossible to build a lookup table of actions. How many states are there in an Atari 2600 game, or for a three-dimensional, first-person adventure game? How many actions for any given state? Certainly, there would be too many to build a lookup table for. In this case (which is true for all healthcare cases), we build deep learning models that approximate the Q function. This turns out to work remarkably well. There are many variations of this approach, and this is an active area of research.

Early Examples of Reinforcement Learning in Healthcare

Researchers are actively investigating whether reinforcement learning can be used for individual customization of treatment approaches in healthcare, learning from observational data. In general, these investigations focus on a narrow action space that is mathematically tractable. The *action space* is the set of choices that a clinician (or reinforcement learning agent) can make at any given time—and the choice of action space is

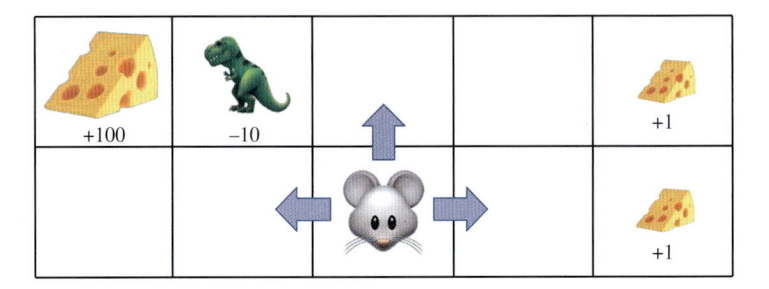

Rules:
(1) Move once per turn.
(2) Can move up or sideways, not diagonally.
(3) Mice like cheese: +1 for small cheese and +100 for giant cheese.
(4) Mice don't like T-Rexes. T-Rexes can't eat mice (due to their short little arms), but they are very scary (so, −10 if you run into a T-Rex).
(5) T-Rexes sometimes (20% of the time) jump into adjacent squares if they see mice there, so the squares next to a T-Rex are (randomly) dangerous, too.

Figure 17-11 • A simple game: Environmental rewards and reinforcement learning.

an important simplification of the real clinical environment. For example, Lin and colleagues studied heparin dosing in the intensive care unit (ICU).[39] They used reinforcement learning to identify an optimal policy for heparin dosing. The action space was the dose of heparin, adjusted over time, and the reward function was designed to reward time in the goal partial thromboplastin time (PTT) range. They found that how much clinicians varied from the learned policy of heparin dosing was associated with anticoagulation-related complications.

Komorowski and colleagues evaluated reinforcement learning in the care of ICU patients with sepsis.[40] They simplified hemodynamic management of patients into just two treatments: fluids and "vasopressors." Each of these treatments was discretized into five categories: no treatment, and then quartiles by dose. This meant that the action space had a total of 25 choices. They chose a reward function of survival (and a very low discount rate, meaning that they valued early and late deaths very similarly). They used reinforcement learning to learn an optimal policy for managing fluids and vasopressors. They then used a held-out set of patients to assess how much clinicians' decisions that varied from the learned policy affected clinical outcomes. (This is called *off-policy evaluation*.) In general, they found that clinicians in this data set gave more fluids, and fewer vasopressors, than the policy would have recommended. In their validation cohort, they found that patients who actually received fluid and vasopressor dosing that matched the policy had the lowest mortality rate.

We think that it's worth noting that none of these approaches has undergone prospective evaluation, and we have some concern about whether any of them will validate prospectively. Reinforcement learning works well in video games because your agent can make actual changes in the environment through its actions and can get feedback about rewards as well. In our opinion, it remains unclear about whether—in healthcare—off-policy retrospective learning will have the same efficacy in determining optimal clinical actions.

PITFALLS IN USING MACHINE LEARNING IN HEALTHCARE

It's easy to get swept up in the hype about machine learning. It seems like there's a new story every day about machine learning doing something that seemed nearly impossible just a year or two ago.

In this context, it's absolutely critical to remember that machine learning is math, not magic.

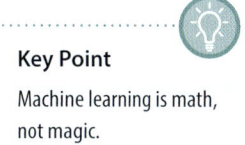

Key Point

Machine learning is math, not magic.

That sounds almost trivial, but it's important. Machine learning is subject to all the fallacies and problems of traditional epidemiology—missing data, biases in data collection, confounding, and others. Here are a few things to keep in mind:

- **Evaluation and validation.** Machine learning models need strong approaches to evaluation and validation, just as traditional predictive models do. Be particularly attentive when evaluating models that predict rare outcomes—the area under the receiver operating characteristics (AUROC) curve can have high numbers solely because of this class imbalance. That means that you cannot assume that a model is good enough to use just because of a high AUROC when events are rare. In this case, many advocate for using the area under the precision-recall (AUPRC) curve instead. See Leisman's very approachable, clinically oriented review for more on this issue.[41]

- **Fairness, disparities, and bias in the data.** We live in a world replete with bias and disparity. Healthcare data record these biases in practice, which are well documented and the subject of substantial research. Therefore, any predictive model (or classification model) is at risk of simply learning these biases. This is true of logistic regression as much as it is of more sophisticated machine learning models. How does this work? Imagine that you are building a model to predict who should be seen first in an overbooked clinic, and you use that health system's historical data to build the model. Then imagine that the health system has historically been more likely to see wealthier patients, or those of a particular race, more quickly than other patients. Unless you pay attention to these issues, your model would tend to learn these patterns of treatment—and then to predict or recommend them. There are both technical and policy approaches to using machine learning to promote fairness in healthcare: this is an important topic that deserves attention throughout the process of model building, implementation, and follow-up. See Rajkomar's approachable, clinically oriented review for more details.[42]

- **Real-time data may look different from historical data.** When you build a model, you always train on historical data. These data almost always look different than data that occur in real time. This results in something called *training-serving skew,* where the model behaves differently in practice than in training. For example, if you are using EHR data, you probably receive them from a data warehouse.

Caution

Machine learning models require strong approaches to evaluation and validation, just as traditional predictive models do.

Caution

Be attentive to techniques that assess and promote fairness in model development, whether using traditional models or machine learning. It is easy to inadvertently learn biases that are inherent in healthcare data.

CHAPTER 17 | PREDICTIVE MODELING 3.0: MACHINE LEARNING

How do they differ from real-time data? First, they have undergone various transformations as they move from transactional systems into these archival systems (e.g., from one database format to another). Second, there are sometimes cleanups as part of extracting the data from the warehouse. For example, a heart rate of 1,000 might be suppressed because it is physiologically impossible. Third, there are real-world corrections that happen before the data ever get to the warehouse. A nurse might inadvertently switch respiratory rate (RR) and oxygen saturation (O_2 sat) in a flowsheet, for example—resulting in an entry with RR = 97 and an O_2 sat = 18. A few minutes later, the nurse may notice the error and correct it (to RR=18 and O_2 sat = 97). Your training data will only include RR = 18 and O_2 sat = 97, but in real time, your model will see RR = 97 and O_2 sat = 18. (If a patient actually had those vital signs, she is really in trouble!). Fifth, the underlying data may change in ways that the model never had the opportunity to see. For example, the lab may move from a single-purpose lab test (e.g., *C. diff* toxin assay) to a multipurpose lab test (e.g., a gastrointestinal multiplex PCR that also includes *C diff* as one of many outputs).

Because your model has never seen this lab before, it doesn't know the relationship to what you're trying to predict. The introduction of new medications into practice is another example. Finally, the relationship of specific predictors to specific outcomes commonly changes over time. Maybe care generally gets better, and length of stay is shorter and mortality lower than when the model was trained (this happened to APACHE, a traditionally built ICU predictive model). Or perhaps new treatments change outcomes. For example, in one study in Alberta performed in 1986 (before highly active antiretroviral therapy), the mortality rate of patients with human immunodeficiency virus (HIV) disease peaked at about 20% per year. By 2003, the mortality rate fell to about 2% per year—a 10-fold difference. In another study from 1996 to 2004, mortality rates fell from 7.0 to 1.3 per 100 person-years—a reduction of > 80%.[43,44] Clearly, models trained in one era would not predict well in another.

> **Caution**
> Beware of training-serving skew: When real-time data look different from historical data, models will perform differently.

- **Causality? Not so fast.** We all want to identify the best treatment for patients, and we want to be able to do so more quickly and with more personalization than randomized controlled trials allow. Just like with traditional clinical models, you should be extremely cautious in conflating correlation and causality. Causal inference is a tricky subject, and it is an area of active research in both traditional biostatistics (propensity scores and instrumental variables, among others) and machine learning (reinforcement learning, off-policy evaluation).

> **Caution**
>
> Be especially cautious about causal inference from observational data, whether from traditional or machine learning models. This is a specialized, challenging, and difficult area.

When evaluating either traditional or machine learning models that make assertions about identifying optimal treatments, it is worth revisiting Sir Bradford Hill's 1965 insights about causality from observational data (now routinely called the *Bradford Hill criteria*, and the paper recently has been republished[45]) and some of their recent updates.[46] For readers interested in this challenging topic, there are a number of outstanding full-length books on the topic of causal inference.[47,48] We will begin to tackle some of this material in Chapter 20.

THE FUTURE

Today is an exciting and transformational time for the use of machine learning in healthcare. Things that seemed impossible just a few years ago now routinely get accomplished, and some of these are moving into practice. The literature is replete with commentaries about how AI and machine learning will dramatically transform healthcare for the better.[49,50]

We generally share this optimism, though with a bit of caution about how fast it will occur. Our impression is that a confluence of factors—the digitization of healthcare, combined with new capabilities of AI, among others—means that we are likely to be at a turning point … one where healthcare will overcome the productivity paradox that has plagued health information technology so far.[51] But it is important to remember that implementing new technology in the delivery of healthcare is a complicated, difficult endeavor and seems likely to take years or decades to reach full fruition. Does this mean that health system leaders should ignore machine learning? Absolutely not. As Bill Gates said,

> [W]e always overestimate the change that will occur in the next two years and underestimate the change that will occur in the next 10. Don't let yourself be lulled into inaction.[52]

KEY POINTS

- Artificial general intelligence (AGI), a computerized intelligence that can learn, handle any task that a human intelligence can take on, and become self-improving, does not exist today, though it is an area of active research.
- Specific (or narrow) AI focuses on one particular task. It may have outstanding (and even superhuman) performance on that one task, but its skills cannot be generalized to other problems. This kind of AI exists and is used today.

- The key insight about machine learning is that computers can learn from examples, rather than being specifically programmed with detailed instructions.
- Deep learning is a particular kind of machine learning that has generated impressive results in many domains.
- In healthcare, machine learning has already been shown to meet or exceed physician-level performance in a number of specific domains, such as identifying diabetic retinopathy, classifying skin lesions, and identifying cancer in pathology images, but numerous challenges remain for machine learning to reach its full impact in healthcare.

REFERENCES

1. Gulshan V, Peng L, Coram M, et al. Development and validation of a deep learning algorithm for detection of diabetic retinopathy in retinal fundus photographs. *JAMA*. 2016;316(22):2402–2410.
2. Krause J, Gulshan V, Rahimy E, et al. Grader variability and the importance of reference standards for evaluating machine learning models for diabetic retinopathy. *Ophthalmology*. 2018;125(8):1264–1272.
3. McCarthy J. *What Is Artificial Intelligence?* 2007. Accessed November 23, 2018, from http://www-formal.stanford.edu/jmc/whatisai/node1.html.
4. Samuel AL. Some studies in machine learning using the game of checkers. *IBM J Res Dev*. 1959;3(3):210–229.
5. Greenemeier L. 20 years after Deep Blue: how AI has advanced since conquering chess. *Sci Am*. June 2, 2017. Accessed April 28, 2019, from https://www.scientificamerican.com/article/20-years-after-deep-blue-how-ai-has-advanced-since-conquering-chess/.
6. Silver D, Huang A, Maddison CJ, et al. Mastering the game of Go with deep neural networks and tree search. *Nature*. 2016;529(7587):484–489.
7. Silver D, Schrittwieser J, Simonyan K, et al. Mastering the game of Go without human knowledge. *Nature*. 2017;550(7676):354–359.
8. Turing AM. I.—Computing machinery and intelligence. *Mind*. 1950;LIX(236):433–460.
9. McCarthy J, Minsky ML, Rochester N, Shannon CE. A proposal for the Dartmouth summer research project on artificial intelligence, August 31, 1955. *AI Magazine*. 2006;27(4):12.
10. Lim M. History of AI Winters. *Digital Actuaries*. 2018. Accessed November 6, 2018, from https://www.actuaries.digital/2018/09/05/history-of-ai-winters/#_edn2.
11. Markoff J. Behind artificial intelligence, a squadron of bright real people. *The New York Times*. 2005. Accessed May 31, 2019, from https://www.nytimes.com/2005/10/14/technology/behind-artificial-intelligence-a-squadron-of-bright-real-people.html.
12. Rumelhart DE, Hinton GE, Williams RJ. *Learning internal representations by error propagation* (No. ICS-8506). Institute for Cognitive Science, University of California at San Diego. 1985.

13. Hinton GE. Learning distributed representations of concepts. In *Proceedings of the Eighth Annual Conference of the Cognitive Science Society* 1986 (August);1:12.
14. LeCun Y, Boser B, Denker JS, Henderson D, Howard RE, Hubbard W, Jackel LD. Backpropagation applied to handwritten zip code recognition. *Neural Comp*. 1989;1(4): 541–551.
15. Erhan D, Bengio Y, Courville A, Manzagol PA, Vincent P, Bengio S. Why does unsupervised pre-training help deep learning? *J Mach Learning Res*. 2010;11(Feb):625–660.
16. Amodei D, Hernandez D. *AI and Compute*. OpenAI Blog. 2018. Accessed November 6, 2018, from https://blog.openai.com/ai-and-compute/.
17. Jha AK, DesRoches CM, Campbell EG, et al. Use of electronic health records in U.S. hospitals. *N Engl J Med*. 2009;360(16):1628–1638.
18. IDC and EMC. *Vertical Industry Brief: The Digital Universe: Driving Data Growth in Healthcare*. 2014. Accessed February 23, 2017, from https://www.emc.com/analyst-report/digital-universe-healthcare-vertical-report-ar.pdf.
19. Beam AL, Kohane IS. Big Data and machine learning in health care. *JAMA*. 2018;319(13):1317–1318.
20. Rumelhart DE, Hinton GE, Williams RJ. Learning representations by back-propagating errors. *Nature*. 1986;323(6088):533.
21. Vanfleteren LE, Spruit MA, Groenen M, et al. Clusters of comorbidities based on validated objective measurements and systemic inflammation in patients with chronic obstructive pulmonary disease. *Am J Respir Crit Care Med*. 2013;187(7):728–735.
22. Seymour CW, Kennedy JN, Wang S, et al. Derivation, validation, and potential treatment implications of novel clinical phenotypes for sepsis. *JAMA*. 2019;321(20):2003–2017.
23. Fonarow GC, Adams KFJr, Abraham WT, et al. Risk stratification for in-hospital mortality in acutely decompensated heart failure: classification and regression tree analysis. *JAMA*. 2005;293(5):572–580.
24. James G, Witten D, Hastie T, Tibshirani R. *An Introduction to Statistical Learning*. New York, NY: Springer; 2013.
25. Hsich E, Gorodeski EZ, Blackstone EH, Ishwaran H, Lauer MS. Identifying important risk factors for survival in patient with systolic heart failure using random survival forests. *Circ Cardiovasc Qual Outcomes*. 2011;4(1):39–45.
26. Rajpurkar P, Irvin J, Zhu K, et al. Chexnet: Radiologist-level pneumonia detection on chest x-rays with deep learning. *arXiv preprint arXiv:171105225*. 2017.
27. Esteva A, Kuprel B, Novoa RA, et al. Dermatologist-level classification of skin cancer with deep neural networks. *Nature*. 2017;542(7639):115–118.
28. Liu Y, Kohlberger T, Norouzi M, et al. Artificial intelligence-based breast cancer nodal metastasis detection. *Arch Pathol Lab Med*. 2018.
29. Pascanu R, Mikolov T, Bengio Y. *On the Difficulty of Training Recurrent Neural Networks*. Paper presented at International Conference on Machine Learning, Atlanta. June 2013.
30. Hochreiter S, Schmidhuber J. Long short-term memory. *Neural Comput*. 1997;9(8):1735–1780.

31. Liu Z, Yang M, Wang X, et al. Entity recognition from clinical texts via recurrent neural network. *BMC Med Inform Decis Mak*. 2017;17(suppl 2):67.
32. Mirshekarian S, Bunescu R, Marling C, Schwartz F. Using LSTMs to learn physiological models of blood glucose behavior. *Conf Proc IEEE Eng Med Biol Soc*. 2017;2017:2887–2891.
33. Tsiouris K, Pezoulas VC, Zervakis M, Konitsiotis S, Koutsouris DD, Fotiadis DI. A Long Short-Term Memory deep learning network for the prediction of epileptic seizures using EEG signals. *Comput Biol Med*. 2018;99:24–37.
34. Jiang Z, Zhao C, He B, Guan Y, Jiang J. De-identification of medical records using conditional random fields and long short-term memory networks. *J Biomed Inform*. 2017;75S:S43–S53.
35. Rajkomar A, Oren E, Chen K, et al. Scalable and accurate deep learning with electronic health records. *NPJ Digital Medicine*. 2018;1(1):18.
36. Mnih V, Kavukcuoglu K, Silver D, et al. Human-level control through deep reinforcement learning. *Nature*. 2015;518(7540):529–533.
37. Kober J, Bagnell JA, Peters J. Reinforcement learning in robotics: A survey. *International Journal of Robotics Research*. 2013;32(11):1238–1274.
38. Shachter RD. Evaluating influence diagrams. *Operations Research*. 1986;34(6):871–882.
39. Lin R, Stanley MD, Ghassemi MM, Nemati S. A deep deterministic policy gradient approach to medication dosing and surveillance in the ICU. *Conf Proc IEEE Eng Med Biol Soc*. 2018;July:4927–4931.
40. Komorowski M, Celi LA, Badawi O, Gordon AC, Faisal AA. The artificial intelligence clinician learns optimal treatment strategies for sepsis in intensive care. *Nat Med*. 2018;24(11):1716–1720.
41. Leisman DE. Rare events in the ICU: an emerging challenge in classification and prediction. *Crit Care Med*. 2018;46(3):418–424.
42. Rajkomar A. Ensuring fairness in machine learning to advance health equity. *Ann Intern Med*. 2018;169(12):866–872.
43. Palella FJJr, Baker RK, Moorman AC, et al. Mortality in the highly active antiretroviral therapy era: changing causes of death and disease in the HIV outpatient study. *J Acquir Immune Defic Syndr*. 2006;43(1):27–34.
44. Krentz HB, Kliewer G, Gill MJ. Changing mortality rates and causes of death for HIV-infected individuals living in southern Alberta, Canada, from 1984 to 2003. *HIV Med*. 2005;6(2):99–106.
45. Hill AB. The environment and disease: association or causation? 1965. *J R Soc Med*. 2015;108(1):32–37.
46. Fedak KM, Bernal A, Capshaw ZA, Gross S. Applying the Bradford Hill criteria in the 21st century: how data integration has changed causal inference in molecular epidemiology. *Emerg Themes Epidemiol*. 2015;12:14.
47. Pearl J, Glymour M, Jewell NP. *Causal Inference in Statistics: A Primer*. Chichester, West Sussex, UK: John Wiley & Sons; 2016.
48. Hernán M, JM R. *Causal Inference*. 2018 Boca Raton, FL: Chapman & Hall/CRC (forthcoming). Accessed June 11, 2019, from https://www.hsph.harvard.edu/miguel-hernan/causal-inference-book/.

49. Hinton G. Deep learning—a technology with the potential to transform health care. *JAMA*. 2018;320(11):1101–1102.
50. Obermeyer Z, Lee TH. Lost in thought—the limits of the human mind and the future of medicine. *N Engl J Med*. 2017;377(13):1209–1211.
51. Wachter RM, Howell MD. Resolving the productivity paradox of health information technology: a time for optimism. *JAMA*. 2018;320(1):25–26.
52. Gates B. Bill Gates' new rules. *Time*. April 19, 1999. Accessed June 11, 2019, from http://content.time.com/time/world/article/0,8599,2053895,00.html.

WHAT EVERYONE SHOULD KNOW ABOUT RISK ADJUSTMENT 18

Risk adjustment in medicine and healthcare is a story of convergent evolution. On one hand, risk adjustment has a history that emerged with the creation of health insurance in the United States in the 20th century. The "risk" is the risk assumed by the insurance company to insure each individual person. In this setting, it represented an estimate of how chronically ill a particular person is, and therefore, how costly that person is to insure.[1] On the other hand, similar efforts were underway at the hospital level to create methods to compare one hospital with another; risk adjustment allows comparisons by understanding the variation in the probability of adverse or favorable outcomes based on patient characteristics versus hospital-driven outcomes.

Why do we need to understand risk adjustment as healthcare delivery scientists? We will spend this chapter discussing the origins of risk adjustment and several current examples in healthcare financing. Then, armed with the tools discussed in Chapters 16 and 17, we will discuss methods of evaluating risk adjustment strategies. We will return to an example of using risk adjustment work in local healthcare delivery science at a single institution and how you can employ risk adjustment techniques. Finally, we will discuss what can go wrong with risk adjustment.

WHAT IS RISK ADJUSTMENT, AND WHY WE SHOULD CARE?

Risk Adjustment Designed by Insurers

Risk adjustment in healthcare financing began as a method for health insurance companies to estimate the cost of insuring a person. A 25-year old man who does not smoke and exercises regularly is unlikely to use much healthcare. But a 64-year old man who formerly smoked, is overweight, and already suffers from hypertension, chronic obstructive pulmonary disease (COPD) on home oxygen therapy, and type 2 diabetes is likely to require multiple healthcare interactions in the coming year. If given a choice, insurance companies would only enroll the first man, charge him health premiums, and never have to pay any of those costs. But if it has to insure both, the insurance company wants to identify which patient is which and then charge more to provide insurance to the second man because he is likely to cost the company more. Joe Newhouse described the insurance company in a similar scenario as walking through the produce aisle of the grocery store, squeezing each apple, and trying to pick only the best ones.[1] Apples have a single cost whether you grab a bad or a good apple, so you will want to pay for the good apple only if you can figure out which one that is. Insurers want to try to figure out which patients are the good apples and only enroll them in their plans, if they can. If they can't choose the healthy from the sick up front, they will want to try to hedge their bets by getting the pricing right—charging the sick person more for insurance.

Before World War II, a single insurance company, Blue Cross, offered one price for all patients when it created the field of health insurance (the apples in Newhouse's analogy all cost the same). But in the face of a commercial market that emerged, the company recognized the heterogeneity of patients and was forced to abandon a one-premium-for-all model.[1] If the insurance company planned to offer different rates to customers, however, the next challenge was to get customers to estimate their own likelihood to need services through offering high- and low-premium plans (or more- or less-expensive plans). When a customer judged himself to be low risk, the insurer would offer low premiums but high costs for use, with high-premium plans offering the reverse. The result, however, was a disproportionate number of sicker people using the higher-cost plan, thereby creating a selection bias in the more expensive plan and concentrating the risks to the insurance company in one place.[2]

The result of this selection bias is that insurers will try to limit customer access to only the high-premium plans. In the absence of workable risk adjustment strategies, insurance companies will try to run from the "bad apples" and offer their plans to only the good, nonbruised ones. Further, insurance companies may start marketing to attract the low-risk patients, leaving less-healthy patients without options.[3] Although the market has evolved, with employer-based plans, and there are numerous regulatory requirements mandating insurance eligibility today, understanding risk adjustment remains important.

Risk adjustment is necessary, from an insurance standpoint, to align the amount of money that a patient will need to pay for healthcare with what the insurer (or the federal government in the form of Medicare) should budget, so that the insurer can know what to charge and still make a profit. But even a very good risk adjuster can never completely predict healthcare expense. For example, a 75-year-old patient with diabetes and atrial fibrillation but who does not take a blood-thinning medication is estimated to have a 4% risk of a stroke per year.[4] Whether that patient actually *has* a stroke has some component of luck, which no risk adjuster will be able to accommodate. But we can think of the pieces of risk adjustment as similar to methods that we learned about in Chapter 16—random and linear fixed effects models. There are *fixed effects*, which raise the risk of everyone in that group (e.g., chronic diseases like hypertension). There are *time-varying effects*, which increase or decrease the risk of harm over time (e.g., age). And there are *random effects*, which incorporate luck.[3] Whether or not the risk adjuster in question incorporates each of these components gets at the reason behind and the quality of the risk adjustment. The story of risk adjustment does not end here. Risk adjusting is central to whether we can compare similar patients, practices, or hospitals, as well as understanding the shortcomings of any of those comparisons.

Risk Adjustment to Compare Hospitals

During much of the same time that insurers were building risk adjustment strategies, so too were researchers, states, and business groups. All became interested in comparing hospitals to one another, and risk adjustment is crucial to the ability to compare hospitals to others like them. The purpose here, different from insurance markets, is to allow us to remove variations in patient outcomes between hospitals that result from the patients themselves, leaving behind patient outcomes that result from high- versus low-quality care at that hospital.[5] Early researchers began developing severity-of-illness measures for a variety of reasons—to respond to state regulators, understand patients' experiences, and evaluate state Medicaid programs—but all relied on the limited data available from patients' charts and expert opinion.[5-8] The intersection with the concerns of the insurer markets emerged with Medicare's use of Diagnosis-Related Groups (DRGs), followed by several state-based or regional initiatives to compare hospitals' outcomes, particularly in light of growing interest in public reporting.[9-13] However, while the risk adjustment strategies continued to grow in terms of access to data and sophistication of different models, the cost of data generation continued to be prohibitively high. Further, multiple risk adjustment models continued to have variable accuracy in predicting mortality by diagnosis.[5]

In the current hospital market, there are multiple efforts to compare hospitals to one another. For example, if a consumer is interested in which of two hospitals in his or her city would be the right place to receive

> **Key Point**
>
> Hospitals are ranked using many tools, but rarely do ranking systems identify the same high-performing hospitals.

subspecialty care in oncology or cardiology, that person can look to a range of published lists, such as those of *U.S. News and World Report* and HealthGrades; business-led consortiums like the Leapfrog Group; and the Hospital Compare program of the Center for Medicare and Medicaid Services (CMS).[14] However, many of these ranking systems have variable performance when it comes to reliably identifying (or even consistently identifying) high-performing hospitals.[15–17] Further, ranking systems do not take into account performance variation based on chance alone.[18] (See also Chapter 12.)

Risk Adjustment to Compare Interventions

One major reason why we should care about risk adjustment in healthcare delivery science concerns how we should use adequate risk adjustment to ensure that, when we are studying the effect of an intervention to improve patient flow or to deliver care more effectively and equitably, we are able to understand our own data. As with other reasons for using risk adjustment, we want to be able to distinguish between patient outcomes due to how sick a patient is (risk adjustment), as opposed to patient outcomes that are due to our intervention. Said another way, if we're interested in understanding how much benefit a patient will receive from our intervention, we should compare similar patients to each other. As discussed in Chapter 16, using multivariable analysis allows us to ask, "For all patients of the same severity of illness, what is the benefit of our exposure?"

Consider the following example of an effort to improve nutrition and facilitate patient flow among patients admitted with pancreatitis. Let's say that a multidisciplinary group of physicians, nurses, and surgeons gets together to improve the care provided to patients admitted with pancreatitis. They decide that, based on prior data, patients with pancreatitis do well and are discharged sooner with the reintroduction of early enteral feeding, so they want to develop a new pathway for pancreatitis patients.[19] The intervention is a patient-focused plan of care, given to all patients, which identifies which day they will start drinking clear liquids, which day they will eat full diets, how much they should walk around the hospital floor, and what day they are expected to go home. This patient progression plan is given to all patients admitted with pancreatitis once the program is up and running, and the plan is to perform a before-and-after study with two outcomes: time to full diet and length of stay. However, we would expect that patients who are sicker will take longer to eat a full diet or to be discharged from the hospital. Because we would want to understand any benefit from our intervention, we would want to make sure that we controlled for patient severity of illness on admission (and potentially other comorbidities) so that we could distinguish between the effect of the illness and the effect of the intervention.

WHAT RISK ADJUSTMENTS ARE AVAILABLE, AND HOW SHOULD WE ASSESS THEM?

First, as Lisa Iezzoni challenged us in her landmark paper, "The Risks of Risk Adjustment," we have to ask—the risk of what?[5] If we are interested in predicting the cost of care by building a risk adjustment strategy designed to encompass severity of illness, the *most* severely ill patients will die rapidly with relatively less expensive hospitalizations.[20] Predicting resource use may not always serve as a prediction of how sick patients are. Alternatively, if we are interested in understanding who the sickest people in the hospital are, we can fall back on a common strategy of trying to predict the risk of dying in the hospital or dying within 30 days of hospitalization. The most common risk prediction strategies do just that.

Several scoring systems have been derived for predicting the risk of death for critically ill patients in order to better align needed resources with the sickest patients. The Acute Physiology and Chronic Health Evaluation (APACHE) score uses patient age, diagnosis, admission location, and acute and chronic variables, and it has several iterative variations (versions I through IV).[21-24] For version IV, data extraction time is estimated at about 37 minutes—a good deal longer than many other scoring systems.[25] APACHE scores typically require software to perform as the categorical variables then are entered into the logistic regression to obtain the predicted mortality for the patient, which limits their bedside utility as well.

Other scoring systems that have transformed their logistic regression coefficients into ordinal scores (a method of transforming logistic regression models into scores that was described in Chapter 16) include the Simplified Acute Physiologic Score (SAPS)[26-29] and the Mortality Prediction Model (MPM0).[29-31] Organ dysfunction scores have also been used to quantify severity of illness. Examples include the Sequential Organ Failure Assessment (SOFA),[32,33] the Logistic Organ Dysfunction Score (LODS),[34] and the Multiple Organ Dysfunction Score (MODS).[35] Several others have been built for general hospitalized patients using a range of methods, including tools from machine learning.[36-39] Many of these scores, such as the SOFA or MPM, are intended to be calculated within a specific, initial time period for the patient.

How should we choose between these types of scores? First, let's consider the statistical considerations of each of their utility: discrimination, calibration, and generalizability. These concerns apply to all risk adjustment and risk prediction models, whether they are from traditional models or machine learning.

Discrimination

Discrimination describes any model's ability to divide the population into two groups: individuals with the outcome of interest and individuals without the outcome of interest.[40] In many of our risk adjustment models, *discrimination* would refer to a model that accurately identified which patients would die in the hospital and which would not. The most common statistic reported is the *C statistic,* referring to the concordance between the event that is predicted and what actually happens. The value of the C statistic ranges from 0.5 (random) to 1.0 (perfect prediction).[40] This value is equivalent to the area under the receiver operating characteristic (ROC) curve, which itself is a plot of the proportion of high-risk patients with the event of interest (sensitivity) against the proportion of patients without the event, but who were predicted to have high risk (1 − specificity).[41] The C statistic's major shortcoming is that it does not assign a value to misclassification errors. For example, let's imagine that we built a model that predicts in-patient death in an intensive care unit (ICU) and releases a score. The misclassification errors can go in two directions: very sick patients could be assigned a low-risk score, or very well patients could receive a high-risk score. In the first example, we would actively miss sick patients. In the second example, we would sound an unnecessary alarm. These two errors are not equivalent, but the C statistic of our imaginary model would treat them both the same. Other methods derived from decision analysis create weights for different outcomes.[42]

Calibration

In contrast to discrimination, *calibration* measures the ability of a model to assign the correct level of risk of our outcome to each group of patients.[43] In our model, we would want to make sure that when we said a patient was at very high risk of death (let's say that our model predicted a 95% chance of death), they really did have a very high risk of death. Measures of calibration help us make sure that *high* really means high.

The most common method used in the healthcare literature is the Hosmer-Lemeshow test.[44] In this test, we divide all of our predicted risks into equal quantiles, or equally spaced buckets of data; deciles are often standard in statistical packages. We then compare each quantile of events with the number of patients in each group who actually experienced that event. If our model is well calibrated, the two quantiles should not be statistically different from one another. Put another way, all our predictions should have sorted the patients into the right buckets in terms of what actually happened. We can test this with the Hosmer-Lemeshow goodness-of-fit test, which asks if these buckets are statistically different from one another (they shouldn't be). Like any test that relies on statistical significance, though, large models are at risk of false-positive tests (more inclined toward a type I error), which in our case would mean that the model would look poorly calibrated simply because of the huge underlying size of the population. For this reason, especially when you have very large sample sizes, visual inspection of the calibration plots is very important. Smaller populations (estimated to be 500 or less) are at risk of just the opposite, appearing well calibrated when they are not.[43]

Generalizability

Fundamentally, *generalizability* requires that the model or study results can be applied outside the setting of the study itself. Biomedical research has wrestled with the challenges of generalizability for some time, deciding whether information we learn about from animal models teaches us about human health based on decisions about whether the biomedical pathway under study or the effect of the drug is universal across all organisms or unique to that individual animal. If we derive a risk prediction strategy for the Medicare population, is that group of patients similar enough to all patients, who might be younger?

This question returns to the concept of bias, as introduced in Chapter 13. If our population differs from another population due to a systematic sampling error (e.g., only elderly Medicare enrollees) or due to the data that we used (e.g., only billing-related electronic information), we may have created a biased result. Similarly, confounding may also be at work. If we are using prior Medicare billing data to predict the use of hospital resources at 30 days, we may be excluding important information (like family support) that may be associated with both prior and future healthcare use—a confounder.

To begin to test the generalizability of our model, we can attempt to replicate our results. There are several methods to do this within the development of risk adjustment. We can start with internal validation, which requires us to draw a new population from within our original population in some way. The first way we can do this is to exclude some people from our original data set, thereby creating a validation data set on which to test our risk adjustment strategy. This can be done in a random or nonrandom way. If we leave out a number of patients in a random way, then the two data sets are statistically likely to be identical, which is less useful for understanding the generalizability of our risk adjustment or predictive model.

Alternatively, we can create a validation set in a nonrandom way. This might include creating a model in one year and then testing the model in the subsequent year. Finally, another method is to use a bootstrapping method, wherein multiple new data sets are created from the original data set, with the predictive strategy repeatedly tested on each subsequent data set.[45] Bootstrapping is further discussed in Chapter 17. *External validation* is even more helpful, which refers to testing a predictive rule or risk adjustment strategy on a new sample from a different location or center.

EXAMPLES OF RISK ADJUSTMENT GONE AWRY

How can using risk adjustments in healthcare delivery fail us? To start, consider the impact that risk adjustment has on pay-for-performance and public reporting for physicians and hospitals.[46] Risk models that fail to account for case volume frequently misrepresent variation due to chance as predictive descriptions of quality and performance. However, models that do account for case volume of individual procedures and use hierarchical strategies in their risk adjustment may make as many as 90% of low-quality performers and all high-quality performers look average, thereby penalizing hospitals that use pay-for-performance programs.[47]

Take as a very specific example the question of whether nationally reported readmission rates between hospitals should be adjusted for the socioeconomic status of their patient populations. Currently, readmission programs are adjusted for patient-level clinical factors, but not for characteristics such as income or housing. Those who oppose adjusting quality measures by socioeconomic characteristics of patients say that hospitals should not be permitted to provide lower-quality care to poorer patients. However, as Ashish Jha and others have pointed out, failing to take into consideration in any risk adjustment strategy that some hospitals take care of large numbers of poorer patients, while others take care of very few, lumps the between-hospital variation (in terms of quality outcomes) together with the within-hospital variation (in terms of outcomes stratified by socioeconomic status). The result is that hospitals caring for larger number of poorer patients are penalized in national reporting strategies. We are left not knowing the quality of care delivered at either type of hospital, whether it be those who care for patients with lower socioeconomic statuses or those who do not.[48] This has been demonstrated in mortality rates reported by hospitals[49] and in the value-based modifier program.[50]

USING RISK ADJUSTMENT IN LOCAL HEALTHCARE DELIVERY SCIENCE

Returning to the reason behind using risk adjustment in local healthcare delivery science, we would highlight three major purposes: controlling for patient risk, stratifying by risk, and using risk adjustment as the intervention itself.

Using Risk Adjustment as a Confounder

Whenever we implement an intervention to improve patient care or want to study an aspect of healthcare delivery, we are fundamentally interested in the incremental benefit or harm of the exposure itself, not the variation that can be attributed to patient characteristics. Many healthcare services increase in use when patients are sicker, particularly for hospitalized patients. Let's say we are interested in studying the number of lab draws per day per patient. We anticipate that some patients get unnecessary labs, potentially because some physicians overuse certain types of labs like routine bloodwork, while other physicians are more parsimonious. However, patients who are sicker in the hospital are likely to have frequent lab draws. If we were to conduct a logistic regression exploring the relationship of lab draws and in-hospital death, we would find that the two are associated. Unfortunately, because we didn't adjust for confounding by severity of illness, we can't know what contribution to lab use is due to patient illness and what is due to physician variation. We would need a strong method of risk adjustment to be able to ask and answer the question we want.

Using Risk Adjustment as an *Effect Modifier*

Effect modification, as described in Chapter 16, is the idea that two variables of interest do not have an additive effect on one another, but instead a multiplicative effect to understand the true association with the outcome of interest. As an example, patients who are over 65 years old and women may have a significantly greater rate of a certain disease than could be accounted for by looking at the association of the disease among women, controlling for age, or of the disease among those over 65 years old, controlling for gender.

To that end, healthcare delivery scientists may want to consider stratifying by patient risk, so as to apply limited healthcare resources to those who need it most, or for whom a delivery method would be most effective. In our example of our program bringing early enteral feeding to pancreatitis patients, perhaps we find that the program works very well for patients with mild pancreatitis, but poorly for patients with severe pancreatitis.

> **Key Point**
> Consider many ways to use risk adjustment in healthcare delivery interventions. Sometimes we want to control it away; other times, it's the star of the show.

Instead, we might risk-stratify our pancreatitis patients from the start of our implementation strategy and plan to understand the population for whom our program would be most useful.

Using Risk to Guide Intervention

Finally, another approach to risk adjustment may be to guide the intervention itself, as a prediction strategy. Consider a plan to implement a new rapid response system, whereby a team of critical care providers and respiratory therapists will be deployed based on a patient's risk of clinical decline. The University of Chicago hospital system did just this.[51] With an electronic risk prediction tool, the institution developed and then tested using a rapid response team activation instead of a more traditional system triggered by abnormal vital signs.

Risk adjustment, as in any aspect of modeling, asks a lot of us as healthcare delivery scientists. We must decide which model to use, what compromises we are willing to make with our models, and how we want to use our risk adjuster. As risk adjustment models are often used to capture the knowable confounders of patient sickness or severity of illness, the shortcoming of each model means that we have to accept even more degrees of uncertainty in the output produced from our analyses. However, in our efforts to bring research-quality methods to the study of healthcare delivery, we are at least armed with tools to decide on the most appropriate risk adjustment model.

KEY POINTS

- Risk adjustment is used broadly in the fields of health insurance, research, and healthcare delivery science.
- Multiple patient-level risk adjustment tools exist, but buyer beware—they vary in the population in which they were derived, their functionality, and their availability in data.
- All risk adjustment tools should be evaluated for their discrimination, calibration, and generalizability to the population in your research question.
- Risk adjustment fails frequently. This chapter describes examples where it overstated variation due to chance, where all values were shrunk to the average eliminating variation of interest, and where it actively penalized one group of hospitals over another.
- Risk adjustment can be used locally, with care, to remove variation across patients due to patient characteristics, to stratify any intervention to the patients who will most benefit, and as the exposure itself to direct limited resources.

REFERENCES

1. Newhouse JP. Patients at risk: health reform and risk adjustment. *Health Aff (Millwood)*. 1994;13(1):132–146.
2. Welch WP. Restructuring the Federal Employees Health Benefits Program: the private sector option. *Inquiry*. 1989;26(3):321–334.
3. Newhouse JP, Buntin MB, Chapman JD. Risk adjustment and Medicare: taking a closer look. *Health Aff (Millwood)*. 1997;16(5):26–43.
4. Lip GY, Nieuwlaat R, Pisters R, Lane DA, Crijns HJ. Refining clinical risk stratification for predicting stroke and thromboembolism in atrial fibrillation using a novel risk factor-based approach: the euro heart survey on atrial fibrillation. *Chest*. 2010,137(2):263–272.
5. Iezzoni LI. The risks of risk adjustment. *JAMA*. 1997;278(19):1600–1607.
6. Horn SD. Validity, reliability and implications of an index of inpatient severity of illness. *Med Care*. 1981;19(3):354–362.
7. Brewster AC, Karlin BG, Hyde LA, Jacobs CM, Bradbury RC, Chae YM. MEDISGRPS: a clinically based approach to classifying hospital patients at admission. *Inquiry*. 1985;22(4):377–387.
8. Gonnella JS, Louis DZ, McCord JJ. The staging concept—an approach to the assessment of outcome of ambulatory care. *Med Care*. 1976;14(1):13–21.
9. Hannan EL, Kilburn H Jr., Racz M, Shields E, Chassin MR. Improving the outcomes of coronary artery bypass surgery in New York State. *JAMA*. 1994;271(10):761–766.
10. Edwards N, Honemann D, Burley D, Navarro M. Refinement of the Medicare diagnosis-related groups to incorporate a measure of severity. *Health Care Financ Rev*. 1994;16(2):45–64.
11. O'Connor GT, Plume SK, Olmstead EM, et al. Multivariate prediction of in-hospital mortality associated with coronary artery bypass graft surgery. Northern New England Cardiovascular Disease Study Group. *Circulation*. 1992;85(6):2110–2118.
12. Markson LE, Nash DB, Louis DZ, Gonnella JS. Clinical outcomes management and disease staging. *Eval Health Prof*. 1991;14(2):201–227.
13. Chassin MR, Hannan EL, DeBuono BA. Benefits and hazards of reporting medical outcomes publicly. *N Engl J Med*. 1996;334(6):394–398.
14. Howell MD. A 37-year-old man trying to choose a high-quality hospital: review of hospital quality indicators. *JAMA*. 2009;302(21):2353–2360.
15. Jha AK, Orav EJ, Ridgway AB, Zheng J, Epstein AM. Does the Leapfrog program help identify high-quality hospitals? *Jt Comm J Qual Patient Saf*. 2008;34(6):318–325.
16. Werner RM, Bradlow ET. Relationship between Medicare's hospital compare performance measures and mortality rates. *JAMA*. 2006;296(22):2694–2702.
17. Krumholz HM, Rathore SS, Chen J, Wang Y, Radford MJ. Evaluation of a consumer-oriented internet health care report card: the risk of quality ratings based on mortality data. *JAMA*. 2002;287(10):1277–1287.
18. Dimick JB, Welch HG. The zero mortality paradox in surgery. *J Am Coll Surg*. 2008;206(1):13–16.

19. Vaughn VM, Shuster D, Rogers MAM, et al. Early versus delayed feeding in patients with acute pancreatitis: a systematic review. *Ann Intern Med.* 2017;166(12):883–892.
20. Freeman JL, Fetter RB, Park H, et al. Diagnosis-related group refinement with diagnosis- and procedure-specific comorbidities and complications. *Med Care.* 1995;33(8):806–827.
21. Zimmerman JE, Kramer AA, McNair DS, Malila FM.Acute Physiology and Chronic Health Evaluation (APACHE) IV: hospital mortality assessment for today's critically ill patients. *Crit Care Med.* 2006;34(5):1297–1310.
22. Varghese YE, Kalaiselvan MS, Renuka MK, Arunkumar AS. Comparison of acute physiology and chronic health evaluation II (APACHE II) and acute physiology and chronic health evaluation IV (APACHE IV) severity of illness scoring systems, in a multidisciplinary ICU. *J Anaesthesiol Clin Pharmacol.* 2017;33(2):248–253.
23. Knaus WA, Wagner DP, Draper EA, et al. The APACHE III prognostic system. Risk prediction of hospital mortality for critically ill hospitalized adults. *Chest.* 1991;100(6):1619–1636.
24. Knaus WA, Zimmerman JE, Wagner DP, Draper EA, Lawrence DE. APACHE-acute physiology and chronic health evaluation: a physiologically based classification system. *Crit Care Med.* 1981;9(8):591–597.
25. Kuzniewicz MW, Vasilevskis EE, Lane R, et al. Variation in ICU risk-adjusted mortality: impact of methods of assessment and potential confounders. *Chest.* 2008;133(6):1319–1327.
26. Poncet A, Perneger TV, Merlani P, Capuzzo M, Combescure C. Determinants of the calibration of SAPS II and SAPS 3 mortality scores in intensive care: a European multicenter study. *Crit Care.* 2017;21(1):85.
27. Metnitz PG, Moreno RP, Almeida E, et al. SAPS 3—From evaluation of the patient to evaluation of the intensive care unit. Part 1: Objectives, methods, and cohort description. *Intensive Care Med.* 2005;31(10):1336–1344.
28. Le Gall JR, Loirat P, Alperovitch A, et al. A simplified acute physiology score for ICU patients. *Crit Care Med.* 1984;12(11):975–977.
29. Lemeshow S, Teres D, Pastides H, Avrunin JS, Steingrub JS. A method for predicting survival and mortality of ICU patients using objectively derived weights. *Crit Care Med.* 1985;13(7):519–525.
30. Carson SS, Kahn JM, Hough CL, et al. A multicenter mortality prediction model for patients receiving prolonged mechanical ventilation. *Crit Care Med.* 2012;40(4):1171–1176.
31. Castella X, Gilabert J, Torner F, Torres C. Mortality prediction models in intensive care: acute physiology and chronic health evaluation II and mortality prediction model compared. *Crit Care Med.* 1991;19(2):191–197.
32. Ferreira FL, Bota DP, Bross A, Melot C, Vincent JL. Serial evaluation of the SOFA score to predict outcome in critically ill patients. *JAMA.* 2001;286(14):1754–1758.
33. Vincent JL, de Mendonca A, Cantraine F, et al. Use of the SOFA score to assess the incidence of organ dysfunction/failure in intensive care units: results of a multicenter, prospective study. Working group on "sepsis-related problems" of the European Society of Intensive Care Medicine. *Crit Care Med.* 1998;26(11):1793–1800.

34. Le Gall JR, Klar J, Lemeshow S, et al. The Logistic Organ Dysfunction system. A new way to assess organ dysfunction in the intensive care unit. ICU Scoring Group. *JAMA*. 1996;276(10):802–810.
35. Marshall JC, Cook DJ, Christou NV, Bernard GR, Sprung CL, Sibbald WJ. Multiple organ dysfunction score: a reliable descriptor of a complex clinical outcome. *Crit Care Med*. 1995;23(10):1638–1652.
36. Subbe CP, Kruger M, Rutherford P, Gemmel L. Validation of a modified Early Warning Score in medical admissions. *QJM*. 2001;94(10):521–526.
37. Gardner-Thorpe J, Love N, Wrightson J, Walsh S, Keeling N. The value of Modified Early Warning Score (MEWS) in surgical in-patients: a prospective observational study. *Ann R Coll Surg Engl*. 2006;88(6):571–575.
38. Escobar GJ, Gardner MN, Greene JD, Draper D, Kipnis P. Risk-adjusting hospital mortality using a comprehensive electronic record in an integrated health care delivery system. *Med Care*. 2013;51(5):446–453.
39. Churpek MM, Yuen TC, Winslow C, Meltzer DO, Kattan MW, Edelson DP. Multicenter comparison of machine learning methods and conventional regression for predicting clinical deterioration on the wards. *Crit Care Med*. 2016;44(2):368–374.
40. Pencina MJ, D'Agostino RB Sr. Evaluating discrimination of risk prediction models: the C statistic. *JAMA*. 2015;314(10):1063–1064.
41. Hanley JA, McNeil BJ. The meaning and use of the area under a receiver operating characteristic (ROC) curve. *Radiology*. 1982;143(1):29–36.
42. Vickers AJ, Elkin EB. Decision curve analysis: a novel method for evaluating prediction models. *Med Decis Making*. 2006;26(6):565–574.
43. Meurer WJ, Tolles J. Logistic regression diagnostics: understanding how well a model predicts outcomes. *JAMA*. 2017;317(10):1068–1069.
44. Hosmer DW, Lemeshow S, Sturdivant RX. *Applied Logistic Regression*. 3rd ed. Hoboken, NJ: Wiley; 2013.
45. Altman DG, Royston P. What do we mean by validating a prognostic model? *Stat Med*. 2000;19(4):453–473.
46. Doherty RB. Goodbye, sustainable growth rate—hello, merit-based incentive payment system. *Ann Intern Med*. 2015;163(2):138–139.
47. Glance LG, Li Y, Dick AW. Quality of quality measurement: impact of risk adjustment, hospital volume, and hospital performance. *Anesthesiology*. 2016;125(6):1092–1102.
48. Jha AK, Zaslavsky AM. Quality reporting that addresses disparities in health care. *JAMA*. 2014;312(3):225–226.
49. Kim Y, Oh J, Jha A. Contribution of hospital mortality variations to socioeconomic disparities in in-hospital mortality. *BMJ Qual Saf*. 2014;23(9):741–748.
50. Roberts ET, Zaslavsky AM, McWilliams JM. The Value-Based Payment Modifier: program outcomes and implications for disparities. *Ann Intern Med*. 2018;168(4):255–265.
51. Kang MA, Churpek MM, Zadravecz FJ, Adhikari R, Twu NM, Edelson DP. Real-time risk prediction on the wards: a feasibility study. *Crit Care Med*. 2016;44(8):1468–1473.

19 MODELING PATIENT FLOW: UNDERSTANDING THROUGHPUT AND CENSUS

Every day, medical directors and administrators of all varieties worry about throughput, census, and patient flow. This concern may show up in many guises, across all care settings:

- "There are no new patient appointment slots in primary care for the next six weeks."
- "We have no urgent care slots in cardiology left open this week."
- "The emergency department is backing up, and our average wait time is 6 hours."
- "Patients are waiting in the operating room because the recovery room is full. We can't get patients out of the recovery room because the hospital floor is full."
- "The intensive care units (ICUs) are full, and cardiac surgery is backing up. A patient just got intubated on the general medicine floor. There are 10 ICU patients ready to go to the floor, but the floor is full so we can't move them. How did it get like this?"

There are many approaches to improving patient flow, most of which do not require sophisticated analytics. A number of effective techniques are reviewed in Chapter 9, which focuses in particular on Lean production/Toyota Production System (TPS) approaches to improvement. In addition, the Institute of Healthcare Improvement (IHI), the National Health Service, and others have both practical advice and courses on improving patient flow.

However, sometimes understanding patient flow in a detailed and more quantitative way can be remarkably helpful. For this purpose, we turn to a different set of modeling tools than we've discussed so far. These come out of the field known as *operations research*. These kinds of tools are particularly well suited to characterizing the dynamic aspects of patient flow. In spite of their relative lack of uptake, their potential value has been recognized for more than a decade. In 2005, the Institute of Medicine and the National Academy of Sciences collaborated to develop

---

External Resource

The Institute for Healthcare Improvement's white paper *Achieving Hospital-wide Patient Flow* is available at http://www.ihi.org/resources/Pages/IHIWhitePapers/Achieving-Hospital-wide-Patient-Flow.aspx.

They also have in-person coursework available, with information at http://www.ihi.org/education/InPersonTraining/Hospital-Flow-Professional-Development-Program/Pages/default.aspx

External Resource

NHS England's *Good Practice Guide: Focus on Improving Patient Flow* is available at https://improvement.nhs.uk/resources/good-practice-guide-focus-on-improving-patient-flow/

a joint report, *Building a Better Delivery System: A New Engineering/ Health Care Partnership*.[1] This document highlighted the usefulness of operations research—a topic that would come up again in subsequent National Academy reports focusing on developing and engineering a learning health system. Operations research is a field that developed over the past century. Its tools—including one of its oldest branches, queuing theory—help provide us a mathematical foundation with which we can understand, quantify, and predict patient flow across the healthcare system.

WHY DOES UNDERSTANDING PATIENT FLOW MATTER?

It is easy to mistake patient flow, census, and throughput as simply bureaucratic problems—things that help determine revenue and that make administrators happy, but nothing else. Patient flow certainly influences these things (it is one of the most important levers for revenue in many settings), but in fact it has a direct impact on patient safety, providers' well-being, and the overall functioning of whatever healthcare setting you're working in.

Key Point

Problems with patient flow can have direct, negative patient safety impacts.

Patient Safety and Quality

Perhaps the easiest way to see the patient safety impacts of patient flow is to think about a hospital's emergency department (ED). It is tempting to think of crowding in the ED as just an ED problem. In fact, the ED is the canary in the coal mine for hospital-level flow problems. ED overcrowding is obvious when you see it: the waiting room backs up and is filled with people, and the wait time for patients goes up. What is less obvious is that one of the most important contributors to ED crowding is so-called *access block*, which occurs when inpatient beds are full and there is no physical space in the hospital for patients to move from the ED to a bed in the hospital.[2]

Key Point

Crowding in the ED is the canary in the coal mine for problems with overall hospital flow.

What is the impact of flow problems on patient safety? The most dramatic example is that patients have died in ED waiting rooms while waiting to receive care, leading to headlines like "Family Sues Bronx Hospital After Father Dies Following 9-Hour ER Wait,"[3] "Man Dies in New York Hospital Waiting Room, Found Hours Later,"[4] and "Investigation as Patient Dies in A&E Waiting Room at Russells Hall Hospital."[5]

These are not just isolated anecdotes. More systematic investigations have found that ED overcrowding is associated with delayed assessment and care, poorer adherence to guidelines, reduced patient satisfaction, and increased mortality.[2,6] This also turns out to be true in many other healthcare environments in which problems with flow have been studied. For example, in ICUs, capacity strain changes the way that intensivists provide prophylactic medications[7] and practice end-of-life care,[8] and in sum, it appears to increase mortality.[9] For inpatient wards, hospital capacity strain worsens health outcomes and increases mortality as well.[10] Although less well studied, problems with patient flow also affect care in the outpatient setting, as well. Regardless of how good your medical care is, it is low quality if you cannot access it. A U.S. Department of Veterans Affairs assessment found average wait times for new patient primary care appointments to be 43 days. A Massachusetts study found average wait times of 50 days for internal medicine physicians and 39 days for family medicine physicians.[11] Taken together, these suggest significant delays in care—which worsens the overall experience of care, and perhaps outcomes.

Provider-Level Consequences

Poor patient flow leads to surges and lulls in patient demand, as well as more wasted time in the process of care. Burnout among primary care providers was found to be strongly associated with time pressure and a chaotic work environment in the Minimizing Error, Maximizing Outcome (MEMO) study.[12] In another study of Veterans Affairs primary care providers, larger patient loads, lower staffing, and staffing turnover were all strongly predictive of provider burnout.[13] Murray and Berwick described the lived experience as follows:

> *Two cardinal goals of primary care are accessibility and continuity of care. Many primary care practices are struggling to achieve these goals, engulfed by seemingly overwhelming demand for patient visits and chaotic procedures for triaging patients into crammed office schedules. Too often, patients are unable to see their own primary care physician in a timely fashion, resulting in delays in care and disruption of patient-physician continuity.*[14]

In the inpatient setting, problems with flow manifest as episodic surges in patient census, which effectively worsens the provider-to-patient ratio. This increases nursing stress (and worsens nurse-patient ratios), which in turn worsens patient outcomes and increases burnout.[15,16] For hospitalists, workload is associated with significantly reduced job satisfaction[17] and probably with increased burnout.[18] For intensivists, increases in workload are also strongly associated with increased prevalence of burnout.[19]

System-Level Consequences: The Danger of Going Solid

Healthcare is a complex adaptive system (see Chapter 2), which means that it can have profoundly nonlinear responses. For patient flow, this nonlinearity can be quite profound—so much so that it is sometimes called *going solid,* a phrase introduced to healthcare by Cook and Rasmussen.[20] (*Going solid* is a term adapted from nuclear power safety, though it describes the lived experience in healthcare quite well.) Cook and Rasmussen describe this as follows:

> *Practitioners are familiar with "bed crunch" situations where a busy unit such as a surgical intensive care unit (ICU) becomes the operational bottleneck within a hospital. Other units in the hospital usually buffer the consequences of a localized bed crunch by absorbing workload, deferring transfers, etc. We have observed situations where an entire hospital is saturated with work, creating a system wide bed crunch. The result is a dramatic change in workplace operational characteristics that creates new demands for coordination of work across the facility and increases the stakes for practitioner decisions and actions. [...] Such situations create opportunities for incidents and accidents ...*

As a hospital gets more and more full, the buffering capacity of different operating units (e.g., floors) goes away. This changes the system from being loosely coupled to being tightly coupled, which dramatically reduces the options for managing the problem. Imagine one of those puzzles with wooden squares, each with a number on it, where your job is to put all the numbers in order. (Most commonly, there are 15 squares, and one empty spot, in a 4×4 grid.) It is much easier to get the numbers in order if you have three or four empty slots than if you have only one. The same thing is true in hospital operations, managing an operating room, and running a clinic. As patient flow degrades, the problem can feed on itself and create increasingly worse challenges and risks.

Key Point

At high levels of patient census, hospitals can "go solid," which increases the risk of accidents and patient safety problems.

UNDERSTANDING PATIENT FLOW CONCEPTUALLY

The path that patients take as they interact with healthcare is almost fractally complex: at each level, you find more details as you dig deeper. Nonetheless, some simplifications are helpful, and having an overview provides a framework for digging deeper.

Inpatient Patient Flow

It is critical to understand that census and patient flow in different areas of the hospital are linked. Figure 19-1 provides a simplified view of patient flow related to a hospital. Mapping any patient flow must begin somewhere. Conceptually, any patient flow has only three components: inflow, time in the system, and outflow. In this case, patients begin at home, in postacute care (e.g., a nursing home), or in other hospitals. Many enter the hospital via the emergency room, but some are admitted directly to the floor or to the ICU. Patients can also flow back and forth between areas in the hospital (e.g., from the floor to the operating room, from the ICU to the floor). Most of the flows are two-way, but some are one-way. For example, patients move from the ED to the patient floor, but not vice versa. Finally, patients leave the hospital. They may return home, go to postacute care, or to other hospitals. (Some patients may die in the hospital as well.) The ability to leave the hospital is determined partly by the patient's condition, partly by the hospital's processes, and partly by the ability of future sites of care to accept the patient. It is also worth noting that, within each box in Figure 19-1, there are many other types of patient flows.

Figure 19-2 gives some examples of how prototypical patients might flow through the system. The first patient (Figure 19-2A) is perhaps the

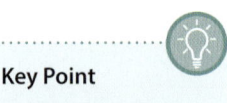

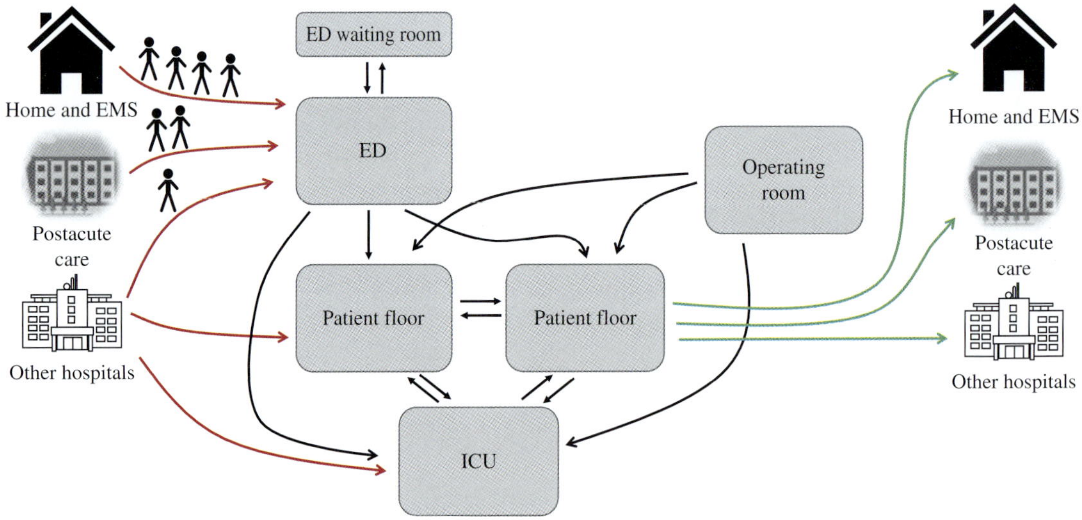

> **Key Point**
>
> Hospitals are systems, and patient flow is coupled between and among different floors and units. Problems in one area often manifest in others.

Figure 19-1 • A highly simplified diagram of patient flow in an inpatient setting. Red arrows represent patient inflow. Green arrows indicate patients leaving (outflow). Black arrows indicate within-hospital transfers. It is worth noting that most hospitals have more floors than represented here. In addition, several flows are omitted here for visual clarity (e.g., both patient floors and the ICU probably discharge patients to all locations).

A

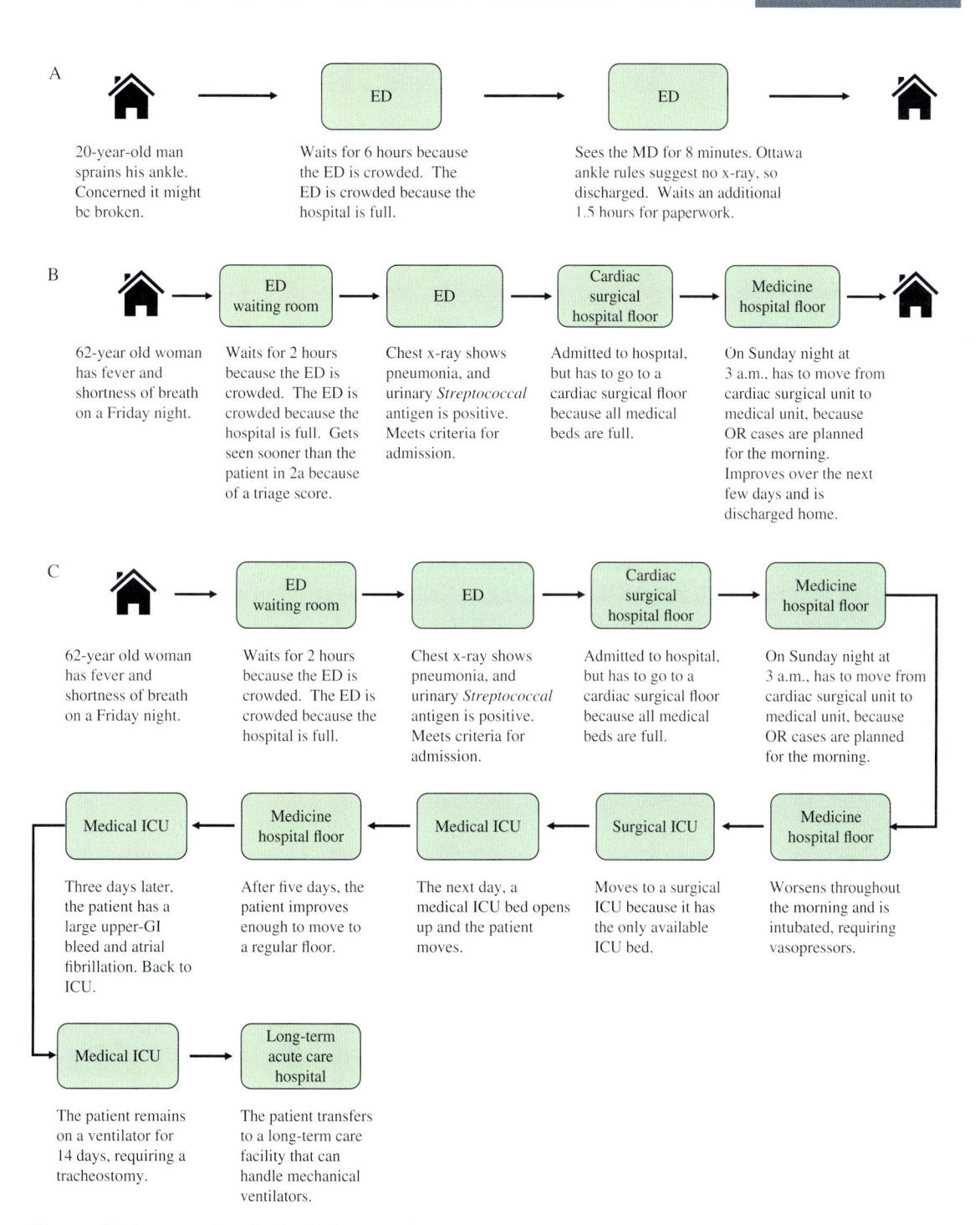

20-year-old man sprains his ankle. Concerned it might be broken. → ED: Waits for 6 hours because the ED is crowded. The ED is crowded because the hospital is full. → ED: Sees the MD for 8 minutes. Ottawa ankle rules suggest no x-ray, so discharged. Waits an additional 1.5 hours for paperwork. → home

B

62-year old woman has fever and shortness of breath on a Friday night. → ED waiting room: Waits for 2 hours because the ED is crowded. The ED is crowded because the hospital is full. Gets seen sooner than the patient in 2a because of a triage score. → ED: Chest x-ray shows pneumonia, and urinary *Streptococcal* antigen is positive. Meets criteria for admission. → Cardiac surgical hospital floor: Admitted to hospital, but has to go to a cardiac surgical floor because all medical beds are full. → Medicine hospital floor: On Sunday night at 3 a.m., has to move from cardiac surgical unit to medical unit, because OR cases are planned for the morning. Improves over the next few days and is discharged home.

C

62-year old woman has fever and shortness of breath on a Friday night. → ED waiting room: Waits for 2 hours because the ED is crowded. The ED is crowded because the hospital is full. → ED: Chest x-ray shows pneumonia, and urinary *Streptococcal* antigen is positive. Meets criteria for admission. → Cardiac surgical hospital floor: Admitted to hospital, but has to go to a cardiac surgical floor because all medical beds are full. → Medicine hospital floor: On Sunday night at 3 a.m., has to move from cardiac surgical unit to medical unit, because OR cases are planned for the morning. → Medicine hospital floor: Worsens throughout the morning and is intubated, requiring vasopressors. → Surgical ICU: Moves to a surgical ICU because it has the only available ICU bed. → Medical ICU: The next day, a medical ICU bed opens up and the patient moves. → Medicine hospital floor: After five days, the patient improves enough to move to a regular floor. → Medical ICU: Three days later, the patient has a large upper-GI bleed and atrial fibrillation. Back to ICU. → Medical ICU: The patient remains on a ventilator for 14 days, requiring a tracheostomy. → Long-term acute care hospital: The patient transfers to a long-term care facility that can handle mechanical ventilators.

Figure 19-2 • Examples of individual patient flows.

most straightforward possible interaction: a patient comes to the ED, waits, is seen, and goes home. But even this example begins to give us some insight into how patient flows are interlinked. Why does this patient with a sprained ankle have to wait in the waiting room for 6 hours? Because the ED is full. Why is the ED full? Because the hospital floors are full, and the ED has many patients who are waiting for beds.

The second patient (Figure 19-2B) has a relatively typical hospital admission. She has pneumonia and needs admission to the hospital. However, all the medical beds are full, so she is admitted to a cardiac surgical floor (which often decompresses over the weekend). She has the unpleasant experience of being transferred in the middle of the night not because of her clinical condition, but because her bed is needed for a surgical patient on Monday morning.

The third patient (Figure 19-2C) has a more complicated, though by no means rare, admission. The admission begins the same way, but the patient decompensates after a couple of days in the hospital, and she requires ICU admission. The medical ICU is full, so she goes to the surgical ICU. She is subsequently transferred to the medical ICU, improves, and goes to the medical floor. However, she subsequently has a large gastrointestinal (GI) bleed and returns to ICU. Her stay is prolonged, and she eventually requires tracheostomy and long-term care.

Patient Flow in Other Contexts, Such as Outpatient Clinics, Procedure and Infusion Suites, and Operating Rooms

Hospitals are 24/7 operations, and except in extreme circumstances, they are never completely empty. Additionally, there is only a limited ability to schedule patients in most hospitals, since substantial demand is created by urgent and emergent demand from the community. There are, though, many other contexts than the inpatient one: outpatient clinic, oncology infusion suites, cardiac catheterization labs, GI procedure suites, and operating rooms are some examples. The rest of this section will refer to "clinics," but the approach applies for the other areas as well.

In these kinds of contexts, different management levers for optimizing flow exist. First, a clinic usually empties out every night and some on weekends as well. This means that tools like Little's Law (discussed later in this chapter) don't work well in this context because you don't reach steady state. Second, most clinics schedule patients into appointment blocks. There are tremendous variations in the kinds and lengths of appointments (sometimes in the hundreds or thousands at a given practice). This provides the opportunity for improvement in capacity utilization by scheduling optimization.

Figure 19-3 provides an example of this. In this figure, patients have different lengths of visits—some short, some long. In Figure 19-3A, which shows what might be a fairly typical use of a small clinic or operating room, there are numerous unused blocks. These empty blocks may arise because of no-shows, because of physician preferences, or by things like *block scheduling* in an operating room (where periods of time are scheduled in advance to specific surgeons, even if that time is not filled). Rearranging these appointments into a more optimal configuration (Figure 19-3B) effectively creates an additional 1.5 rooms of capacity—with no capital expense.

ANALYTICAL APPROACHES TO UNDERSTANDING PATIENT FLOW

Process mapping (Chapter 3) and value-stream mapping (Chapter 9) provide tools for qualitative understanding of patient flow. Tools from statistics, epidemiology, and especially operations research can help us understand patient flow in a more quantitative manner.

Everyday Analytics for Understanding Patient Flow

Routine analysis of length of stay (LOS) and patient flow can often be helpful in planning and management. Run charts, and their more sophisticated cousins, statistical process control charts, are often remarkably helpful with understanding patient flow, as are standard statistical tests (see Chapters 13 and 14).

A Deeper Dive into *Length of Stay (LOS)*

Perhaps the most common metric of patient flow (at least for inpatients) is length of stay (LOS). However, there are several important caveats for understanding this seemingly simple measure. It is remarkable how often these cause problems:

1. **LOS ≠ LOS, Part 1: Hours, days, or "days"?** LOS can be calculated in numerous ways. These can have quite different results, but always seem to be called the same thing (LOS). When dealing with large numbers of patients over a long period of time, these average out—but when performing detailed analytics, they often matter. Perhaps the most common is "days," where a "day" is defined as crossing a midnight. This can lead to some unexpected results. For example, a patient who stays 23 hours (1 a.m.—11 p.m.) could have

Caution

There are many definitions of *length of stay (LOS)*; make sure you know which one you're looking at.

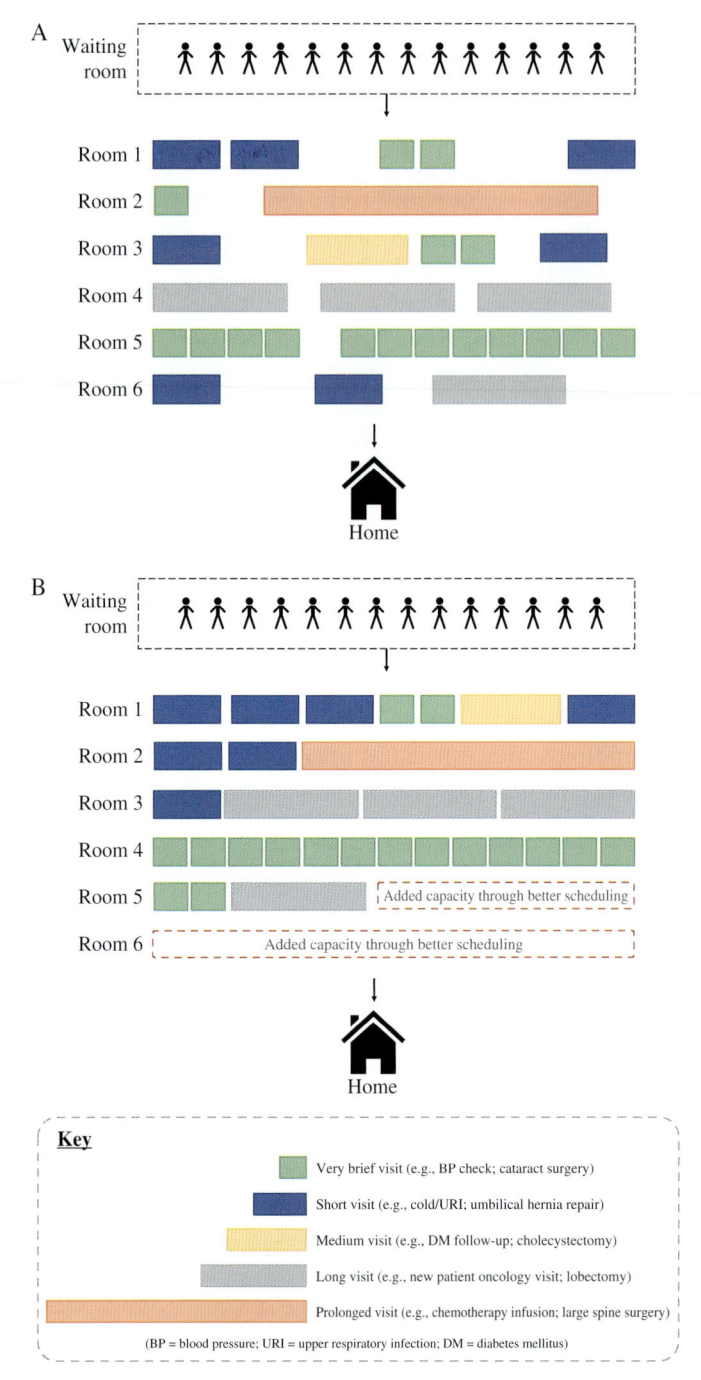

Figure 19-3 • Patient flows in a scheduled context. Patient flows are different in a scheduled context, likes clinics or operating rooms, for several reasons. First, things can decompress overnight, or on the weekend (when clinics or operating rooms may be closed). Second, there are opportunities for efficiency in the way that blocks (appointments) can be ordered and arranged. The figures here could apply to a clinic, an oncology infusion suite, a procedure suite (like a cardiac catheterization lab), or to an operating room. Both figures have precisely the same number and types of visits—the second is just arranged in a more efficient way. An optimized scheduling approach effectively creates 1.5 additional rooms of capacity, without building additional physical capacity.

an LOS = 0 days, while a patient who stays 1 hour (11:30 p.m.–00:30 a.m.) could have an LOS = 1 day, and a patient who stays 24.5 hours (11:45 p.m. on Monday until 00:15 a.m. on Wednesday) could have an LOS = 2 days. An additional complication is that some approaches to LOS calculation round up "0 days" to "1 day." Others count any calendar day that a patient is present (so a patient who is hospitalized from 11 p.m. to 1 a.m. would have an LOS = 2 days). Finally, other approaches simply calculate the actual number of hours or minutes that a patient was in-house (e.g., a patient present from 11 p.m.–1 a.m. would have an LOS of 2.0 hours, or 0.083 days). The critical point is that you should know precisely how LOS is calculated in your data, and that you aren't comparing between two different methods of calculation.

2. **LOS ≠ LOS, Part 2: Patient-centered, or time-centered**. The methods described in point 1 all focus on the patient as the unit of analysis for LOS. This makes clinical sense. On the other hand, often you want to know the average length of stay (ALOS) for your hospital (or for a ward, or a service). This is typically reported as "monthly ALOS." However, because you are calculating and reporting on a monthly basis (or weekly, or daily), what do you do with patients who are in the hospital at the time that you are calculating LOS?

   - **Approach 1 (patient-centered):** Attribute an admission, and all the days of a patient's stay, to the day of discharge.
   - **Approach 2 (month-centered):** Calculate the ALOS for the month as the number of patient-days, divided by the number of admissions that month.

   Approach 2 is commonly used for financial and regulatory reporting. Approach 2 has the advantage that it smooths variation. It has the disadvantage that there is no concept of a single patient's LOS (and that conceptually no patient can have an LOS longer than the time period being assessed. Over long periods of time (e.g., a year) and over large numbers of patients, these approaches result in essentially identical estimates of ALOS. However, as you slice and dice your analysis more, these numbers may diverge by quite a large amount. For example, if you built a report that allowed decision-makers to stratify weekly LOS by service and by patient floor, these factors would almost certainly come into play. Figure 19-4 provides a thought experiment with a worked example where LOS estimates diverge by almost 300%. Although this is an extreme example, it illustrates the point. In many hospital reports, these two methods of calculating LOS are conflated, and called the same thing. Again, the critical point is that you should know

Task: Calculate average LOS for January and February

Scenario for thought experiment: Imagine you have a hospital that admits six patients across the two months. These patients' admission and discharge dates are shown below.

Admissions & Discharges

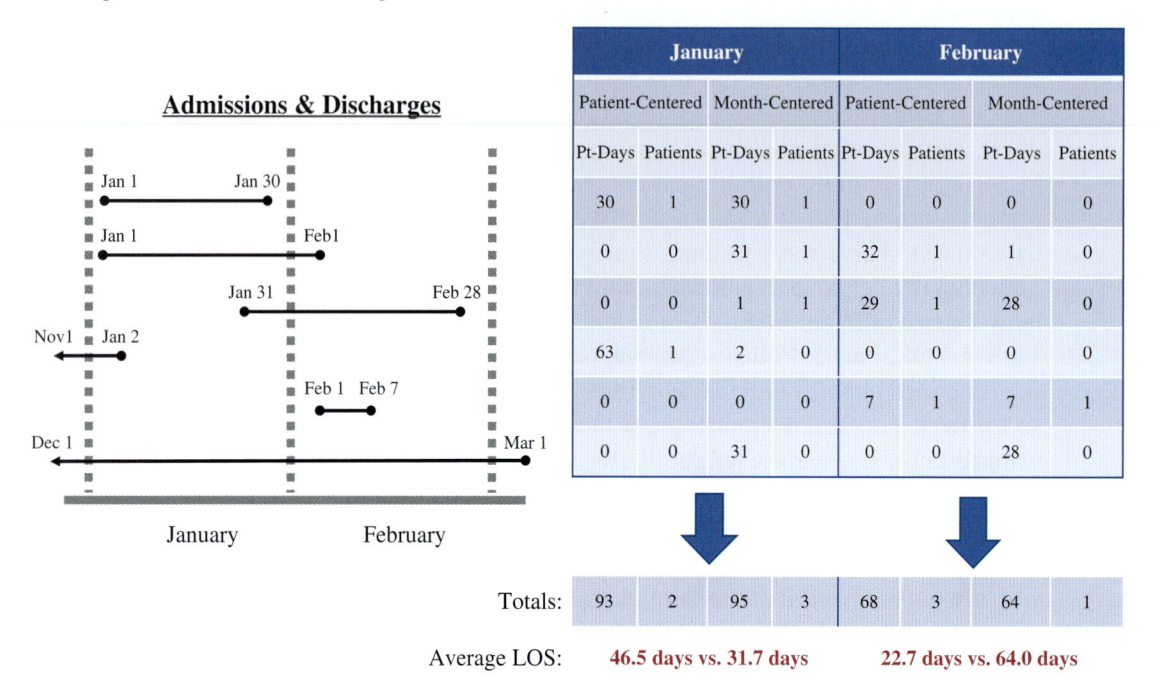

	January				February			
	Patient-Centered		Month-Centered		Patient-Centered		Month-Centered	
	Pt-Days	Patients	Pt-Days	Patients	Pt-Days	Patients	Pt-Days	Patients
Jan 1 – Jan 30	30	1	30	1	0	0	0	0
Jan 1 – Feb 1	0	0	31	1	32	1	1	0
Jan 31 – Feb 28	0	0	1	1	29	1	28	0
Nov 1 – Jan 2	63	1	2	0	0	0	0	0
Feb 1 – Feb 7	0	0	0	0	7	1	7	1
Dec 1 – Mar 1	0	0	31	0	0	0	28	0
Totals:	**93**	**2**	**95**	**3**	**68**	**3**	**64**	**1**
Average LOS:	**46.5 days vs. 31.7 days**				**22.7 days vs. 64.0 days**			

Figure 19-4 • How patient-centered and time-centered LOS calculations can differ.

precisely how LOS is calculated in your data, and that you aren't comparing between two different methods of calculation.

3. **ALOS ≠ ALOS** A particular problem with LOS analysis is that very-long-stay patients can swing a month's average LOS by a meaningful amount. A cursory example of your hospital's LOS data will show that it is *not* normally distributed. Rather, LOS (and also healthcare costs) are almost always right-skewed. Figure 19-5 shows this using nationally representative U.S. hospital data. Why is this important? It means that it is easy to be seriously misled when using *means* because the movement of one or two very-long-stay patients can dramatically affect mean lengths of stay. (Just imagine if a patient with a 150-day LOS is discharged in 1 month!) In many cases, comparing medians is a simple way to overcome that problem. Nonetheless, the most common measure of LOS for a hospital is ALOS, which stands for "average (mean) LOS."

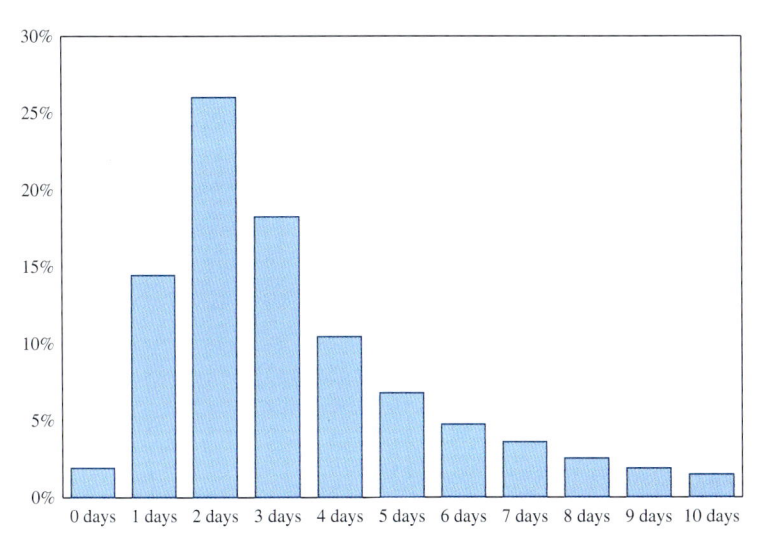

Figure 19-5 • Hospital LOS is not normally distributed. This chart shows the LOS in U.S. hospitals up to 10 days. This is a good example of right-skewed data: LOS typically has a Weibull, lognormal, or more complex distribution. Data are from the AHRQ National Inpatient Sample, 2016 (https://www.hcup-us.ahrq.gov/db/nation/nis/tools/stats/MaskedStats_NIS_2016_Core_Weighted.PDF).

Little's Law: Simple but Remarkably Useful

In the early 1960s, John Little articulated a mathematical proof of what came to be called *Little's Law*[21]—an arithmetic tautology that lets you calculate how long something (an item, a person, an email, etc.) will remain in a *queuing process*. Little showed that—given certain conditions—the average number of items waiting in the queue is exactly equal to the mean arrival rate multiplied by the mean time that items are in the system. This formula (which turns out to be pretty useful operationally) is

$$L = \lambda W$$

where L is the average number of items in the queuing system, W is the mean waiting time, and λ is the mean number of items that arrive (per unit time).

It's easier to understand this if you think about your email inbox. (Little himself gave this example in a 2008 piece.)[22] If you get 50 email messages a day ($\lambda = 50$) and the average size of your inbox is 150 (L = 150), then that means it takes you an average of three days to return (and then archive or delete) an email (W = 3). $L = \lambda W \rightarrow$ 150 messages in inbox = 50 email messages per day × 3-day response time.

Table 19-1 LITTLE'S LAW AND HOSPITAL OPERATIONS

Little's Law Formula	L	=	λ	×	W
Meaning	Average number of items in the system	=	Average number of items that arrive per unit time	×	Average time spent in the system by each item
Translation to hospital operations	Average daily census	=	Average number of daily admissions	×	ALOS

Table 19-1 translates this into terms familiar to hospital operations. This leads to some pretty interesting conclusions, which turn out to be useful for estimating important aspects of hospital operations:

- ADC = ADM × ALOS. Given the number of admissions per year (ADM), and the ALOS, we can calculate average daily census (ADC). (We have to remember to divide by 365 because one of these is a yearly value and one is a daily value.)
- ADM = ALOS / ADC. If we know the ALOS, and the average daily census, we know the average number of daily (or yearly) admissions.
- How many extra admissions can we handle if we reduce LOS?

> **Key Point**
> Little's Law is remarkably useful. It describes the relationship between admissions, census, and LOS.

> **Key Point**
> Little's Law (L = λW) can be translated into hospital operations terms as Average Daily Census = Average Daily Admissions × ALOS.

How might you use Little's Law in the real world? First, Little's Law turns out to be very useful for quickly double-checking estimates about patient flow, capacity, and census. For example, if someone presents a report saying that your 500-bed hospital admitted 1.1 million inpatients last year, you can quickly assess whether that's possible. (The answer is "no"—ALOS in that case would be just 4 hours if you kept 100% capacity 24 × 7 × 365, which is obviously wrong.) Second, Little's Law lets you estimate the impact of changes in things like LOS. Case 19-1 walks through a concrete example of this. While the case itself has a number of simplifications, it is still a realistic problem that Little's Law is quite useful to address.

However, there are some mandatory conditions for Little's Law to hold. First, the system needs to be at *steady state,* meaning that things aren't rapidly changing. That means that Little's Law is really useful only

CHAPTER 19 | MODELING PATIENT FLOW

Case 19-1 CASE STUDY 1: USING LITTLE'S LAW

Susan is the chief operating officer of Arbitrary Regional General Hospital (ARGH), a 500-bed hospital. ARGH is persistently full, routinely running at 99% capacity, and patients often have to wait in the ED for more than 12 hours for a bed. Recently, ARGH has turned away potential transfers, and last week, it even had to delay some elective surgeries.

The Management Question

The LOS task force has proposed adding five case managers to help facilitate discharges for long-stay patients. This will obviously cost a nontrivial amount of money to do. Will it pay for itself?

The Facts and Beliefs

- Susan believes that there is adequate demand in the community: If ARGH could take more patients, the demand would be there.
- She also knows that her hospital is almost exclusively paid on a Diagnosis-Related Group (DRG) basis (one payment per hospitalization), and that the average DRG payment is $15,000 per hospitalization.
- Over the past year, ARGH's ALOS was 5.0 days.
- Also over the past year, ARGH's average daily census was 500. (In practice, even when completely full, average daily census will be somewhat lower than capacity because patients are being admitted and discharged, and census is usually lower on weekends.)

Questions

- How many patients did ARGH admit last year?
- If ARGH reduced ALOS by 0.1 days, how many additional patients could they care for?
- If they filled all these slots, how much revenue would this generate?

Using Little's Law to Answer these Questions

Little's Law can help you easily answer these questions.

How Many Patients did ARGH Admit Last Year?:
Little's Law is $L = \lambda \cdot W$.
This translates to healthcare: ADC = # admissions per day · ALOS
500 = (# admissions per day) · 5.0

> \# admissions per day = 500 / 5.0 = 100 admissions per day
> \# admissions per year = 100 · 365 = 36,500 admissions per year
>
> *If ARGH Reduced ALOS by 0.1 Days, How Many Additional Admissions Could They Care For?*
> Little's Law is $L = \lambda \cdot W$.
> This translates to healthcare: ADC = # admissions per day · ALOS
> 500 = (# admissions per day) · 4.9
> \# admissions per day = 500 / 4.9 = 102.04 admissions per day
> \# admissions per year = 102 × 365 = 37,244 admissions per year
> How many additional admissions are that? 37,244−36,500 = 744 additional admissions per year
>
> *How much revenue would this generate?*
> In a DRG-based system…
> Revenue = average payment × number of discharges
> Revenue = $15,000 × 744 = $11,160,000 per year
>
> *Comment:*
> There are obviously many simplifications in this example, but Little's Law still provides a very useful way to reality check more sophisticated estimation techniques.

Caution

Little's Law requires that things be at steady state, and it doesn't work if things are rapidly changing. For example, if your number of admissions is rising month-to-month, Little's Law may not hold.

External Resource

A full-length book focused on patient flow, with more detail on queuing theory and simulation, among other topics, is Hall R. *Patient Flow: Reducing Delay in Healthcare Delivery*. Vol. 206: Springer Science & Business Media; 2013. https://link.springer.com/book/10.1007/978-0-387-33636-7.

over a longer period of time, not usually over short periods (like hourly fluctuations in the census). Second, you must be able to account for how every patient leaves the system … they cannot just disappear from the system. Third, you need to make sure that you're dealing with units correctly. For example, if you measure LOS in days, then you have to be careful that you're counting admissions in admissions per day, not admissions per year. Otherwise, though, Little's Law is pretty resilient to assumptions.

Little's Law is also decomposable in some useful ways. For example, different segments of patient flow are additive, as shown in Figure 19-6. This allows you, for example, to quantify waiting time, and then to estimate the impact of reducing wait time on patient flow and census.

More Advanced Methods

Little's Law is remarkably useful for being so simple. However, more complex approaches are sometimes needed. We will provide an overview of some of these here, recognizing that more in-depth works will be useful for those who wish to explore these methods.

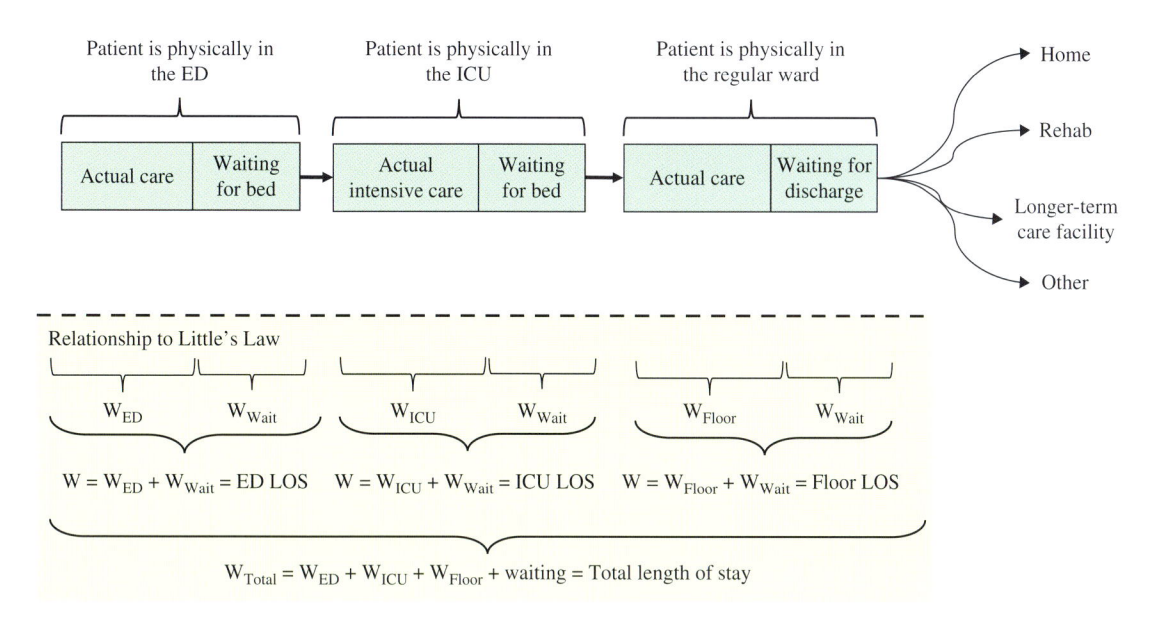

Figure 19-6

Figure 19-6 • Breaking down Little's Law. Patient flow can be broken down into many components. In this example, a patient comes to the ED, is admitted to the ICU, goes to the regular hospital floor, and is finally discharged. This allows you, for example, to understand the impact of waiting times on throughput throughout the system.

Relationships shown:

$$W = W_{ED} + W_{Wait} = \text{ED LOS}$$
$$W = W_{ICU} + W_{Wait} = \text{ICU LOS}$$
$$W = W_{Floor} + W_{Wait} = \text{Floor LOS}$$
$$W_{Total} = W_{ED} + W_{ICU} + W_{Floor} + \text{waiting} = \text{Total length of stay}$$

Queuing Theory

Little's Law is perhaps the simplest queuing theory model. More complex models teach us new things about patient flow. These models have a few things in common:

- "Customers" arrive. A *customer* could be a person (like a patient), but it could also be an email, a purchase order, or an x-ray. Customers need a *service* provided to them. That could be a physical service (like a meal being served) or it could be a process being accomplished (like an email being read and archived).
- "Servers" provide the service. There can be one server, or many. It takes some amount of time to provide the service.
- Customers who have arrived, but who have not yet been served, form a *queue* while waiting (hence the name of the approach). There can be one queue or many, depending on the model structure. Most queuing models assume that the waiting room for queues is infinitely large.
- *Models* specify the order in which customers in the queue are served. It might be first come first served, or it could be based on another process (such as a triage score in the ED).

Key Point

Queueing models are mathematical representations of what happens when more patients show up than there are servers (physicians, beds, clinic rooms, etc.) to take care of them at the moment they arrive. These models use strong mathematical assumptions to make operationally useful predictions about the future.

Figure 19-7 • Higher utilization worsens delays. As percent utilization increases, the amount of average delay increases by an increasing amount. This helps account for the phenomenon of going solid, described earlier in the chapter. (Adapted from Green 2006 [37].)

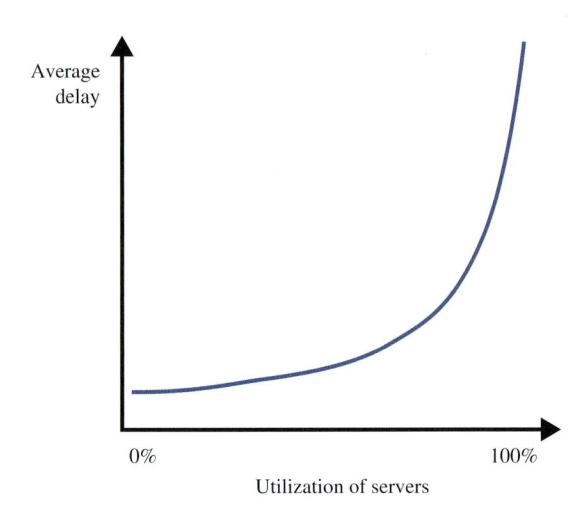

> **Key Point**
>
> As systems get closer to full capacity, delays increase *at increasing rates*. Things get slower as hospitals get fuller.

There are a few principles we learn from queuing models that seem to hold across a wide variety of circumstances:

- As we get closer to full capacity, delays increase … and they do so at an increasing rate (Figure 19-7). This accounts for the phenomenon that moving from 40% capacity to 50% capacity may not change delays much, but moving from 85% to 95% capacity may markedly worsen delays.
- As variability increases, so do delays (Figure 19-8). What does *variability* mean in this context? The term can mean variability in arrivals or in the process/service time. An example would be variation in the number of patients who arrive at the clinic at the same time: a steady rate of arrivals will result in lower average delays than if patients arrive in batches. Similarly, variation in hospital admissions (usually based on surgical scheduling) will cause greater delays than smooth admissions. Variability in process time also causes delays. Therefore, a highly specialized surgery suite that does the same procedure every time will have fewer delays than an operating room with a wide variety of cases. The same holds true in other arenas. For example, creating a "fast track" area in an ED for minor problems reduces waiting time for all patients because it separates variability into two separate queues.[23–25]

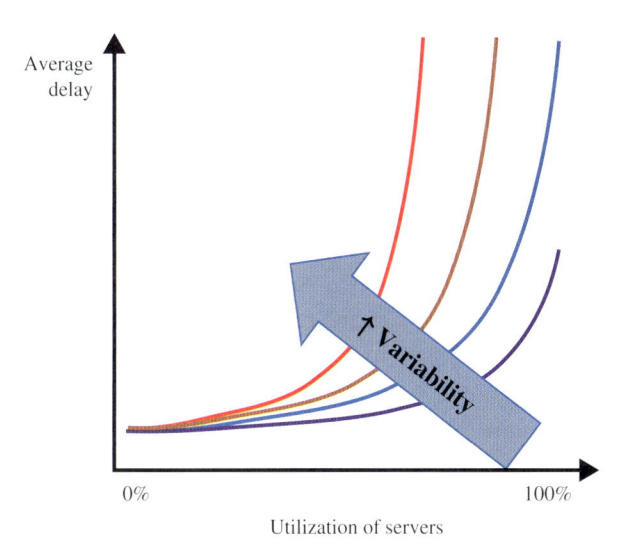

Figure 19-8 • Variability worsens delays. As variability increases, so do delays. Variability can mean variability in arrivals (e.g., patients per hour in the ED) or in the process time (e.g., LOS). What does *variability* mean in this context? An example would be variation in the number of patients who arrive at a walk-in clinic at the same time: a steady rate of arrivals will result in a lower average number of delays than when patients arrive in batches. Similarly, variation in hospital admissions (usually based on surgical scheduling) will cause greater delays than smooth admissions.

Key Point

As variability increases, delays increase too.

An Example of a Common Queuing Model

An advantage of queuing models is that, unlike simulation models, they often require very little empirical data. The tradeoff for this is that they make strong mathematical assumptions. For example, many assume that the timing with which patients arrive is a *Poisson process*. Some characteristics of a Poisson process include that patients arrive one at a time, that one patient's arrival does not influence whether another patient arrives, and that whether a patient arrives is independent of the time. This results in an exponential distribution of delay times. Even though most situations do not strictly meet these criteria, the Poisson distribution has been empirically shown to match average arrivals in a number of healthcare environments. The Poisson simplification is useful because it needs only one parameter (λ) to describe it.

Just as in Little's Law, here λ means the average number of patients arriving per unit time (e.g., patients per day). Given that, you can calculate the probability that the next patient will arrive within a given amount of time: $1 - e^{-\lambda t}$. For example, if on average 2 patients an hour arrive to your walk-in clinic, and one patient just arrived, the probability that a patient will arrive in the next 15 minutes is 39%. On the other hand, if the average

External Resource

Many online and spreadsheet tools for queueing models exist. One example was created by David Ashley[35]. It is available at https://www.stat.ncsu.edu/people/reiland/courses/st501/Q.xls.

arrival rate were 10 per hour, then the probability that a patient will arrive in the next 15 minutes is 92%.

A common queuing model is the *Erlang delay model*, which is also called an *M/M/s model*.* In this model, the arrival process is Poisson and the service time is exponential. While the formulas for these models are quite complicated, there are numerous spreadsheets, programs, and online calculators that make them easy to apply. One only needs to know the average patient arrival rate, the ALOS, and how many servers (beds, physicians, etc.) you have. You can then answer questions like "What is the likelihood a patient will have to wait?" or "What will the average utilization of my beds be?"

Case 19-2 gives a working example of this, applied to a hypothetical planning process for an ICU. It is worth noting that the Erlang delay model is one of the simpler types of queuing models. For example, it assumes that ICU admissions do not vary by time of day or day of week, so it is only useful for long planning periods. Many other types of queuing models exist. Each model has different assumptions, uses, and limitations.

Simulation Methods

Queuing theory starts to be less useful when its assumptions aren't met, or when you need much more granular information about how patient flow plays out. *Simulation methods* provide more flexibility in the questions you can ask, and they can accommodate a wider range of assumptions. This often comes with a tradeoff of increased data requirements to build the model, and increased computational complexity. However, in our experience, simulation models are often easier to explain to clinicians and administrators than models that are based on mathematical theorems. For many people, it is easier to get an intuitive grasp of how something like a discrete-event simulation works than it is to grasp the underlying equations in a queuing model.

There are many types of computational simulation methods. Static simulations, such as Monte Carlo models, are often used to generate a result at a single point in time. Dynamic models may evolve over time, and stochastic models may incorporate additional dimensions of variation.

---

*Kendall's notation is used to describe queuing nodes and models: A/S/c, where A = time between arrivals, S = distribution of service times, and c = the number of servers. The *M*'s in this case refer to a Markovian, or a memoryless exponential process, and the *s* means that the model can vary the number of servers. Kendall's notation has been extended to include parameters for the possible size of the queue (K), the size of the population (N), and the order/discipline in which the queue is served (D), so the full notation A/S/c/K/N/D. When only three parameters are provided in the notation, then by convention $K = \infty$, $N = \infty$ and D = first in, first out.

CHAPTER 19 | MODELING PATIENT FLOW

Case 19-2 CASE STUDY 2: USING A SIMPLE QUEUEING MODEL

The Management Question

Bob is the head of planning for the ICU at a new hospital. He knows that it is dangerous for patients to have to wait when they need an ICU bed. However, he also knows that having an unused ICU bed is expensive. He wants to understand these tradeoffs, and so he uses an Erlang delay model to get an approximation.

The Facts and Beliefs

- Bob's best estimate is that the average number of ICU admissions per day will be 5.
- Bob's best estimate is that the average ICU LOS for these patients will be 3.85 days.
- A plausible planning estimate is between 20 and 40 ICU beds.

Questions

- For each bed capacity, what is the probability that a patient will be delayed?
- For each bed capacity, what is the predicted utilization?

Using a Queueing Model to Answer these Questions

Bob uses an Erlang delay model (i.e., an M/M/1 queueing model) to quantify the relationship between the number of beds, ICU bed utilization, and the likelihood that patients who need ICU admission will experience delays:

Beds	Average Admissions Per day	ALOS (days)	Probability that a Patient Seeking ICU Admission will have to wait	Utilization of ICU Beds
20	5	3.85	81%	96%
22	5	3.85	44%	87%
25	5	3.85	15%	77%
27	5	3.85	7%	71%
30	5	3.85	1.5%	64%
32	5	3.85	0.5%	60%
35	5	3.85	0.1%	55%

> **Comment**
>
> While this model makes a number of simplifications, it demonstrates the profound nonlinearity of the relationship between bed capacity, bed utilization, and the likelihood that patients will have to wait.
>
> Many other types of queuing models exist. Each model has different assumptions, uses, and limitations.

Two approaches that warrant particular comment are *discrete-event simulation* and *agent-based modeling*.

Discrete-event simulation is a method that has been used for decades in operations research. This type of simulation is especially useful for answering what-if questions. What if we added five physicians to afternoon clinics? What if we built a 20-bed labor-and-delivery (L&D) unit instead of a 30-bed L&D? What would happen to inpatient capacity if we smoothed the operating room schedule across the week? A discrete-event simulation takes the organization, or system, as its target of simulation (this will distinguish it from agent-based models, which model individuals). How does it work? This type of simulation gets its name because the system that is defined in the simulation changes only when events occur—it is static otherwise (hence the name *discrete event*). It is also *stochastic*, meaning that there are several random variables whose distributions are drawn from real data.

A very simple simulation might ask the question: "how many people will be in my urgent care clinic's waiting room?" This simulation will just have a waiting room and a single person working at the front desk. (For the sake of simplicity, we'll assume that there are infinite rooms and doctors in the back.) Everything starts empty. The simulation has a clock, and the clock ticks forward. We have determined (ideally from real data) what the statistical distribution is of how patients arrive. We might have measured the average number of patient arrivals over a given time period, as well as the shape of that distribution (undoubtedly right-skewed and truncated at 0), and we might have learned that the time of day matters in the probability of patient arrivals. For example, there might be more patients who come to urgent care during lunch hours. Let's say our clock runs at 1-minute increments. For a given minute increment, the simulation generates a random number. We compare that number to the probability distribution of patient arrivals and find out whether 0 patients arrived, 1 patient arrived, or more. (We could also limit to single-patient arrivals with fine time slices.)

The patient comes into the waiting room. If the front desk is empty, the patient goes to the front desk. We will also have estimated the service time: how long does it take to check in? (Again, we will have estimated the *distribution* of this time because these times can vary.) Another random number is generated, and that patient's time at the front desk is calculated. As the clock ticks forward, the front desk is occupied for however long that patient requires. If other patients arrive into the waiting room at that time, they wait until the front desk is cleared. (We assume, for simplicity, that patients go back immediately to see the doctor after checking in.) As the simulation runs forward, the waiting room fills and empties. The simulation records the state of the waiting room at every time increment, and at the end of the simulation—as a manager—you can find out how often your waiting room is empty, how often is has <5 people, etc. You can also calculate the average waiting time of patients.

That simulation is obviously a toy problem—too simple to be useful. But intuitively, you can imagine what might come next. You could add further steps in the simulation that model a clinic that has four doctors. You could add another constraint of there being only four rooms. Now, if your waiting room is full all the time, you can ask some interesting questions about *where* the bottlenecks are. What if I gave every doctor an extra room? Would that help? Not if the bottleneck is the front desk! What if I added an extra check-in station? More doctors? Each of these can be modeled using discrete-event simulation.

There are numerous other complexities (and variations) on discrete-event simulation. However, it is a generally intuitive method for clinicians, and there is deep experience with it in healthcare. In fact, the technique has been used broadly enough that there are now systematic reviews of its application in healthcare, and we refer the reader to those for an accounting of the many and varied ways the technique finds use in healthcare.[26–28] For those interested in applying the technique, special software packages exist to help. In addition, in 2019, Bean and colleagues published their experience using discrete-event simulation for healthcare management education,[29] and they took the additional step of open-sourcing the discrete-event simulator they built.

Agent-based modeling is a technique that more recently has moved from research to practice. Its building block, from a modeling perspective, is an autonomous agent. (An *agent* could be a doctor, a nurse, a patient ... or in other domains could be an animal, or a virus, or even other cellular

External Resource

Bean et al.'s paper[29] on discrete-event simulation in healthcare management education is available at https://stel.bmj.com/content/5/1/46, and the open-source implementation of the simulator is at https://khp-informatics.github.io/patient-flow-simulator.

components). Agents can perceive some of their environment, and they also have an internal *state,* represented as a set of variables, that sets the conditions for their decision-making. Then, agents also have a set of decision-making rules. These rules can be simple, or they can be extremely complex and be intended to represent true cognitive decision-making processes. Finally, agents exist in an environment with which they interact, and which contains other agents. (In this sense, there are obvious parallels to our discussion of reinforcement learning in Chapter 17.)

These rules can be macro decisions ("Should I open a new hospital?") or micro decisions ("Should I put an intravenous catheter in this patient in the ED?") depending on the goals of the simulation. Then, a clock runs and agents act based on their rules and the rules of the environment. The properties of the health system (e.g., waiting time, patient flow) usually emerge from the interactions of the individual autonomous agents rather than being directly programmed in.

Agent-based models are increasingly used in healthcare. For example, systematic reviews of agent-based models now exist for issues as diverse as malaria transmission,[30] noncommunicable diseases like heart disease and diabetes,[31] and emergency medicine topics such as triage, scheduling, and workflow.[32] One of the important aspects of agent-based models as a technique is that they can function across scales—moving from the microscopic to the individual to systems of care.[33,34] For those who wish to explore more, numerous texts, courses, and tools are available.

External Resource

Grimm and Railsback's book[36] on agent-based learning is a common reference for introductory courses in the field, and is implemented using Netlogo, which is an open-source agent-based modeling software package. The book is available at http://www.railsback-grimm-abm-book.com/, and Netlogo is available at https://ccl.northwestern.edu/netlogo/.

SUMMARY

Patient flow is of critical importance for healthcare delivery scientists. It has a direct impact on patient outcomes, patient experience, provider experience, and on financial performance. Tools for understanding patient flow range from the simple (Little's Law) to the complex (queuing theory and simulation methods). The usability of these tools has improved in recent years, making them increasingly accessible and practical for everyday use.

KEY POINTS

- Problems with patient flow can have direct, negative patient safety impacts. They also directly affect financial performance.
- At high levels of patient census, hospitals can "go solid," which increases the risk of accidents and patient safety problems.

- Little's Law, which describes the relationship between admissions, census, and LOS, is remarkably useful. Its formula (L = λW) can be translated into hospital operations terms as Average Daily Census = Average Daily Admissions × ALOS.
- An insight from queueing theory is that as systems get closer to full capacity, delays increase *at increasing rates*. Things get slower as hospitals get fuller. As variability increases, delays increase too.
- Queuing theory, discrete-event simulation, and agent-based models are more sophisticated tools that help model and understand patient flow.

REFERENCES

1. Reid PP, Compton WD, Grossman JH, Fanjiang G. *Building a Better Delivery System: A New Engineering/Health Care Partnership.* Vol. 15. Washington, DC: National Academies Press; 2005.
2. Morley C, Unwin M, Peterson GM, Stankovich J, Kinsman L. Emergency department crowding: A systematic review of causes, consequences and solutions. *PLoS One.* 2018;13(8):e0203316.
3. Burkett NJ. Family sues Bronx hospital after father dies following 9-hour ER wait. ABC7NY News. 2017. Accessed December 31, 2018, from, https://abc7ny.com/health/family-sues-hospital-after-father-dies-following-9-hour-wait/2457458/.
4. Shaw ME. Man dies in New York hospital waiting room, found hours later. *Atlanta Journal-Constitution.* January 27, 2014.
5. Leather H. Investigation as patient dies in A&E waiting room at Russells Hall Hospital. *Express and Star (Wolverhampton, England, UK).* January 4, 2018.
6. Bernstein SL, Aronsky D, Duseja R, et al. The effect of emergency department crowding on clinically oriented outcomes. *Acad Emerg Med.* 2009;16(1):1–10.
7. Weissman GE, Gabler NB, Brown SE, Halpern SD. Intensive care unit capacity strain and adherence to prophylaxis guidelines. *J Crit Care.* 2015;30(6):1303–1309.
8. Hua M, Halpern SD, Gabler NB, Wunsch H. Effect of ICU strain on timing of limitations in life-sustaining therapy and on death. *Intensive Care Med.* 2016;42(6):987–994.
9. Gabler NB, Ratcliffe SJ, Wagner J, et al. Mortality among patients admitted to strained intensive care units. *Am J Respir Crit Care Med.* 2013;188(7):800–806.
10. Eriksson CO, Stoner RC, Eden KB, Newgard CD, Guise JM. The association between hospital capacity strain and inpatient outcomes in highly developed countries: a systematic review. *J Gen Intern Med.* 2017;32(6):686–696.
11. Institute of Medicine. *Transforming Health Care Scheduling and Access: Getting to Now.* Washington, DC: National Academies Press; 2015. Accessed June 2, 2019, from https://doi.org/10.17226/20220.
12. Rabatin J, Williams E, Baier Manwell L, Schwartz MD, Brown RL, Linzer M. Predictors and outcomes of burnout in primary care physicians. *J Prim Care Community Health.* 2016;7(1):41–43.

13. Helfrich CD, Simonetti JA, Clinton WL, et al. The association of team-specific workload and staffing with odds of burnout among VA primary care team members. *J Gen Intern Med.* 2017;32(7):760–766.
14. Murray M, Berwick DM. Advanced access: reducing waiting and delays in primary care. *JAMA.* 2003;289(8):1035–1040.
15. Litvak E, Buerhaus PI, Davidoff F, Long MC, McManus ML, Berwick DM. Managing unnecessary variability in patient demand to reduce nursing stress and improve patient safety. *Jt Comm J Qual Patient Saf.* 2005;31(6):330–338.
16. Vahey DC, Aiken LH, Sloane DM, Clarke SP, Vargas D. Nurse burnout and patient satisfaction. *Med Care.* 2004;42(2 suppl):II57–66.
17. Hinami K, Whelan CT, Wolosin RJ, Miller JA, Wetterneck TB. Worklife and satisfaction of hospitalists: toward flourishing careers. *J Gen Intern Med.* 2012;27(1):28–36.
18. Wachter RM. Hospitalist workload: the search for the magic number. *JAMA Intern Med.* 2014;174(5):794–795.
19. Embriaco N, Azoulay E, Barrau K, et al. High level of burnout in intensivists: prevalence and associated factors. *Am J Respir Crit Care Med.* 2007;175(7):686–692.
20. Cook R, Rasmussen J. "Going solid": a model of system dynamics and consequences for patient safety. *Qual Saf Health Care.* 2005;14(2):130–134.
21. Little JDC. A proof of the queuing formula: $L = \lambda W$. *Operations Research.* 1961;9(3):383–387.
22. Little JDC, Graves SC. Little's Law. In: Chhajed D, Lowe TJ, eds. *Building Intuition: Insights from Basic Operations Management Models and Principles (International Series in Operations Research & Management Science)*. New York: Springer; 2008:81–100.
23. Devkaran S, Parsons H, Van Dyke M, Drennan J, Rajah J. The impact of a fast-track area on quality and effectiveness outcomes: a Middle Eastern emergency department perspective. *BMC Emerg Med.* 2009;9:11.
24. Sanchez M, Smally AJ, Grant RJ, Jacobs LM. Effects of a fast-track area on emergency department performance. *J Emerg Med.* 2006;31(1):117–120.
25. Chan TC, Killeen JP, Kelly D, Guss DA. Impact of rapid entry and accelerated care at triage on reducing emergency department patient wait times, lengths of stay, and rate of left without being seen. *Ann Emerg Med.* 2005;46(6):491–497.
26. Zhang X. Application of discrete event simulation in health care: a systematic review. *BMC Health Serv Res.* 2018;18(1):687.
27. Salleh S, Thokala P, Brennan A, Hughes R, Dixon S. Discrete event simulation-based resource modelling in health technology assessment. *Pharmacoeconomics.* 2017;35(10):989–1006.
28. Mohiuddin S, Busby J, Savovic J, et al. Patient flow within UK emergency departments: a systematic review of the use of computer simulation modelling methods. *BMJ Open.* 2017;7(5):e015007.
29. Bean DM, Taylor P, Dobson RJB. A patient flow simulator for healthcare management education. *BMJ Simul Technol Enhanc Learn.* 2019;5(1):46–48.
30. Smith NR, Trauer JM, Gambhir M, et al. Agent-based models of malaria transmission: a systematic review. *Malar J.* 2018;17(1):299.

31. Nianogo RA, Arah OA. Agent-based modeling of noncommunicable diseases: a systematic review. *Am J Public Health*. 2015;105(3):e20–e31.
32. Adleberg JM, Catlett CL, Rothman RE, Lobner K, Hsieh YH. Novel applications of agent-based modeling in emergency medicine research—a systematic literature review. *Am J Emerg Med*. 2017;35(12):1971–1973.
33. An G. Integrating physiology across scales and formalizing hypothesis exploration with agent-based modeling. *J Appl Physiol (1985)*. 2015;118(10):1191–1192.
34. Cockrell C, An G. Sepsis reconsidered: Identifying novel metrics for behavioral landscape characterization with a high-performance computing implementation of an agent-based model. *J Theor Biol*. 2017;430:157–168.
35. Ashley DW. An introduction to queuing theory in an interactive text format. *INFORMS Transactions on Education*. 2002;2(3):96–98.
36. Grimm V, Railsback S. *Agent-Based and Individual-Based Modeling: A Practical Introduction*. Princeton, NJ: Princeton University Press; 2011.
37. Green L. Queueing analysis in healthcare. In: *Patient Flow: Reducing Delay in Healthcare Delivery*. Springer; 2006:281–307.

20 PROGRAM EVALUATION
How to Tell If Something Worked in the Real World

We have covered a lot of ground so far in this book, reviewing multiple methods ranging from medical research to automotive manufacturing to machine learning. Our goal is to improve, measure, and evaluate changes in healthcare delivery. But fundamentally, we are interested in whether a change in the care we provide *benefits* patients and is not merely *associated with* a benefit. Does the availability of board-certified intensivists improve the care of the critically ill at night?[1] Does the introduction of an electronic health record (EHR) improve or harm the care of patients?[2] How can we know when our interventions have actually made a difference to our patients?

Unlike other fields of research, healthcare delivery only occasionally lends itself to a randomized control trial. To randomize patients to one type of care-delivery strategy requires that we have equipoise, which is to say that we must be truly uncertain about the benefit of our intervention if we are administering it to only a fraction of our study population. It is hard to argue against efforts to improve the sterility of central line insertion[3] or same-day primary care appointments.[4] How would we respond if we were asked to enroll our aging and critically ill mother in a randomized study where, in one arm, she'd be cared for overnight in the intensive care unit (ICU) by a first-year resident and, in the other arm, she'd be cared for by a board-certified intensivist with at least seven years of post-medical-school training?[1] Would we allow her to participate in that study? Healthcare delivery interventions that use randomization also require huge commitments of resources, including the staff, implementation, and leadership for two different care pathways, which could almost never be blinded to one another. But as healthcare delivery scientists, we have to remain open to the idea that what seems like the obviously correct path of care may turn out to be a very wrong path of care for patients. (See Chapter 1 for some examples.) Maybe, as it turns out, having a board-certified intensivist present in the hospital does not meaningfully change a patient's care overnight and, as a downside, is incredibly expensive. Maybe we could have enrolled our mom in that trial, and it wouldn't have harmed her at all.

Fortunately (and unfortunately), the care we provide in hospitals and in the outpatient setting is often random in nature. While unnecessary variation can be frustrating and wasteful, it does have an upside. Variation in care provides us opportunities to study what we do and attempt to draw true causal inferences from our care. For example, suppose that we are interested in whether the use of a transthoracic echocardiogram within 2 hours of admission with shock improves inpatient mortality. We could imagine that transthoracic echocardiograms are available only to patients admitted during the weekday business hours in our hospital. Essentially, knowing whether a patient comes into the hospital on a weekend or a weekday could serve as a way of randomizing patients to early or late echocardiograms in shock, and help us ask if this tool is beneficial to improve in-patient mortality. Whether we receive timely cardiac interventions in the setting of an acute myocardial infarction may be determined by how far our home is from a hospital, which can help us study if those interventions improve care.[5] Whether we receive a particular vasopressor medication may be determined by whether the hospital that we go to is experiencing an active shortage for that particular drug; this unfortunate event gives an opportunity to help us study which vasopressor is best for shock.[6] Despite our efforts to control unnecessary, nonclinical variation in healthcare, it surrounds us every day, providing multiple opportunities to study different patients who are essentially randomized to different care pathways.

In this chapter, we will discuss what is meant by *causal inference,* a field of statistics that draws causal conclusions from observational data. This will take us from all the methods we've used so far to ask about what's going on in the real world. Next, we will present a series of methods that exploit random variations in care to identify the effect of different care pathways on patients who are otherwise similar at baseline. These methods, which build on the work we've already done in both predictive modeling and statistical process control, will afford us a new level of flexibility in our analytics in order to help understand the consequences of the care we provide.

CAUSAL METHODS

Thus far, this book has discussed how to determine if variables are associated with one another: within a limited population (e.g., patients admitted to our hospital) what can we say about the overlapping distribution of variables, assuming that conditions always remain the same? But we already know that these models, such as linear regression models, require major assumptions and bring with them shortcomings and restrictions. When we discussed confounding, we described the definition of confounding as a variable that has an effect on both the exposure and the outcome. For example, age is a confounder for the risk of hypertension and death—the older you are, the more likely you are to have high blood pressure, and the older you are, the more likely you are to die. If we fail to control for age in our study, we will overstate the relationship between hypertension and risk of death. However, in any observational study, we can never come up with all possible confounders. This limits us from ever knowing the true relationship between our exposure and our outcome. We can never know true unbiased effects when we work with measures of association.

Into this realm of uncertainty comes *causal methods*. Causal methods or causal inference were largely put forward in both philosophy and statistics in the past 50 years, and they push the boundaries of how to use observational data to understand true causal relationships.[7–10] Causal reasoning, unlike some of the statistical models described earlier in this book, already comes naturally to the human mind. Causal models require the identification of and reflection on the counterfactual—the imaginary example of what would have happened if the conditions were different—so that then we can make claims about the relationship between the exposure and the outcome. While you may not know the counterfactual by that name, you likely are already familiar with the concept on a daily basis, expressed in statements such as: "If only I hadn't missed the bus, I would have made my dentist appointment on time." "If only he hadn't smoked, he'd still be alive." "If that car was $10,000 cheaper, I'd buy it tomorrow." The philosopher David Lewis raised this idea in his 1973 book *Counterfactuals*, which took this idea to a magical extreme and imagined a series of alternative worlds where the counterfactual became you living out your alternative life: making the dentist appointment on time, never smoking, and purchasing the car.[8]

Several statisticians and mathematicians brought the concept of causal inference into the light in the past 50 years, including Donald Rubin and Judea Pearl; the latter won the Turing Award for his body of work. Pearl, in his accessible book, *The Book of Why*, spells out the transformation from Bayesian thinking and modeling to causal models, as well as the formal assumptions spelled out by Rubin.[7] We will start with causal models, as these require us to take a different approach to confounding, which in turn becomes essential to understanding the assumptions underpinning causal methods.

Key Point

What is a counterfactual? Critical to causal methods, a counterfactual is what would have happened to our study participants if they had been in the opposite study group. If our patient had been in the intervention arm, what would his or her outcome have been in the control arm?

Causal models are visual. They require us to hypothesize the causal relationships between our exposure, our outcome, and other variables. By drawing these out in the way we'll describe, we then begin to see how to design a meaningful study to answer our question of interest (and the risks of unfettered adjustment in our models!). Causal models use arrows to demonstrate the direction of the relationship. Pearl describes the variables as "listening" to those variables that connect to it with arrows. To start with the basics, let's draw an isolated causal diagram:

$$A \rightarrow B$$

In this model, B listens only to A. Let's use Pearl's example and imagine that A is a fire and B is the alarm going off. A causes B: The alarm goes off because of a fire.

Now let's add in another variable, C. That variable can live on the causal pathway or along the chain of causation:

$$A \rightarrow C \rightarrow B$$

In this instance, C serves as a *mediator*. C listens to A; B listens to C; B listens to A only through C. In Pearl's *fire* → *alarm* relationship, C could be smoke. Smoke should cause the alarm to go off, with or without fire, at the same rate.

Pearl has us imagine *wiggling* a variable and, in turn, holding different variables constant (or controlling for a variable), and seeing what happens to the other variables. In the case of our initial causal relationship, if we wiggle A, we have a result in B. In the case of a mediator, if we wiggle A, we will wiggle B through C. Now imagine what would happen if we held C constant. We are controlling for C. Functionally, we are looking only at cases where there was no smoke (or only smoke). If we wiggled A, B wouldn't wiggle because C would be held still. If there's no smoke, the alarm won't ever go off. If there's only smoke, the alarm will always go off. This would be a terrible result. Now it would look like there was no relationship between A and B, *fire* and *alarm*. This is particularly important: this is why simply controlling for every possible variable may be harmful to our study. In the case of a mediator, like smoke, when we control for it, we break the relationship between our exposure and our outcome. We control away our relationship of interest—the very thing we want to study!

Returning to our various types of models, let's reverse the direction of the first arrow. Now the model becomes a *fork,* or a common cause of

A and B, and it will make A and B correlated even though there is no direct relationship between the two:

$$A \leftarrow C \rightarrow B$$

For example, we could imagine C as old age, A as living in an assisted-living facility, and B as death. In the case of a fork, if we control for C, and there is no separate relationship between A and B, we will see that there is no relationship. If we control for age in our study, we should remove the association of living in a skilled nursing facility and death (we can hope that the assisted living facility isn't killing off its residents!). In this instance, we are not harming our study; in fact, we are bringing the truth to light.

And finally, if we reverse both arrows, we have a collider, where A and B are both related to C, but not to each other:

$$A \rightarrow C \leftarrow B$$

Pearl cites Felix Elwart and Chris Winship's example of Talent → Celebrity ← Beauty as an example of a collider in daily life.[7] In the case of a collider, if you control for C, you will suddenly open up a spurious association between A and B. Talent and beauty will suddenly look related. Now if we go about controlling for everything, we may actually generate a biased result.

A confounder, U, is frequently defined in the following relationship, which highlights the benefit of controlling for U to try to identify the relationship between X and Y:

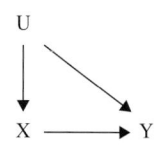

$$\begin{array}{c} U \\ \swarrow \searrow \\ X \longrightarrow Y \end{array}$$

But Pearl highlights a different definition from Greenland and Robins, which draws again on the idea of the counterfactual, *exchangeability*. In this definition, the researcher first must imagine all the members of the treatment group, then imagine that everyone who was treated did not actually receive the treatment, and finally determine if they would have had the same outcome as all of the actually untreated participants. In other words, we must ask ourselves: Could the unexposed participants be considered the counterfactual of the treatment group? If yes, then we will not have confounding in our study. While difficult to achieve, we will see, in the methods of quasi-experimental design that we will discuss in the remainder of this chapter, that we seek exchangeability.

To practice our causal diagrams, consider the following (an illustration that we will come back to):

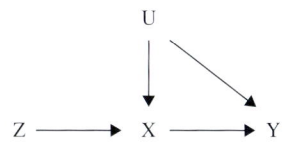

```
          U
          |  \
          ↓   ↘
    Z ──→ X ──→ Y
```

In this diagram, X is a mediator, U is an unmeasured confounder, Z is our exposure of interest, and Y is our outcome. What would happen if we control for X? Perhaps we didn't recognize that it was a mediator of the relationship between Z and Y. If so, we would control for X and think that we had uncovered the true relationship between Z and Y. In fact, we opened up X as a collider and now we're reporting the relationship between Z and Y, confounded by U. We will capitalize on this model later in the chapter when we get to instrumental variable (IV) analysis.

Armed with this approach to study design, let's turn to the three fundamental assumptions of causal inference that also overlay our subsequent methods:

- **Stable Unit Treatment Value Assumption (SUTVA)**—This assumption requires that an exposure, or treatment, should have the same effect on all participants. If I take a medication, it should have the same effect on me that it would on the person next to me.
- **Consistency**—In this assumption, we presume that if the same treatment or exposure was offered in an experimental design, the effect would be the same, or consistent, as in the quasi-experimental design we use. If I give my daughter acetaminophen when she has a fever and is home from school, the medication should have the same effect on her whether she is in a clinical trial of acetaminophen or not (which suggests there is no placebo effect—something I cannot be certain of with regard to my daughter when acetaminophen tastes like bubble gum).
- **Ignorability**—The final assumption deals with the relationship of a confounder (U), the exposure, and the outcome—and this is the hardest to understand. We need to assume that the assignment of any participant to the exposed group or the unexposed group at each level of the confounder U is independent of the outcome. In the case of a randomized control trial, where each measured and unmeasured confounder is balanced, we can assume ignorability. In quasi-experimental designs, whether we meet this assumption can be challenging because of unmeasured confounders and biases in the data.

QUASI-EXPERIMENTAL DESIGNS—CAUSAL INFERENCE IN OBSERVATIONAL DATA

In the remainder of this chapter, we will expose you to four methods that draw on our earlier discussion of causal analysis to ask questions of observational data. These methods can be grouped as quasi-experimental, as they take advantage of the variation and randomness of life to exploit these natural experiments. We would recommend that readers use these methods with caution and to seek the assistance of statisticians with a background in econometrics and causal inference. Each method requires that the three assumptions given previously are met, and then adds restrictions and requirements that can make drawing false conclusions a very real risk. That said, they are also exceedingly powerful when effective. And an awareness of the conditions of when they can be used can set up readers to make important causal discoveries in existing, real-world data.

Interrupted Time Series (ITS)

Interrupted time series (ITS) analysis is a powerful tool that capitalizes on the longitudinal nature of data when a natural experiment has taken place in time, such as a new national- or state-level policy, or a new intervention put in place in a hospital or clinic. To use it, we use the linear trend that was present before the intervention took place (the time series) and then examine what happens when the pre-intervention trend is *interrupted* at the point of the intervention. If we assume that the intervention had no effect, the preexisting trend should continue unchanged despite the interruption. If we see changes in the linear trend, or a break in the trend, after the intervention, we can assume that the intervention had an effect.

To use this design, the intervention itself must have a clear pre-period and post-period and an outcome that, ideally, is relatively short term or rapid onset, which can be seen soon after the intervention takes place. Data need to be available both before and after the study; fewer time points make the estimate less stable. Power in ITS increases with the number of time points. To identify the right model for the statistical design, we must put forward a hypothesis of how the intervention is likely to change the outcome. Is the outcome likely to lead to a change in slope of the pre-intervention trend? Or a change in the y-intercept of the line (the level)? Or both? Should we expect a lag in the effect? To derive the right model for the analysis, we need to have an initial understanding of how we expect the intervention to change our outcome.

Figure 20-1 provides an example of how ITS can work. We propose a hypothetical research study: What would happen to hospital rates of

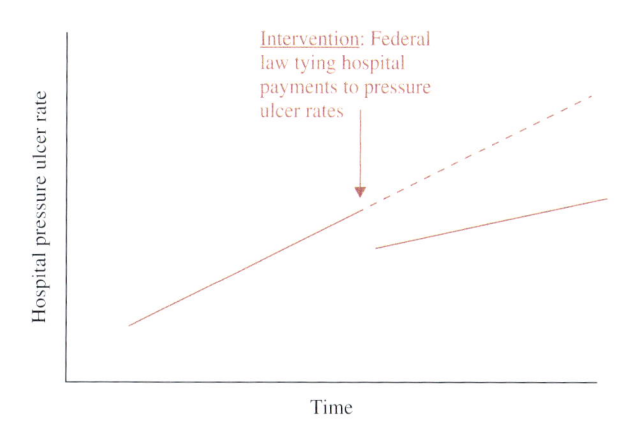

Figure 20-1 • A hypothetical example of an interrupted time series that explored the effect on hospital pressure ulcer rates (i.e., outcome) of a federal law that tied hospital payments to pressure ulcer rates (i.e., intervention or interruption). After the law takes effect (the postintervention phase), hospital pressure ulcer rates decline in both the slope and the y-intercept of the graph.

pressure ulcers if a law were put in place to tie hospital reimbursements from Medicare to whether a pressure ulcer develops—something that the Centers for Medicare and Medicaid Services (CMS) already does! We can imagine that the preintervention trend was linear (a requirement for ITS), as shown in Figure 20-1. Now, to explore the effect of the law on our pressure ulcer rates, at its most straightforward, we would design a model with three variables: time (T); a variable to indicate the intervention period (X, coded as 0 in the preperiod and 1 in the postperiod); and our outcome of pressure ulcer rates (Y). The model uses a segmented regression model that looks like the following:

$$Y_t = \beta_0 + \beta_1 T + \beta_2 X + \beta_3 T * X.$$

In this equation, β_0 is the rate of pressure ulcers at T = 0 in the preintervention period, before the law started; β_1 is the slope of the rate of change of pressure ulcers before the law; β_2 is the change in intercept (or the level change) after the law; and β_3 is the slope change following the law. ITS is flexible to use linear, logistic, or count data to accommodate the type of outcome of interest.

ITS does fall prey to seasonality, particularly because we are required to have large amounts of data over time. If we have short periods of time, such as only winter in the pre-period and summer in the post-period, seasonality may affect our results, as we cannot assume that our preintervention and post-intervention trends are actually the same (if the interruption never happened). We can solve this particular problem with

> **Caution**
>
> Always look for seasonality or other threats to linear pretrends in interrupted time series (ITS) analysis. If these trends are not linear, you will need to use extensions of ITS to handle them.

more data. However, seasonality can still foil us. One month may be more correlated with its neighboring months than more distant months, which would fundamentally invalidate our linear assumption in the pre-period. Other statistical transformations can be made to correct for this problem, such as stratifying by calendar month; but at the very least, seasonality or other examples of autocorrelation need to be addressed in the design.

If you find that the relationship between time and your outcome of interest is not linear, there are several extensions of standard interrupted time series that can be used to address nonlinearity, seasonal variation, and other problems.[11,12] The technical aspects of these methods are beyond the scope of this chapter, but understanding the linear time-series approach will serve as an important foundation as you explore these methods.

ITSs are some of the most common quasi-experimental designs to be used in medicine, health policy, and healthcare delivery science. Walley and colleagues used an ITS design to study whether distribution of bystander naloxone rescue kits (an opioid antidote) changed the rates of fatal opioid overdoses and hospital admissions.[13] Serumaga and colleagues asked whether a national pay-for-performance program in the United Kingdom concerning care for patients with high blood pressure changed the frequency of blood pressure monitoring among patients.[14] Grundy et al. demonstrated that the introduction of 20-mph speed limits in London were associated with a 42% reduction in road casualties.[15] Having caught on in the medical literature, we have cited other examples from the literature, primarily descriptive, so the reader may explore this method further.[16–22]

Difference in Differences (DiD)

Difference in differences (DiD) is a similar strategy to ITS, in that it is a quasi-experimental design that uses observational data over time. The method, however, adds a new element: we now compare the population exposed to the intervention to a control group not exposed to the intervention over the entire time period.

The assumptions of DiD are the following:

- The intervention was not related to or determined by the outcome at baseline.
- There is limited to no spillover between the exposed population and the control population.
- The composition of the two groups are similar.
- The intervention and control groups meet the parallel trends assumption, described next.

The parallel trends assumption says that the difference between the treatment and the control group should be the same (i.e., parallel) over time. If the two trends started to differ before the intervention occurred, the estimate of the effect of the intervention would be wrong.[23]

Figure 20-2 illustrates a hypothetical example of a DiD program, building on the example from Figure 20-1. We now test a hypothetical state-level law that ties hospital payments to pressure ulcer rates of the hospital. We can now compare hospitals in the state that does have the law (the intervention group) to hospitals in states that do not have it (the control, or counterfactual group). In Figure 20-2, the blue line is the control data; the red line is the intervention data. If the law had not been passed, pressure ulcer rates would have been similar over time between hospitals in the control states and intervention state. After the intervention takes place, we can see how much of an effect the intervention had on rates, based on how much the line diverges from its original trend (labeled the "intervention effect").

Law et al. used the DiD method to study a state law and its effect on critically ill patients. The state of Massachusetts put in place a law that required ICUs to limit the nurse-to-patient ratio to 2:1 or 1:1, depending on how sick the patients were. Law and colleagues had all

> **Caution**
>
> Difference-in-differences (DiD) requires that the intervention and control trends be parallel.

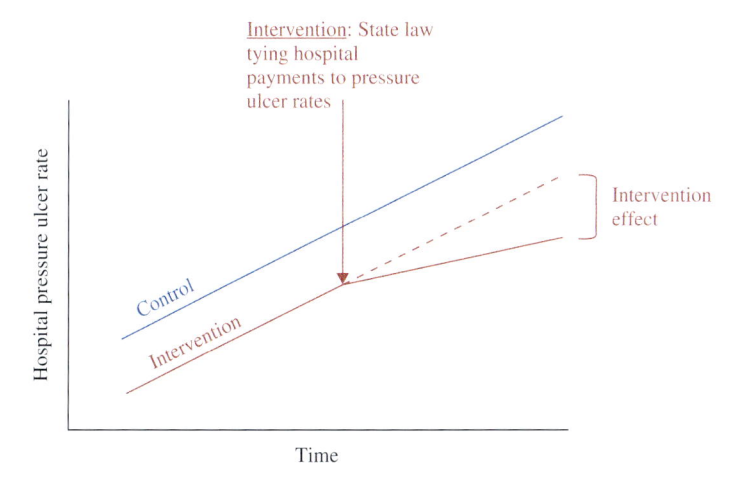

Figure 20-2 • Building on Figure 20-1, this proposes a hypothetical set of results of a difference-in-differences study of a state law tying hospital payments to pressure ulcer rates. The blue line represents the hospital pressure ulcer rates in states not exposed to the new law; the red line represents hospital pressure ulcer rates in states exposed to the new law after the intervention point. The two lines are parallel, and if the law had not been put in place, the difference between the two groups would have remained the same over time. That allows us to conclude that the intervention effect is due to the law, not due to trends that had already been in place.

the elements necessary for a DiD. First, the intervention was put in place at a specific time. Second, it was a statewide law in Massachusetts, which made other patients in ICUs in states outside Massachusetts a ready-made control group. And finally, the intervention group and control group met the parallel trends assumption. The study found that the law had no influence on in-hospital mortality or other hospital-acquired infections and complications that could be related to nurse availability.[24]

There are a number of additional DiD studies that the interested reader can use to explore the models and see examples of their use in the healthcare delivery science literature, ranging from women's health to Medicare payment innovations to drug shortages.[6,25–28]

Regression Discontinuity (RDD)

Regression discontinuity (RDD) takes advantage of pseudorandomization around an arbitrary cutoff in a continuous score. A cutoff to a continuous scale, such as severity of illness score, a series of exam results, or continuous laboratory values, means that people who fall just on either side of the arbitrary cutoff are essentially randomized to the exposure and can be followed to monitor their outcomes. The major shortcomings of RDD include the need to have a particularly large sample size and uncertainty about whether one can generalize away from the treatment threshold.

Take as an example a study that looked at an arbitrary cutoff of CD4 counts and antiretroviral therapies. The researchers noted that patients with CD4 counts at or below 200 cells/μL received antiretroviral therapy, while those above that level did not. Patients with CD4 counts of 201 cells/μL were unlikely to be meaningfully different in both measurable and unmeasurable confounders than those with counts of 199 cells/μL, but they received vastly different treatment strategies. Patients were noted to have a 35% lower risk of death with CD4 counts below 200 cells/μL because they underwent treatment.[29]

In their discussion of RDD in the healthcare literature, Walkey et al. proposed several healthcare delivery ideas of how to use the technique. For example, imagine a hospital that deploys a pressure ulcer prevention team to evaluate patients admitted to the hospital with high risk of in-hospital pressure ulcers. To employ RDD, the hospital could develop a risk score, target different harm prevention efforts for patients who score above an arbitrary cutoff, and then evaluate whether there is any change. Figure 20-3 illustrates a successful set of results of such a program. Walkey et al. put forth several other candidate examples, including efforts

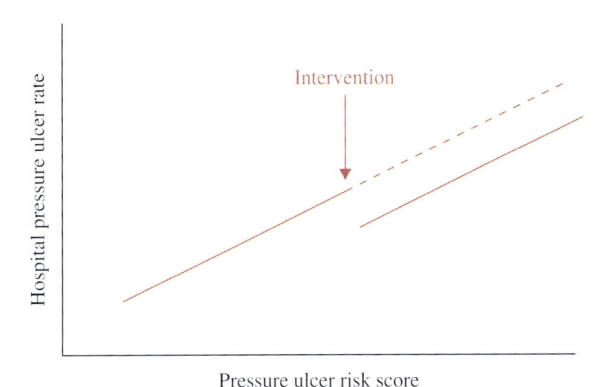

Figure 20-3 • Example of regression discontinuity design and an intervention to reduce pressure ulcers. When patients score above an arbitrary pressure ulcer risk score, they receive a visit from the pressure ulcer prevention team (Intervention). Based on these graphs, we would conclude the intervention was successful. Patients on either side of the cutoff for the risk score should be similar to those immediately below the cutoff. And yet, note that there is a downward shift in the number of patients who develop pressure ulcers. In fact, those on the intervention side of the cutoff have a significantly reduced risk of harm.

to reduce ICU readmissions with a risk score and cutoff or an evaluation of a program to increase referrals of patients with chronic obstructive pulmonary disease to pulmonary rehabilitation using a cutoff from the 6-minute walk tests.[17]

Instrumental Variable (IV) Analysis

In 2009, the Tea Party was rapidly gaining momentum in the United States. A libertarian movement that was organized to protest public investment to stabilize the economy during the 2008 financial crisis, the group organized national protests on tax day, April 15, 2009. People have long believed that participation in organized protests change the political conversation, and that larger protests are more likely to be influential than smaller ones. However, this has not been empirically proven. A straightforward regression of a protest size on policy outcomes is at risk to unmeasured confounders, such as political preferences, and this method is unable to draw a true causal link between the size of a protest itself and change. *Instrumental variable (IV) analysis,* our final causal method (and the one most difficult to do correctly), can help us answer whether protest size is causally related to a change in policy outcomes, rather than simply associated with one.

IV analysis is derived from the economics and education literature. In a randomized control trial, we control the function of randomization (the assignment of each participant to exposure or control) and thereby create groups that are balanced in their measured and unmeasured confounders. We can assume that the counterfactual of each participant exists in each group, which allows us to compare whether there is any true effect of the exposure on the outcome. Fundamentally, IV analysis takes advantage of the randomness of other parts of life. An *instrument* is something that is associated only with the exposure but itself has no association with the outcome, except through the exposure. The analysis exploits this instrument, which itself acts to have randomized participants.[30–34]

The power of such a method is exciting. As we have noted throughout this book, our work is constantly riddled with bias and confounding. We face confounding by indication when providers give different treatments to patients based on features of the patients themselves (e.g., if a medication is given only to the sickest, most frail patients, a regression of that medication will look harmful because more of the patients who receive it do worse than those who do not). We also face healthy user/compliance bias, whereby patients who are more health conscious are more likely to seek an exposure, which may make the intervention look more beneficial than it actually is (e.g., patients who get influenza vaccines may take better care of themselves in general than those who do not, so that an analysis of the effect of influenza vaccines makes them look like they work better than they really do). IV analysis offers a way to essentially randomize patients to our exposure and functionally eliminate these threats to the validity of our study question.

However, IV analysis has three significant assumptions that must be met for the study to be valid:

1. The instrument Z has a causal effect on X.
2. The instrument Z has an effect on Y, but *only* through X.
3. The instrument Z also does not have a relationship with Y in either measured or unmeasured ways.

We can see this using the causal diagram from the earlier part of the chapter:

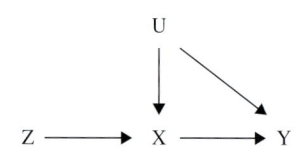

$$Z \rightarrow X \rightarrow Y$$
$$U \rightarrow X,\ U \rightarrow Y$$

Here, Z represents the instrument, X the exposure, and Y the outcome. U represents both measured and unmeasured confounders, which are shared between X and Y. Note that we are using slightly different words for the variables than what we did previously, but the same concepts apply. X becomes a mediator between Z and Y. Assumption 3 indicates that there are no unmeasured or measured confounders shared between Z and Y, such that treatment assignment is exchangeable, as described previously.

Returning to our example of political protests and their influence on political outcomes, Madestam et al. identified a very powerful instrument: rainfall.[35] They noted that rainfall on April 15 (Z) was likely to influence the size of a political protest in that region (X). The only way that rainfall could be related to the Republican turnout (Y) in November 2010 could be through X. First, they proved that rainier days were associated with 50% lower protest turnout than sunny days (Z → X). Further, nonrainy districts were found to increase the Republican voting share by 1.6 percentage points (Z → Y), and every 0.1 percentage point increase in protesters increased Republican vote share by 1.8 percentage points (X → Y). They further pushed their assumptions to see if rainfall on other historical days in April and in other years between 1980 and 2008 changed voting behaviors, and they found the results on April 15, 2009, to be a significant outlier in the relationship between rainfall and political outcomes. Protest size in 2009 made a difference in the congressional elections in 2010 (X → Y).

There are far fewer examples of how IV analysis has been used in healthcare because the true challenge of these analyses is identifying an instrument that meets the three assumptions. McClellan et al. asked about the benefit of cardiac catheterization in the setting of a myocardial infarction. They used the instrument of distance of patients from hospitals, noting that patients who lived closer to hospitals that performed cardiac catheterizations were likely to be taken there by emergency services and undergo the procedure.[5] Kahn et al. examined the distance between home and hospital, and also looked at the volume-outcome relationship of mechanical ventilation and in-hospital mortality.[36] Valley and colleagues utilized the same IV to explore the benefit of ICU admission for mortality from pneumonia.[37] Brookhart et al. used variation in physician prescribing patterns to look at the relationship of COX-2 inhibitors and complications from gastrointestinal bleeding, finding no benefit from COX-2 inhibitors.[38]

Why hasn't IV analysis swept through healthcare? First, it is hard to find good instruments that meet all of the assumptions above. Second, IV analysis often yields results that require some additional work for readers to understand them. The method relies on another assumption that we make in other types of analyses implicitly: treatment-effect homogeneity, also described as *consistency* earlier in the chapter, or that all populations should receive the same effect from the exposure. The method also provides information on the so-called marginal participant, or the participant who is fully compliant with the treatment assignment. For example, in McClellan's study of distance, cardiac catheterization, and outcomes, the marginal patient was the patient who lived close to the cardiac catheterization facility and got assigned there to have a catheterization. The estimate derived from the results of their study does not inform us about the patient who lived far from the hospital but who underwent a cardiac catheterization anyway. This represents a departure from the typical analysis seen in the medical literature, which gives the reader an average effect between treatment groups.

The shortcomings or risks of IV analyses rest largely with the downsides of having weak instruments. *Weak instruments,* or instruments that are associated with the exposure in only a limited way, subsequently generate a large standard error, which can lead to an imprecise estimate of the effect. IV analyses also do poorly with time-varying exposures, which are common in healthcare. The largest challenge in IV analyses is identifying an instrument that actually meets the assumptions described in this section.

EVALUATIONS IN THE REAL WORLD

Causal analyses bring with them significant power to ask whether our healthcare innovations matter in the real world. Did it matter to patient wait times that we changed the design of the emergency room (a question that we could ask with ITS)? Did our intervention, piloted on some of but not all our hospital floors, reduce length of stay as we had planned (a question that we could ask with DiD)? Did any of these interventions matter with regard to cost of care or quality-adjusted life years (QALYs), a measure defined as 1 year in perfect health and which, more generally, serves as a measure that balances longevity versus quality of life (see https://www.nice.org.uk)? As we continue to push healthcare delivery science and ask rigorous research questions of the care we provide to patients, we can use these tools to draw truly causal conclusions.

KEY POINTS

- Consider the counterfactual in your daily life when planning your study designs.
- Causal methods are incredibly powerful tools that can let us ask if our healthcare delivery interventions have really made a difference to patients.
- However, these methods are among the most difficult to get right, so they should be done in collaboration with a statistician.
- Several assumptions in causal methods can be proven, but others cannot be and require careful study design from the beginning.
- Presenting the results of causal methods can be challenging in the medical literature, as healthcare has not used these methods extensively. The most straightforward (ITS, DiD) can be explained easily; the most challenging (RDD, IVA) can more difficult.

REFERENCES

1. Wallace DJ, Angus DC, Barnato AE, Kramer AA, Kahn JM. Nighttime intensivist staffing and mortality among critically ill patients. *N Engl J Med.* 2012;366(22):2093-2101.
2. Ash JS, Sittig DF, Poon EG, Guappone K, Campbell E, Dykstra RH. The extent and importance of unintended consequences related to computerized provider order entry. *J Am Med Inform Assoc.* 2007;14(4):415-423.
3. Pronovost P, Needham D, Berenholtz S, et al. An intervention to decrease catheter-related bloodstream infections in the ICU. *N Engl J Med.* 2006;355(26):2725-2732.
4. Murray M, Bodenheimer T, Rittenhouse D, Grumbach K. Improving timely access to primary care: case studies of the advanced access model. *JAMA.* 2003;289(8):1042-1046.
5. McClellan M, McNeil BJ, Newhouse JP. Does more intensive treatment of acute myocardial infarction in the elderly reduce mortality? Analysis using instrumental variables. *JAMA.* 1994;272(11):859-866.
6. Vail E, Gershengorn HB, Hua M, Walkey AJ, Rubenfeld G, Wunsch H. Association between US norepinephrine shortage and mortality among patients with septic shock. *JAMA.* 2017;317(14):1433-1442.
7. Pearl J, Mackenzie D. *The Book of Why: The New Science of Cause and Effect.* New York: Basic Books; 2018.
8. Lewis DK. *Counterfactuals.* Oxford: Blackwell; 1973.
9. Halpern JY. *Actual Causality.* Cambridge, MA: MIT Press; 2016.
10. Hernan MA, Robins JM. Estimating causal effects from epidemiological data. *J Epidemiol Community Health.* 2006;60(7):578-586.
11. Bernal JL, Soumerai S, Gasparrini A. A methodological framework for model selection in interrupted time series studies. *J Clin Epidemiol.* 2018; 103:82-91.

12. Kantz H, Schreiber T. *Nonlinear Time Series Analysis*. Cambridge, UK: Cambridge University Press; 2004.
13. Walley AY, Xuan Z, Hackman HH, et al. Opioid overdose rates and implementation of overdose education and nasal naloxone distribution in Massachusetts: interrupted time series analysis. *BMJ*. 2013;346:f174.
14. Serumaga B, Ross-Degnan D, Avery AJ, et al. Effect of pay for performance on the management and outcomes of hypertension in the United Kingdom: interrupted time series study. *BMJ*. 2011;342:d108.
15. Grundy C, Steinbach R, Edwards P, Green J, Armstrong B, Wilkinson P. Effect of 20 mph traffic speed zones on road injuries in London, 1986–2006: controlled interrupted time series analysis. *BMJ*. 2009;339:b4469.
16. Kontopantelis E, Doran T, Springate DA, Buchan I, Reeves D. Regression based quasi-experimental approach when randomisation is not an option: interrupted time series analysis. *BMJ*. 2015;350:h2750.
17. Walkey AJ, Drainoni ML, Cordella N, Bor J. Advancing quality improvement with regression discontinuity designs. *Ann Am Thorac Soc*. 2018;15(5):523–529.
18. Wagner AK, Soumerai SB, Zhang F, Ross-Degnan D. Segmented regression analysis of interrupted time series studies in medication use research. *J Clin Pharm Ther*. 2002;27(4):299–309.
19. Smith DH, Perrin N, Feldstein A, et al. The impact of prescribing safety alerts for elderly persons in an electronic medical record: an interrupted time series evaluation. *Arch Intern Med*. 2006;166(10):1098–1104.
20. Feldstein AC, Smith DH, Perrin N, et al. Reducing warfarin medication interactions: an interrupted time series evaluation. *Arch Intern Med*. 2006;166(9):1009–1015.
21. Kirkland KB, Homa KA, Lasky RA, Ptak JA, Taylor EA, Splaine ME. Impact of a hospital-wide hand hygiene initiative on healthcare-associated infections: results of an interrupted time series. *BMJ Qual Saf*. 2012;21(12):1019–1026.
22. Craig P, Katikireddi SV, Leyland A, Popham F. Natural Experiments: An overview of methods, approaches, and contributions to public health intervention research. *Annu Rev Public Health*. 2017;38:39-56.
23. Dimick JB, Ryan AM. Methods for evaluating changes in health care policy: the difference-in-differences approach. *JAMA*. 2014;312(22):2401–2402.
24. Law AC, Stevens JP, Hohmann S, Walkey AJ. Patient outcomes after the introduction of statewide ICU nurse staffing regulations. *Crit Care Med*. 2018;46(10):1563–1569.
25. Etzioni DA, Wasif N, Dueck AC, et al. Association of hospital participation in a surgical outcomes monitoring program with inpatient complications and mortality. *JAMA*. 2015;313(5):505–511.
26. Schwartz AL, Chernew ME, Landon BE, McWilliams JM. Changes in low-value services in year 1 of the Medicare Pioneer Accountable Care Organization Program. *JAMA Intern Med*. 2015;175(11):1815–1825.
27. Stevenson AJ, Flores-Vazquez IM, Allgeyer RL, Schenkkan P, Potter JE. Effect of removal of Planned Parenthood from the Texas Women's Health Program. *N Engl J Med*. 2016;374(9):853–860.
28. Desai S, Hatfield LA, Hicks AL, Chernew ME, Mehrotra A. Association between availability of a price transparency tool and outpatient spending. *JAMA*. 2016;315(17):1874–1881.

29. Bor J, Moscoe E, Mutevedzi P, Newell ML, Barnighausen T. Regression discontinuity designs in epidemiology: causal inference without randomized trials. *Epidemiology*. 2014;25(5):729–737.
30. Martens EP, Pestman WR, de Boer A, Belitser SV, Klungel OH. Instrumental variables: application and limitations. *Epidemiology*. 2006;17(3):260–267.
31. Hernan MA, Robins JM. Instruments for causal inference: an epidemiologist's dream? *Epidemiology*. 2006;17(4):360–372.
32. Rassen JA, Brookhart MA, Glynn RJ, Mittleman MA, Schneeweiss S. Instrumental variables I: instrumental variables exploit natural variation in nonexperimental data to estimate causal relationships. *J Clin Epidemiol*. 2009;62(12):1226–1232.
33. Harris KM, Remler DK. Who is the marginal patient? Understanding instrumental variables estimates of treatment effects. *Health Serv Res*. 1998;33(5 Pt 1):1337–1360.
34. Newhouse JP, McClellan M. Econometrics in outcomes research: the use of instrumental variables. *Annu Rev Public Health*. 1998;19:17–34.
35. Madestam A, Shoag D, Veuger S, Yanagizawa-Drott D. Do political protests matter? Evidence from the Tea Party movement. *Quarterly Journal of Economics*. 2013;128(4):1633–1685.
36. Kahn JM, Ten Have TR, Iwashyna TJ. The relationship between hospital volume and mortality in mechanical ventilation: an instrumental variable analysis. *Health Serv Res*. 2009;44(3):862–879.
37. Valley TS, Sjoding MW, Ryan AM, Iwashyna TJ, Cooke CR. Association of intensive care unit admission with mortality among older patients with pneumonia. *JAMA*. 2015;314(12):1272–1279.
38. Brookhart MA, Wang PS, Solomon DH, Schneeweiss S. Evaluating short-term drug effects using a physician-specific prescribing preference as an instrumental variable. *Epidemiology*. 2006;17(3):268–275.

21 HOW TO EMBED HEALTHCARE DELIVERY SCIENCE INTO YOUR HEALTH SYSTEM

INTRODUCTION

At this point, you've reached the end of *Understanding Healthcare Delivery Science*, and the obvious question is "Now what?" How do you begin to make this real so that it affects your work and improves the care that you give your patients? How do you scale your healthcare delivery science work so that it has an impact beyond your particular patients, beginning to affect all the patients in your institution, or even beyond? This can happen in at least a few ways: in your own work, in your interactions with others, and even by changing your health system, if you're a healthcare leader. Another important approach is by building a national and international community of healthcare delivery scientists.

The purpose of this chapter is to give some practical strategies for accomplishing this, so you can begin to embed healthcare delivery science into your health system. We first start with the question of how to join (or build) a community of healthcare delivery science. We then turn to the question of how to embed healthcare delivery science into your health system. How you do this depends on *your* context. Perhaps you're a medical student or a resident, considering this as a career. Maybe you're done with training, and you're working in a health system as a frontline nurse, physician, or other provider, or you've just taken your first job in healthcare administration. On the other hand, you may be even further along in your career, with a significant leadership position in your health system. In each of these cases, you have opportunities to help embed healthcare delivery science into your health system.

HOW DO I JOIN (OR BUILD) A COMMUNITY OF HEALTHCARE DELIVERY SCIENCE?

Being part of a community helps all of us grow, succeed, feel welcomed, and thrive. Regardless of whether you are just starting off in healthcare or are a senior leader in a health system, we all need a community.

Because healthcare delivery science is a still-emerging field, however, finding this community can require some effort. In particular, those working on healthcare delivery science tend to be *bridging leaders* between healthcare operations and healthcare research. David Brooks wrote an article in *The New York Times* with the headline "At the Edge of Inside," which focused on exactly this issue. Although Brooks was writing about the political landscape, his words describe the challenges of healthcare delivery science, too. You should read his whole article, but a particularly relevant passage is:[1]

> *In any organization there are some people who serve at the core. These insiders are in the rooms when the decisions are made.... Then there are outsiders. They throw missiles from beyond the walls. They are untouched by internal loyalties ... But there's also a third position in any organization: those who are at the edge of the inside. These people are within the organization, but they're not subsumed by the group think. They work at the boundaries, bridges and entranceways.*

Being at the edge of inside is one of the defining characteristics of healthcare delivery science. It brings challenges, but also benefits. Brooks continues:[1]

> *The person on the edge of inside is ... involved in a process of perpetual transformation, not a belonging system ... There are downsides to being at the edge of inside. .... You may be respected and befriended, but you are not loved as completely as the people at the core, the band of brothers. You enjoy neither the purity of the outsider nor that of the true believer ... But the person on the edge of inside can see reality clearly. The insiders and the outsiders tend to think in dualistic ways: us versus them; this or that. ... The person on the edge of inside is more likely to see wholeness of any situation.*

Building and Growing a Local Community of Healthcare Delivery Science

Building a local community is important for healthcare delivery science practitioners. Our experience is that, when you build your team, you will often find that people outside your specialty or department can be tremendously helpful. Many health systems have a number of people interested in healthcare delivery science, but they are often distributed across departments. As you are building your community, remember to look outside your usual silos. These relationships often turn out to be tremendously rewarding and productive.

A National Community of Healthcare Delivery Science

Taking part in the growing national community of healthcare delivery science is also a way to join and build a community. How do you find this community? There are a few ways:

- **Centers that focus on healthcare delivery science.** Even if your health system does not have a center, other places near you may. Table 21-1 lists many of the current centers, and we will keep an ongoing, updated list at https://www.bidmc.org/research/research-centers/center-for-healthcare-delivery-science/what-we-do/industry-landscape. (We tend to be friendly and welcoming—just reach out!)
- **Training programs in healthcare delivery science.** Another way to connect with the healthcare delivery science community is through educational activities. Master programs, as well as other advanced training opportunities in the field, are emerging at an increasing rate. Table 21-2 lists some of them, and we will keep an updated list at https://www.bidmc.org/research/research-centers/center-for-healthcare-delivery-science/what-we-do/industry-landscape. In addition to formal, longer-term programs, these programs may host seminars and other events, as well as serving as a nucleus of healthcare delivery science talent.
- **Read the journals.** Many specialty journals now include healthcare delivery science articles, reviews, and editorials. The field also has its own journal—*Healthcare: The Journal of Delivery Science and Innovation*
- **National professional societies.** Numerous physician specialty societies are beginning to recognize the importance of delivery science by holding sessions on the topic at national meetings, workshops, and other forums. Other societies also focus more intently on healthcare delivery science. For example:
  - The National Forum on Quality Improvement in Health Care, held by the Institute for Healthcare Improvement (IHI), has an associated Scientific Symposium each year.
  - AcademyHealth, which is the major professional society for health services research, has launched a specific interest group focused on delivery science.

> **External Resource**
> A list of centers and institutes of healthcare delivery science is available at https://www.bidmc.org/research/research-centers/center-for-healthcare-delivery-science/what-we-do/industry-landscape

> **External Resource**
> A list of programs with advanced training in healthcare delivery science is available at https://www.bidmc.org/research/research-centers/center-for-healthcare-delivery-science/what-we-do/industry-landscape

> **External Resource**
> *Healthcare: The Journal of Delivery Science and Innovation* is a peer-reviewed journal focused on healthcare delivery science. It is available at https://www.journals.elsevier.com/healthcare-the-journal-of-delivery-science-and-innovation.

Table 21-1 CENTERS AND INSTITUTES OF HEALTHCARE DELIVERY SCIENCE

Institution	Center/Institute	Web Page
Beth Israel Deaconess Medical Center (Boston)	Center for Healthcare Delivery Science	https://www.bidmc.org/research/research-centers/center-for-healthcare-delivery-science
Brigham and Women's Hospital (Boston)	Center for Healthcare Delivery Sciences	https://www.c4hds.org/
Dartmouth College (Hanover, NH)	Dartmouth Institute for Health Policy and Clinical Practice	https://tdi.dartmouth.edu/education/degree-programs/master-science-healthcare-research/
Eastern Virginia Medical School–Sentara (Norfolk, VA)	Healthcare Analytics and Delivery Science Institute	https://www.evms.edu/research/centers_institutes_departments/healthcare_analytics_and_delivery_science_institute/
Icahn School of Medicine at Mount Sinai (New York)	Institute for Health Care Delivery Science	https://icahn.mssm.edu/research/institute-health-care-delivery
Mayo Clinic (Rochester, MN)	Kern Center for the Science of Health Care Delivery	https://www.mayo.edu/research/centers-programs/robert-d-patricia-e-kern-center-science-health-care-delivery/about
Medical College of Wisconsin (Milwaukee, WI)	Collaborative for Healthcare Delivery Science	https://www.mcw.edu/departments/center-for-advancing-population-science-caps/programs/collaborative-for-healthcare-delivery-science
Nemours Children's Health System (Wilmington, DE)	Center for Healthcare Delivery Science	https://www.nemours.org/pediatric-research/area/health-care-delivery-science.html
New York University Langone Health (New York)	Center for Healthcare Innovation and Delivery Science	https://med.nyu.edu/chids/
University of Chicago Medicine (Chicago)	Center for Healthcare Delivery Science and Innovation	https://hdsi.uchicago.edu/
University of Massachusetts Medical School—Baystate (Springfield, MA)	Institute for Healthcare Delivery and Population Science	https://www.baystatehealth.org/education-research/research/research-centers/institute-for-healthcare-delivery-and-population-science
Weill Cornell Medical College (New York)	Division of Healthcare Delivery Science and Innovation	http://hpr.weill.cornell.edu/divisions/health_systems_innovation/

Table 21-2 PROGRAMS WITH ADVANCED TRAINING IN HEALTHCARE DELIVERY SCIENCE

Institution	Program	Web Page
Arizona State University (Online)	Master of Science in Science of Health Care Delivery	https://asuonline.asu.edu/online-degree-programs/graduate/master-science-science-health-care-delivery
Cedars-Sinai Medical Center (Los Angeles)	Master of Health Delivery Science	https://www.cedars-sinai.edu/Research/Research-Areas/CORE/Masters-Program/
Dartmouth Institute for Health Policy and Clinical Practice (Hanover, NH)	Master of Health Care Delivery Science	http://mhcds.dartmouth.edu/
Eastern Virginia Medical School	Master of Healthcare Delivery Science	https://www.evms.edu/education/masters_programs/healthcare_delivery_science/
Harvard Medical School (Boston)	Master of Healthcare Quality and Safety	https://postgraduateeducation.hms.harvard.edu/masters-degree-programs/master-healthcare-quality-safety
Icahn School of Medicine at Mount Sinai	Master of Science in Health Care Delivery Leadership	https://icahn.mssm.edu/education/masters/health-care-delivery
Kaiser Permanente Division of Research	Delivery Science Fellowship Program	https://divisionofresearch.kaiserpermanente.org/research/fellowship-program
Mayo Clinic	Kern Health Care Delivery Scholars Program	https://www.mayo.edu/research/centers-programs/robert-d-patricia-e-kern-center-science-health-care-delivery/education-training/scholars-programs
University of Chicago Graham School Pritzker School of Medicine	Master of Science in Biomedical Informatics, Healthcare Delivery Science Concentration Pritzker School of Medicine Healthcare Delivery Sciences Track	https://grahamschool.uchicago.edu/academic-programs/masters-degrees/biomedical-informatics/mscbmi-concentrations/healthcare-delivery-science-concentration https://pritzker.uchicago.edu/page/healthcare-delivery-sciences-track
University of Tulsa	MBA in Health Care Delivery Sciences	https://business.utulsa.edu/graduate-business-programs/mba-programs/mbahcds/

HOW TO EMBED HEALTHCARE DELIVERY SCIENCE IN YOUR HEALTH SYSTEM

The tools available to you to promote and encourage healthcare delivery science vary based on your own personal context.

What If I'm a Trainee?

Until very recently, no dedicated training programs in healthcare delivery science existed. Today, these programs are being created at an accelerating rate. If you are participating in one, or considering doing so, this section is for you. But the chances are that you're someone else:

- Perhaps you're a medical student, or a resident.
- Maybe you're a fellow entering your research years.
- You might be a student in a master's program in a health-related field, and you want to bridge scholarship and real-world practice.
- Maybe you are in an earlier stage of your career, studying business in college or university, and you want to focus on the future of healthcare.

It may feel like you have no control over your environment, but in fact students often have profound influence on their teachers and mentors. We recommend doing the following:

- **Treat this book like a survey course.** Use it to identify areas in which you want to develop more skills. You are at a point when you have the gift of time to spend on exploration; take courses and do practicums in those areas that interest you. But also talk to your instructors and make sure that they know that you are interested in healthcare delivery science: not only practice, and not only research—but the intersection of both. Not only are you likely to have a better experience, but you may influence the way that this instructor looks at the world after you have left her or his class.
- **Find people who've done things you're interested in and work with them.** Finding mentors in healthcare delivery science can be challenging, but you will recognize interesting work when you see it. Seek these people out, ask them questions, and work with them.

External Resource

AcademyHealth is an organization that provides information about the current and future needs of healthcare systems. More information about it and its members can be found at https://www.academyhealth.org

And again, be clear that you are interested in healthcare delivery science.
- **Ask questions.** For those of us who have been attending physicians for a while (or have taught in classrooms for a while), questions from our trainees are tremendously important and remarkably powerful. Your questions influence us, affect us, and change the way we think and how we teach. Ask us about our results, and then ask us about the next level of analysis that we didn't show.

What If I'm an Individual Working in a Health System?

Perhaps you're done with training, and you're working in a health system as a frontline nurse, physician, pharmacist, or other provider. Or maybe you've just taken your first job in healthcare administration. How can you help your health system move toward healthcare delivery science?

Up-Level Your Own Work

Leading by example is profoundly powerful. Each of us is often responsible for improvement efforts or performance measurements of some kind. When you are analyzing data so you can make decisions, you can spend the time and effort to have just a bit more rigor (i.e., up-level your work). You almost never truly have time for the perfect analysis, but you can consider what the just-a-little-more-rigorous approach might look like. Thinking about a before-and-after pie chart? A run chart often shows trends over time better than the alternatives. Looking at a run chart? A statistical process control will help you understand when variations are meaningful instead of random. Making a high-stakes decision? Maybe it's worth investing in an interrupted time-series analysis, or something similar. Chapters 11–20 can help with this.

Help Others do Their Best Work

As a frontline provider or administrator, you are in a great position to encourage others to do their best work. One way to do this is, on occasion, to gently and politely ask about the next level of analysis, just as you are beginning to do for your own work. Another powerful action you can take is calling out positive exemplars: When you see others doing the right things, call attention to it, both privately and publicly. This helps reinforce healthcare delivery science in your environment.

What If I'm a Health System Leader?

Leaders come in all shapes and sizes. Some are informal leaders, who are often the most influential in any organization. Others have positional authority—ranging from frontline managers to chief executive officers. Recall that Chapter 7 reviews leadership techniques in the context of implementation science frameworks. How can you use your leadership to help embed healthcare delivery science into your health system? This section discusses some good ideas.

Ask for (and Provide) Just a Little More Rigor Every Day

As a leader, your actions speak volumes. One of the most impactful things you can do is demand just a bit more rigor in analyses that you encounter. Gently and politely, help others to be their best by asking about the next level of analysis. Even more powerful is to walk the walk: When you are responsible for analyzing data that you need to make decisions, spend the time and effort to have just a bit more rigor. Push your analyses to where you can really be proud of your work. Chapters 11–20 can help with this.

Celebrate Positive Exemplars

We all respond to cues from our leaders, whether they have positional authority or informal influence. This means that a key action that you can take is to recognize healthcare delivery science when you see it, and let people know that you value it. Call out positive exemplars both privately and publicly. This helps create a culture where healthcare delivery science is valued.

Invite Speakers

Grand Rounds are a longstanding tradition in healthcare for a reason. You may not have access to experts in healthcare delivery science, but you can begin to build a culture of healthcare delivery science by inviting experts in the field to come and give talks to your staff. This helps demonstrate your organization's awareness of the field, and it also helps trainees and others to begin to build their network. Inviting speakers is also a way to build a potential talent pool as you think about further investment in recruitment efforts. Incorporating speakers into existing conferences is often the easiest, first step. Later, consider having special talks that focus on healthcare delivery science, such as visiting professorships and other keynote-type events.

Help Trainees Find Mentors, Whether in Your Own Health System or in Other Systems

Healthcare delivery science is a bridging field between operations and research-quality methods. It can be really challenging for trainees and junior leaders to find appropriate mentorship. As a leader, your network is likely to be broader than theirs. Help them find mentors from your network and from your network's network. This can be extraordinarily powerful—not only because it improves the quality of healthcare delivery science at your institution, but also because it demonstrates your personal commitment to these future leaders as individuals.

Host a Formal Event, Like a Healthcare Delivery Science Symposium

Both of the editors of this book have witnessed the benefit of hosting formal events focused on healthcare delivery science and related fields—namely, the Silverman Symposium at the Beth Israel Deaconess Medical Center and the Quality and Safety Symposium at the University of Chicago Medicine. A common format for this type of event is to have a Grand Rounds with a well-known external speaker, linked with a poster session that highlights innovation, improvements in quality and safety, and healthcare delivery science. In our experience, these sessions started out being fairly small, but they have since grown to include many hundreds of people from across the health system along with executive leadership and Board members who routinely attend.

Travel Grants

Many people who are getting started in healthcare delivery science do not have access to funds to present their work at relevant national meetings. For example, bedside nurses (or nurses pursuing master's degrees) often do really interesting work in this space, but they may not have professional development funds for travel. The same is true for respiratory therapists, pharmacists, and medical students, among other professionals. Sponsoring a small number of travel grants is a relatively low-cost way to promote scholarship and activity in healthcare delivery science at your institution.

Innovation Grant Programs

Innovation grants are seed funds that help drive an organization's focus on healthcare delivery science. In our experience, we have tended to fund these as one-year grants of up to $50,000. We chose that amount specifically because it parallels the funding level of the National Institutes of

Health (NIH) for one of its smallest grants, the R03, which helps attract true interest from the research community at an organization. Funding one or two of such grants per year clearly requires investment, but the return on this investment has been compelling.

It is important to specify things that you value when making a proposal. For example, we have typically required a multidisciplinary team (not just physicians, and not just researchers). This helps encourage new kinds of collaborations that your organization may not have seen before. Another strategy is to require the grant application's specific aims to explicitly align with the health system's strategic plan or annual operating plan objectives.

A final tactic that, in our experience, has been remarkably valuable is in the review and selection process for the grants themselves. We have used a modified (shorter) NIH format for the applications themselves, and we have included a "study section" for review. The novel approach to grant review that we have used, though, is the following: We have assigned each grant two primary reviewers. One is a senior, respected researcher. The other is a member of the C-suite or other senior leader from the health system. Each completes a review using the NIH scale, and then we meet for 2–4 hours with all reviewers (usually on the order of 10 to 20 people, depending on the number of applications). We can typically review about 10 grants with discussions, and so we use the scores to streamline which ones are considered. We then have a discussion where one primary reviewer may be the hospital's chief operating officer and the other may be an epidemiologist who is a member of the National Academy of Medicine. At the end, we rank the grants because we can usually only fund one or two proposals.

Here's the key reason why this review process is helpful: Many of these people will never have met each other, and so the review process itself helps build a community of healthcare delivery science. It also exposes senior health system leaders to all the ideas that come forth as proposals, and we have seen occasions where a vice president will like a proposal enough that—even though it isn't funded by this process— she or he allocates operational resources that help move the project forward.

Recruit Those Skilled in Healthcare Delivery Science to Join Your Health System

You may be a leader who has personal responsibility for the recruitment of new physicians, new administrators, or other members of your team. Or you may at least have influence over the process. For some fraction of these cases, insist on a diverse slate of candidates that includes people skilled in healthcare delivery science. Just opening these doors can help. But when selecting candidates, you also have the chance to weight accomplishments in healthcare delivery science appropriately. The first time you do this, it will take some courage on your part, because these individuals may not fit traditional multiple-R01-grant phenotypes, nor are they likely to have taken a traditional fully operations-focused career path. However, seeding just one or two experts in the field can dramatically transform your organization's culture.

Launch a Center for Healthcare Delivery Science

If you are a senior leader at a larger health system, you may want to formally organize your efforts in healthcare delivery science by creating a center or an institute. This is definitely a substantial undertaking, but one that is increasingly popular. Just a few years ago, centers of healthcare delivery science were rare. Today, there are more and more of them. Table 21-1 lists many of the current centers, and we will keep an ongoing, updated list at https://www.bidmc.org/research/research-centers/center-for-healthcare-delivery-science/what-we-do/industry-landscape.

> **External Resource**
>
> A list of centers and institutes of healthcare delivery science is available at https://www.bidmc.org/research/research-centers/center-for-healthcare-delivery-science/what-we-do/industry-landscape

Launch a Degree Program for a Master's in Healthcare Delivery Science

Perhaps you are at a university-affiliated health system or a medical school. One of the challenges in the field of healthcare delivery science is that there are relatively limited places to get advanced training today. One powerful action is to help open up the field for future leaders by expanding the opportunity to obtain formal advanced education. A master's program is a very high-leverage action that will influence many future careers. Master's programs, and other advanced training opportunities in the field, are emerging at an increasing rate. Table 21-2 lists some of them, and we will keep an updated list at https://www.bidmc.org/research/research-centers/center-for-healthcare-delivery-science/what-we-do/industry-landscape.

> **External Resource**
>
> A list of programs with advanced training in healthcare delivery science is available at https://www.bidmc.org/research/research-centers/center-for-healthcare-delivery-science/what-we-do/industry-landscape

SUMMARY

Regardless of who you are, there are many practical tools to help you grow, encourage, and promote the practice of healthcare delivery science in your health system.

KEY POINTS

- Being part of a community helps all of us grow, succeed, feel welcomed, and thrive—and this is true for healthcare delivery scientists, too.
- Centers focused on healthcare delivery science are emerging at an increasing rate—as are advanced training programs in healthcare delivery science.
- Increasing the rigor in your own work is an effective way to lead by example in embedding healthcare delivery science into your health system.
- Inviting Grand Rounds speakers, or even hosting a formal event like a healthcare delivery science symposium, can help introduce healthcare delivery science to your health system.
- Innovation grant programs, and travel grant funding, are also ways to encourage healthcare delivery science in your health system.

REFERENCE

1. Brooks D. At the edge of inside. *The New York Times*, June 24, 2016. Accessed April 30, 2019, from https://www.nytimes.com/2016/06/24/opinion/at-the-edge-of-inside.html.

Index

A
A3, 174–175
ACA. *See* Affordable Care Act (ACA)
AcademyHealth, 436, 439
ACC. *See* Accountable care community (ACC)
Access block, 391
Access management, 210
Access to healthcare, 391–393
Accountable care community (ACC), 181b
Accountable care organization (ACO), 52, 229
Achieving Hospital-wide Patient Flow, 390
ACO. *See* Accountable care organization (ACO)
ACTA. *See* Applied cognitive task analysis (ACTA)
Action opportunities, 89
Action rates, 89
Action space, 368
Active attention, 79
Acute Physiology and Chronic Health Evaluation (APACHE), 371, 381
Adaptive Boosting (AdaBoost), 353
ADHERE, 350
Advanced practice providers (APPs), 63. *See also* Primary care providers
Adverse event, 137
Advocacy groups, 184
Affordable Care Act (ACA)
 central pillars, 55
 changes to healthcare delivery, 52
 flawed in both conception and execution, 55
 major expansion in healthcare coverage, 51
 value in healthcare, 55
Agency for Healthcare Research and Quality (AHRQ), 226
Agent-based modeling, 411–412
AGI. *See* Artificial general intelligence (AGI)

AHRQ. *See* Agency for Healthcare Research and Quality (AHRQ)
AHRQ hospital survey on patient safety culture, 112
AHRQ patient safety indicators, 140
AI. *See* Artificial intelligence (AI)
AI winters, 344
Airline incidents (near-misses, etc.), 56
Algorithm development, 210
ALOS. *See* Average length of stay (ALOS)
AlphaGo, 343
Alternate form reliability, 301
Alternative providers, 63. *See also* Primary care providers
AMIA Clinical Informatics program, 206
Analytic techniques, 233–430
 bias, 236–239
 chance, 235–236
 confounding, 239–242
 easy-to-use techniques. *See* Everyday analytics
 overview, 252–253
 survey. *See* Survey-based data
 threats to validity of the analysis, 235–243
 violating the assumptions of your method, 243, 250
Anchoring, 78
Anchoring-and-adjustment heuristic, 80
Anchoring effect, 80–81, 82, 83
APACHE. *See* Acute Physiology and Chronic Health Evaluation (APACHE)
Applied cognitive task analysis (ACTA), 95
Appointment blocks, 396
APPs. *See* Advanced practice providers (APPs)
Area under the precision-recall curve (AUPRC), 370
Area under the receiver operating characteristic curve (AUROC), 327, 370, 382

448 INDEX

Artificial general intelligence (AGI), 341
Artificial intelligence (AI), 64, 342. *See also* Machine learning
Artificial trans fats, 186–187
Ascertainment bias, 78, 83
Ashley, David, 407
Assumptions, 243, 250
Astronomical point, 269
"At the Edge of Inside" (Brooks), 435
Attractors, 29
Attribution error, 78
AUPRC. *See* Area under the precision-recall curve (AUPRC)
AUROC. *See* Area under the receiver operating characteristic curve (AUROC)
Autocorrelation, 251
Automated medication-dispensing system, 74
Automobile manufacturing, 163
Autoregressive covariance matrix, 336
Available working time, 172
Availability bias, 78, 82
Availability heuristic, 80
Average length of stay (ALOS), 399, 400

B

Background chart lines, 267f, 268
Backpropagation of errors, 362n
Backward selection, 321, 322
Bagging, 352
Balancing measures, 217t, 219
Banzett's multidimensional dyspnea profile (MDP), 301
Bar chart, 264t
Basic data governance, 210
Bayes' theorem, 79, 271, 274
Bayesians, 271
"Bed crunch" situations, 393
Behavioral Risk Factor Surveillance System (BRFSS), 291
Bellman equation, 367
Berwick, Don, 7
Beth Israel Deaconess Medical Center, 442
Between-subject variation, 334, 336, 337
Bias
 analytic techniques, 236–239
 ascertainment, 78, 83
 availability, 78, 83
 cognitive, 78–79, 82–83
 commission, 78
 confirmation, 79, 83
 feedback, 83
 hindsight, 81
 information, 238–239
 machine learning, 370
 nonresponse, 306
 perceptron, 357
 selection, 236, 378
 surveillance bias, 239
Biden, Joe, 4
Big-box stores with embedded pharmacies, 185
Big data, 9–12, 58, 62. *See also* Data in healthcare
Billing-based patient safety indicators, 140
Billing codes, 246
Billing data, 212
Binary data, 248
Bioterrorism-related data, 189t
Blameworthy events, 147
Block scheduling, 397
Blood sugar control, 12–14
Blue Cross, 378
Boids, 26
Bone marrow and stem cell transplantation, 6, 37, 48
Book of Why, The (Pearl), 418
Bootstrapping, 324, 351, 351f, 384
Bounded rationality, 79–80
Bradford Hill criteria, 372
Branching logic, 296
BRFSS. *See* Behavioral Risk Factor Surveillance System (BRFSS)
British coal miners, 105
Brooks, David, 435
Building a Better Delivery System: A New Engineering/Health Care Partnership, 391
Building an HDS network. *See* Practical strategies for building an HDS network
Built environment, 43
Bundled Payments Initiative for Medical Conditions program, 46
Burnout, 392
Business intelligence, 210

C

C5. *See* Citywide Coalition for Colorectal Cancer Control (C5)
C. diff, 7–8
c-chart, 283t
C statistic, 382
CAHPS. *See* Consumer Assessment of Healthcare Providers and Systems (CAHPS)
Calibration, 382–383
Capitated care, 57
Car manufacturing, 163
CART. *See* Classification and regression tree (CART)
CAS. *See* Complex adaptive system (CAS)
Categorical data, 248–249
CATS. *See* Communication and teamwork skills (CATS)
Causal inference, 371–372, 417. *See also* Causal methods
Causal methods, 417–421
Cause mapping, 145, 146f
CBOs. *See* Community-based organizations (CBOs)
CDM. *See* Critical decision method (CDM)
Center for Medicare and Medicaid Innovation, 52, 229
Centers for Medicare and Medicaid Services (CMS), 53, 154, 226
Centers of healthcare delivery science, 436, 437t
Central limit theorem, 248
Central line infections, 165
Central line specific wastes, 169
Central line venous catheter, 24
CFIR. *See* Consolidated framework for implementation research (CFIR)
Chance, 235–236
Change management, 132–133
Changover time, 172
Chart lines, 267f, 268
Chartjunk, 265
Cheaper by the Dozen (Gilbreth/Carey), 75
Checking if something worked in real world. *See* Program evaluation
Checklists, 55
Chess, 342–343
Chi-squared statistic, 279
Chi-squared test, 279
Chief analytics officer, 206
Chief data officer, 206
Chimeric antigen receptor (CAR) T-cell therapy, 6
Choice architecture, 158
CI. *See* Confidence interval (CI)
Cicero, Marcus Tullius, 73
CIT. *See* Critical incident technique (CIT)
City-wide diabetes registry, 189, 190b, 191f
Citywide Coalition for Colorectal Cancer Control (C5), 192
Classification and regression tree (CART), 330–332, 349–350
Cleveland Health Quality Choice Program, 14–15, 187
"Cleveland Health Quality Choice Was a Failure, not a Martyr," 15
Clinical monitoring systems, 58
Clinical Process of Care Measures, 227
Closed-ended questions, 305
Clostridium difficile (C. diff), 7–8
Cluster analysis, 349
Clustered data, 333
Clustering, 251, 251n
CMS. *See* Centers for Medicare and Medicaid Services (CMS)
CNN. *See* Convolutional neural network (CNN)
Coefficient of determination (R^2), 317
Cognitive biases, 78–79, 82–83. *See also* Bias
Cognitive reasoning, 77–86
Cognitive task analysis (CTA), 94, 95
Cognitive testing, 296–297
Collider, 420
Collinearity, 329–330
Commission bias, 78
Commission error, 83
Common cause variation, 280
Communication and teamwork skills (CATS), 90
Community and clinical partnerships. *See* Partnering with community organizations
Community-based organizations (CBOs), 183–184

Community-based pharmacies, 185
Complete case analysis, 244–245
Complex adaptive system (CAS)
  common features, 28–29, 34
  components of population not the same, 32
  connections, 28
  defined, 26
  evolving over time, 28, 33
  example (Wikipedia), 29–30
  nondeterministic in nature, 29
  opportunities for evaluation, 31–33
  outliers, 32
  parts of system learning and adapting, 33
  variation over time and space, 31–32
Complex system, 23, 75
Complexity
  complex system/complicated system, compared, 23–24
  data systems, 214
  healthcare delivery, 7–9
  humans having fundamental difficulties dealing with complex systems, 25
  medical care, 5–7, 48
Complicated system, 23–24
Composite scorecards, 226–227
Comprehensive data governance, 210
"Computing Machinery and Intelligence" (Turing), 344
Concurrent validity, 302–303
Confidence interval (CI), 276–278
Confirmation bias, 79, 83
Conflating outcomes and exposures, 237
Confounders, 321
Confounding, 239–242, 418
Confounding by indication, 241
Confounding by severity, 241
Consolidated framework for implementation research (CFIR), 126–127, 130, 131f
Construct validity, 303
Consumer Assessment of Healthcare Providers and Systems (CAHPS), 227, 228
Consumerism, 60–61
Content validity, 302
Context, 120–121
Continuous data, 246–248, 278
Contributing factors analysis, 142
Convenience sample, 305–306
Convergent validity, 303
Convolution, 359, 360f
Convolutional neural network (CNN), 358–362
Conway, John Horton, 27
Core Measures, 227
Core Public Health Functions Steering Committee, 182b
Correlation, 314
Cost function, 348
Costco, 185
Costs of data collection, 225
Counterfactual, 418
Covariance structure, 336
Cox regression, 314
Creating an HDS network. *See* Practical strategies for building an HDS network
Creeping determinism, 81
Crew, 105–106
Crew resource management (CRM), 110–112
Criterion validity, 302
Critical decision method (CDM), 93–95
Critical incident technique (CIT), 92–93
CRM. *See* Crew resource management (CRM)
Cronbach's alpha, 301, 302
Croskerry, Pat, 82, 84, 85
Crossing the Quality Chasm, 40–41, 41t, 220
CTA. *See* Cognitive task analysis (CTA)
Culture change, 117–119
Cumulative frequency, 264t
CVS, 185
Cycle time, 172

D

Data, 245–251. *See also* Data in healthcare
  binary, 248
  categorical, 248–249
  clustered, 333
  continuous, 246–248, 278
  discrete, 279
  missing, 243–245

multicategory, 248–249
structured, 246
unstructured, 246
visual display. *See* Displaying data
Data analytics, 205, 206
Data czar, 212
Data fields, 213
Data governance, 208–211
Data guru, 212
Data in healthcare, 203–215. *See also* Data
   accessing good data, 212–214
   big data, 9–12
   billing data, 212
   chief data officer, 206
   complexity of data systems, 214
   consequences of poorly designed system, 207
   data fields, 213
   data governance, 208–211
   data guru/data czar, 212
   data lineage, 209
   data quality program, 205
   data set, 213, 214
   data table, 213
   data warehouse, 205, 210, 211
   documentation, 213
   fragmented and disjointed environment, 205, 206
   garbage in, garbage out, 205
   good data, defined, 206
   healthcare analytics team, 206
   IT ecosystem, 207
   model of data flow in healthcare, 204f
   multiple sources for same data element, 208
   perfect data?, 214
   questions to ask, 213
   relational databases, 211
Data integration, 211
Data lake, 211
Data lineage, 209
Data mart, 211
Data quality management, 210
Data quality program, 205
Data security, 65
Data set, 188–189t, 213, 214
Data-sharing agreement, 195
Data steward community, 210

Data table, 213
Data warehouse, 205, 210, 211
Daughter node, 331
Death
   causes of death (1912), 47f
   medical error, 41–42
Deep Blue, 342–343
Deep learning, 344, 356
Deep learning models, 356–365
Deep reinforcement learning, 365–369
DeepMind, 343
Defects, 167
Degrees of freedom *(df)*
   chi-square test, 279
   t test, 278
Deming cycle, 157
Dependent variable, 316, 316f
Derivation data set, 324
Deterministic process, 24
df. *See* Degrees of freedom *(df)*
Diagnostic anchoring, 81
Diagnostic momentum, 82
DiD. *See* Difference in differences (DiD)
Difference in differences (DiD), 424–426
Differential misclassification, 236
Dinosaur footprints, 233–235
Discrete data, 279
Discrete event simulation, 319, 410–411
Discriminant validity, 303
Discrimination, 382
Displaying data, 261–268
   bar chart, 264t
   chartjunk, 265
   common mistakes to avoid, 265–268
   cumulative frequency, 264t
   frequency polygon, 264t
   graph, 261
   line graph, 264t
   pie chart, 265–267
   scatter plot, 264t
   strange and distracting eye effects (Moire effect), 265, 266f
   table, 261, 262t, 263t
   three-dimensional graphics, 265, 266f
   too many notes and annotations (unnecessary information), 267–268, 267f
   Tufte's principles of graphical excellence, 262–265

Diversity and group decision-making, 87
Dixon-Woods, Mary, 120, 121
Donabedian, Avedis, 216, 224
Donabedian Structure-Process-Outcome-(Balancing) framework, 216, 217t
Dorner, D., 25, 28
Dot product, 359, 360f
Double-barreled questions, 295, 304
Drop-in clinics in pharmacy chains, 185
Drucker, Peter, 121, 122
Drug overdose deaths, 16–17, 17f

E
Early childhood education interventions, 43–44
Easy-to-implement analytics. *See* Everyday analytics
eCQMs. *See* Electronic clinical quality measures (eCQMs)
Effect modification, 287, 329, 385
EHR. *See* Electronic health record (EHR)
8 wastes, 167–169
Electronic clinical quality measures (eCQMs), 227
Electronic footprints, 235
Electronic health record (EHR), 10f, 58, 66, 205
Electronic patient-safety trigger tools, 141
Electronic "sniffers," 141
Elwart, Felix, 420
Embedding HDS in your health system, 439–444
  celebrating positive exemplars, 441
  finding mentors for trainees and others, 442
  Grand Round speakers, 441
  healthcare delivery science symposium, 442
  hosting a formal event, 442
  individuals working in a health system, 440
  innovation grants, 442–443
  inviting speakers, 441
  launching a center or institute, 444
  launching postgraduate degree program, 444
  leading by example (walking the walk), 441
  recruiting experts, 443–444
  trainees, 439–440, 442
  travel grants, 442
Emergency department (ED) overcrowding, 391
Emergent change management, 132
Emergent themes approach to CDM, 94
Encryption, 65
Ensemble model, 352
Environmental services (EVS), 8
Epidemiological survey, 291
EpiQuery, 190
Equipoise, 416
Ergonomics, 75. *See also* Human factors
Erlang delay model, 408
Ernest Amory Codman Award, 13
Essential public health services, 182b, 183f
Evaluating effectiveness of programs. *See* Program evaluation
"Evaluating the Quality of Medical Care" (Donabedian), 216
Everyday analytics, 256–288
  chi-squared test, 279
  confidence interval (CI), 276–278
  incidence, 275
  mean, 258
  measures of central tendency, 258–259
  measures of comparison, 270–279
  median, 258–259
  mode, 259
  odds ratio (OR), 276, 277
  outliers, 256, 258
  P value, 270–272, 277
  positive/negative predictive value, 274
  power, 271
  prevalence, 275
  range, 259–260
  relative risk (RR), 276
  run chart, 268–270
  sensitivity, 273
  SPC chart. *See* Statistical process control (SPC) chart
  specificity, 273
  standard deviation (SD), 260
  standard error, 260–261

summative measures of data, 257–261
t test, 278
type I error, 271
type II error, 271
understanding patient flow, 397–400
univariate tests of difference, 270–279
visual display of data. *See* Displaying data
Evolutionary psychology, 24
EVS. *See* Environmental services (EVS)
Exabyte, 346
Exchangeability, 420
Exchangeable covariance matrix, 336
Expectation states theory, 87, 88, 109
"Explaining Matching Michigan: An Ethnographic Study of a Patient Safety Program" (Dixon-Woods et al.), 120
Explanatory variable, 315
Exploding gradient, 364
Exploration versus exploitation dilemma, 367
Exposure variable, 315
External validation, 384
Externalizing decision-making process, 85

F
Face validity, 302
Facility billing data, 212
Failure mode, 153
Failure mode effects analysis (FMEA), 151–154
Failure mode effects criticality analysis (FMECA), 151–154
Faith-based organization (FBO), 183
Family Satisfaction in the Intensive Care Unit (FS-ICU) instrument, 302–303
FBO. *See* Faith-based organization (FBO)
Federal public health agencies, 186
Fee-for-service system, 44–45
Feedback bias, 83
Filter, 360, 361f, 362f
Fishbone diagram, 143
Fisher's exact test, 279
Five rules of causation, 147, 149t
5 Whys, 143, 144t

Fixed effects, 379
Fixed effects model, 335, 336–337
Flanagan, John, 92
Flat hierarchy, 113
Flexner report, 5
FMEA. *See* Failure mode effects analysis (FMEA)
FMECA. *See* Failure mode effects criticality analysis (FMECA)
Forced choice, 304
Forcing functions, 84
Forget gate, 364
Fork, 419–420
Forward selection, 321, 322
Framington risk score, 347
Frequency distribution, 261, 262t, 264t
Frequency polygon, 264t
Frequentist theory, 272
FS-ICU. *See* Family Satisfaction in the Intensive Care Unit (FS-ICU) instrument
Fukushima reactor, 328
Full-day kindergarten, 44
Function-based cognitive task analysis (CTA), 95
Fundamental attribution error, 83
Fundamental philosophical shift, 60
Fuzzy join, 211

G
Game of Life (Conway), 27
Garbage in, garbage out, 205
Gates, Bill, 372
Gauss, Carl Friedrich, 247
Gaussian distribution, 247
GEE model. *See* Generalized estimating equation (GEE) model
Gemba walk, 170
Generalizability, 383–384
Generalized estimating equation (GEE) model, 337–338
Generalized linear mixed effects model, 334
Gilbreth, Frank and Lillian, 75
Global Trigger Tool, 42, 140–141
Glycemic control, 13, 219
Go game, 343
Going solid, 393
Going to gemba, 170

Good data, 206. *See also* Data in healthcare
Good-old-fashioned AI, 342–343
Good Practice Guide: Focus on Improving Patient Flow, 390
Goodhart's law, 46, 225
Goodness of fit, 250
GPU. *See* Graphics processing unit (GPU)
Gradient boosting, 353
Gradient descent, 362n
Grand Round speakers, 441
Graph, 261. *See also* Displaying data
Graphics processing unit (GPU), 345
Group decision strategy, 85
Group-designation variables, 336

H
HAC. *See* Hospital-Acquired Conditions (HAC) program
Harm events, 56
Harvard Medical Practice Study, 37–38
Hawthorne effect, 33
HCAHPS. *See* Hospital Consumer Assessment of Healthcare Providers and Systems (HCAHPS)
HDS. *See* Healthcare delivery science (HDS)
Health
  how health is created, 179–180
  influencing factors, 43
  methods of improvement, 43–44
  social determinants, 179, 179f
Health and Retirement Study (HRS), 291
"Health in All Policies" tactic, 181b
Health information exchange (HIE), 191
Health Information Technology for Economic and Clinical Health (HITECH) Act, 9
Health services research, 3, 4f
Healthcare: The Journal of Delivery Science and Innovation, 436
Healthcare analytics team, 206
Healthcare-associated infections, 141
Healthcare data. *See* Data in healthcare
Healthcare data warehousing projects, 205
Healthcare delivery science (HDS), 17–18
  ability to appreciate healthcare system as living organism, 68
  adaptability of, 67
  analytic designs, 34
  benefits of, 60, 67
  centers and institutes, 436, 437t
  conceptual model, 18f
  creating an HDS network. *See* Practical strategies for building an HDS network
  critical role in reaching healthcare of the future, 56
  defined, 76
  human factors. *See* Human factors
  most important feature, 67
  overlap between operational innovation and research, 18, 18f
  training programs, 436, 438t
  why needed, 5–12, 19
Healthcare delivery science symposium, 442
Healthcare Effectiveness Data and Information Set (HEDIS), 228
Healthcare quality improvement tools. *See* Standard quality improvement tools
Healthcare system
  absence of central coordination, 59
  amount of healthcare data, 9–12
  attractors, 29
  complex adaptive system, 18. *See also* Complex adaptive system (CAS)
  complexity, 7
  deployment of assets, 57
  fee-for-service system, 44–45
  influencing factors, 68
  key stakeholders in shaping health, 181–186
  more and more complex and intensive services, 57
  overutilization, 44
  "physician's workshop," 5
  problems with, 18
  quality. *See* Quality and safety in healthcare
  R&D, 3, 4f
  structural gap, 59
  supplier-induced demand, 45

INDEX 455

value, 42, 43f, 53–54
volume-based contracting, 59
what will be required in the future, 67
worker burnout, 168
Healthcare worker burnout, 168
HealthGrades, 380
HEDIS. *See* Healthcare Effectiveness Data and Information Set (HEDIS)
Hemoglobin A1c (HBA1c) registry, 190b, 191f
Henderson, Lawrence, 4
Heuristics, 80–81, 82–83
HIE. *See* Health information exchange (HIE)
Hierarchical linear models, 252
Hierarchy, 86–90
High-reliability practices, 55
Hills, Bradford, 372
Hindsight bias, 81
HITECH. *See* Health Information Technology for Economic and Clinical Health (HITECH) Act
Hollnagel, Erik, 154
Homoscedasticity, 318, 323
Hosmer-Lemeshow test, 327, 382, 383
Hospital-Acquired Conditions (HAC) program, 228
Hospital Compare, 141, 380
Hospital Consumer Assessment of Healthcare Providers and Systems (HCAHPS), 227, 288, 291, 306
Hospital Inpatient Quality Reporting Program, 227
Hospital Outpatient Quality Reporting Program, 227
Hospital Readmissions Reduction Program (HRRP), 228
Hospital Safety Grade (Leapfrog Group), 226
Hospital scorecards, 226
Hospital Stars, 226, 227
Hospital value-based purchasing, 46, 228
Hospitalists. *See* Primary care providers
Hospitals, 379–380, 393
How to Improve, 157
HRRP. *See* Hospital Readmissions Reduction Program (HRRP)
HRS. *See* Health and Retirement Study (HRS)

Human factors, 73–103
 bounded rationality, 79–80
 cognitive biases, 78–79, 82–83
 cognitive reasoning, 77–86
 cognitive task analysis (CTA), 94, 95
 critical decision method (CDM), 93–95
 critical incident technique (CIT), 92–93
 defined, 75, 96
 diversity and group decision-making, 87
 expectation states theory, 87, 88
 externalizing decision-making process, 85
 group decision strategy, 85
 heuristics, 80–81, 82–83
 hierarchy, 86–90
 humans as "intuitive scientists," 79
 intersection of human factors and medicine, 75–76
 knowledge-elicitation techniques, 95
 metacognition, 77, 84
 observable power and prestige order (OPPO), 88–89
 reluctant rationality, 79
 status, 87–88
 strategies to mitigate biases in reasoning, 84
 theories of human decision-making, 79–82
 World Wars I and II, 75
Hyperplane, 354, 354f, 355

I
Idle time, 167
Iezzoni, Lisa, 381
Ignorability, 421
IHI. *See* Institute of Healthcare Improvement (IHI)
ImageNet Large-Scale Visual Recognition Challenge, 344, 345f
Implementation science, 123–133
 choosing the appropriate tool, 132
 consolidated framework for implementation research (CFIR), 126–127, 130, 131f
 defined, 123
 family-on-rounds intervention, 124–125, 130–132
 PARiHS, 127–128
 questions to ask, 124
 RE-AIM, 128–130, 130–131, 131f

Improvement Guide (Nolan et al.), 158
Inception v3, 362
Incidence, 275
Incidence and Types of Adverse Events and Negligent Care (Utah-Colorado study), 38–39
Incidence of Adverse Events and Negligence in Hospitalized Patients (Harvard Medical Practice Study), 37–38
Inclusion/exclusion criteria, 237
Independent observations, 251
Independent variable, 251, 315, 316, 316f
Infant mortality, 37, 38f
Informal data governance, 208
Information bias, 238–239
Inner setting, 126
Innovation burnout, 119
Innovation grants, 442–443
Inpatient patient flow, 394–396
Input gate, 364
Institute of Healthcare Improvement (IHI), 140, 141, 154, 390, 436
Institute of Medicine, 39–41, 204, 390
Institutes of healthcare delivery science, 436, 437t
Instrument, 428, 430
Instrumental variable (IV) analysis, 427–430
Integration of methods, 56
Interaction, 329
Intermediate actions, 150–151t
Intermediate outcomes, 217t, 219–220
Internal consistency reliability, 301
Internal validation, 383
International comparisons, 42–45
  administrative costs, 45
  country with most expensive healthcare (U.S.), 44
  hospital admission, 45
  life expectancy vs. health expenditures, 43f
  pharmaceutical costs, 45
  physician salaries, 45
  social care and healthcare spending, 44f
International Ergonomic Association (IEA), 74
Interobserver reliability, 223

Interquartile range, 260
Interrupted time series (ITS), 422–424
Intervention effect, 425
Interventional model review, 210
Interventions, 380–381
Inventory overages, 167
Ishikawa diagram, 143–144, 145f
IT ecosystem, 207
Item-response theory, 296
ITS. *See* Interrupted time series (ITS)
IV analysis. *See* Instrumental variable (IV) analysis

J

James, William, 79
Japanese earthquake analytics, 328
Jha, Ashish, 384
Jillette, Penn, 77, 84
Joint Commission, 13, 16, 139
Journals, 436

K

Kahneman, Daniel, 80, 81
Kaizen, 163
Kanban, 165
Kasparov, Garry, 342
Kavanaugh, Brian, 13, 219
Kendall's notation, 408n
Kernel, 355, 359
Kernel trick, 355
Knew-it-all-along effect, 81
Knowledge-elicitation techniques, 95

L

Last observation carried forward, 245
Latent failure model, 86
Latent failure (Swiss cheese) model of accidents, 142–143, 142f
Le Guin, Ursula K., 91
Lead time, 172
Leadership, 121–123
  be clear about the vision, 122–123
  building an HDS network. *See* Practical strategies for building an HDS network
  establish urgency and focus, 122
  keep patients as center of what we do, 123
  own the idea of "we," 122
  take responsibility, 122

Leading by example (walking the walk), 441
Lean improvement techniques, 162–177
   A3, 174–175
   8 wastes, 167–169
   going to gemba, 170
   historical overview, 163–164
   process mapping, 170–171
   rules of lean, 165–166
   ThedaCare Improvement System, 164
   Toyota Production System (TPS), 163
   TPS ideal for healthcare, 166
   value stream mapping, 171–173
   Virginia Mason Production System, 164
Leapfrog Group, 380
Leapfrog Group's Hospital Safety Grade, 226
Lee, Tom, 122
Left-skewed distribution, 259
Length of stay (LOS), 397–400
Lewin, Kurt, 132
Lewis, David, 418
Life expectancy, 37, 42, 43f
Lighthill report, 344
Likert, Rensis, 294
Likert-type scale, 246–247, 295–296, 304
Line graph, 264t
Linear and monotonic, 250f
Linear data, 249–250
Linear fixed effects model, 336–337
Linear mixed effects model, 333–336
Linear regression, 250. *See also* Multiple linear regression
Little, John, 401
Little's law, 270, 401–405
Local public health agencies, 186–194. *See also* Public health agencies
LODS. *See* Logistic organ dysfunction score (LODS)
Log-linear relationship, 250
Log-normal distribution, 248
Log-transformed data, 248
Logistic organ dysfunction score (LODS), 381
Logistic regression, 249, 314, 322–323
Logistic/sigmoid function, 357
Long short-term memory (LSTM) network, 364
Longitudinal design, 34
LOS. *See* Length of stay (LOS)
Loss function, 348
LSTM network. *See* Long short-term memory (LSTM) network

M
M/M/s model, 408
Machine learning, 58, 62, 64, 341–376
   artificial general intelligence (AGI) vs. specific AI, 341–342
   artificial intelligence, defined, 342
   bagging, 352
   bootstrapping, 351, 351f
   canonical definition, 342
   causal inference, 371–372
   classification and regression tree (CART), 349–350
   convolutional neural network (CNN), 358–362
   deep learning models, 356–365
   deep reinforcement learning, 365–369
   exploration versus exploitation dilemma, 367
   fairness, disparities, and bias, 370
   historical overview of AI, 344–346
   long short-term memory (LSTM) network, 364
   loss function, 348
   matrix multiplication, 345
   off-policy evaluation, 369
   perceptron, 356–358
   pitfalls, 369–372
   random forests, 351–353
   real-time data vs. historical data, 370–371
   recurrent neural network (RNN), 362–365
   relationship between AI, machine learning, and deep learning, 343f
   supervised/unsupervised learning, 348–349
   support vector machine (SVM), 353–3356
   symbolic AI, 343
   terminology, 347t
   training-serving skew, 370–371
   translating epidemiology to machine learning, 346, 347t
   tree-based models, 349–353

Machine learning models, 348
Machine that Changed the World, The (Womack/Jones), 163
Managing to Learn: Using the A3 Management Process to Solve Problems, Gain Agreement, Mentor, and Lead (Shook), 175
Mann-Whitney U test, 248
Manual, sampled chart review (Global Trigger Tool), 140–141
MAR. *See* Missing at random (MAR)
Marginal average response, 335
Marginal participant, 430
Markov decision process, 366–367
Marx, David, 147
Master data management, 210
Matching Michigan, 120–121
Matrix multiplication, 345
Max pooling, 360
MCAR. *See* Missing completely at random (MCAR)
McCarthy, John, 342, 344
McGlynn study, 39
Mean, 247, 258
Measure databases and aggregators, 226
Measures of central tendency, 32, 258–259
Measures of comparison, 270–279
Measuring quality and safety, 216–232
  balancing measures, 217t, 219
  challenges, 223–225
  common pay-for-performance programs and measure sets, 227–229
  composite scorecards, 226–227
  costs of data collection, 225
  Donabedian model and Six Aims together, 220–221, 221t
  Donabedian Structure-Process-Outcome-(Balancing) framework, 216, 217t
  Goodhart's law, 225
  intermediate outcomes, 217t, 219–220
  measure databases and aggregators, 226
  outcome measures, 217t, 218
  process measures, 217–218, 217t
  Six Aims for Improvement, 220, 221t
  statistical impossibility, 224
  structural measures, 216–217, 217t
  what makes a good measure?, 222–223
Medial frontal negativity (MFN), 88
Median, 247, 258–259, 286
Mediator, 419
Medicaid, 185
Medical director of analytics, 206
Medical error
  appreciation of, prompting introspection and regulation, 55
  deaths from, 41–42
  defined, 138
"Medical Error--The Third-Leading Cause of Death in the US," 42
Medical Expenditure Panel Survey (MEPS), 291
Medicare, 184–185
Medicare Advantage, 51, 229
Medicare overall hospital star rating, 227
Medicare Prescription Drug, Improvement, and Modernization Act, 51
Medicare Shared Savings Program (MSSP), 52
Medicare Stars, 227, 229
Medicare value-based purchasing (for hospitals), 140
MEMO study. *See* Minimizing Error, Maximizing Outcome (MEMO) study
Memory cells, 364
MEPS. *See* Medical Expenditure Panel Survey (MEPS)
Merit-based Incentive Program System (MIPS), 226, 228–229
Metacognition, 77, 84
MFN. *See* Medial frontal negativity (MFN)
Micromotion studies, 75
Miles, Caroline, 289
Million Hearts campaign, 193
Minimizing Error, Maximizing Outcome (MEMO) study, 392
MIPS. *See* Merit-based Incentive Program System (MIPS)
Misclassification error, 236
Missing at random (MAR), 244
Missing completely at random (MCAR), 243–244

Missing data, 243–245
Missing not at random (MNAR), 244
Mixed effects model, 333–336
MNAR. *See* Missing not at random (MNAR)
Mode, 259
Model for Improvement, 156–158
Modeling patient flow, 390–415
　agent-based modeling, 411–412
　discrete-event simulation, 410–411
　Erlang delay model, 408
　examples of individual patient flows, 395f
　external resources, 390
　inpatient patient flow, 394–396
　length of stay (LOS), 397–400
　Little's law, 401–405
　outpatient clinics, procedure suites, operating rooms, 396–397
　patient-centered vs. time-centered LOS calculations, 399–400, 400f
　patient flows in a scheduled context, 398f
　patient safety and quality, 391–392
　provider-level consequences, 392
　queuing theory, 405–410
　simulation methods, 408–412
　system-level consequences, 393
MODS. *See* Multiple organ dysfunction score (MODS)
Moire effect, 265, 266f
Monotonic data, 249, 250f
Monotonic relationship, 249
Moore's law, 346
Mortality prediction model (MPM), 381
MOS 36-item short-form health survey (SF-36), 291, 308
Motion inefficiencies, 168
MPM. *See* Mortality prediction model (MPM)
MSSP. *See* Medicare Shared Savings Program (MSSP)
Multicategory data, 248–249
Multiclass logistic regression, 362n
Multimorbidity, 6
Multinomial logistic regression, 362n
Multiple imputation, 245, 300

Multiple linear regression, 314–322
　assumptions, 318
　coefficient of determination (R^2), 317
　correlation, 314
　fitting a line to the graph, 316, 317, 317f
　forward/backward selection, 321–322
　graph, 316, 316f
　homoscedasticity, 318
　number of variables, 321
　overview, 314
　Pearson correlation coefficient (r), 315
　residuals, 317, 318, 319f, 320f
Multiple logistic regression, 314, 322–323
Multiple organ dysfunction score (MODS), 381

N

Narrow AI, 342
National Academy of Medicine, 40
National Academy of Sciences, 390
National Forum on Quality Improvement in Health Care, 436
National Health and Nutrition Examination Survey (NHANES), 291
National Health Interview Survey (NHIS), 291
National Health Service, 390
National Health Services Corps, 52
National Healthcare Quality and Disparities Report, 45
National Healthcare Safety Network (NHSN), 141, 227
National Information Center on Health Services Research and HealthCare Technology (NICHSR), 190
National Institutes of Health (NIH), 53, 218, 443
National Patient Safety Foundation, 46, 147
National Quality Forum, 139, 226
National Quality Measures Clearinghouse, 226
Natural-language processing, 66
Near-miss, 138
Negative predictive value, 274
Netlogo, 412

Neural networks, 358–362
Neuron, 359
Never events, 139
New York City (NYC)
   city-wide diabetes registry, 189, 190b, 191f
   Citywide Coalition for Colorectal Cancer Control (C5), 192
   demonstration community health worker program, 190b
   EpiQuery, 190
   trans fats, 186–187
Newhouse, Joe, 378
NHANES. *See* National Health and Nutrition Examination Survey (NHANES)
NHIS. *See* National Health Interview Survey (NHIS)
NHSN. *See* National Healthcare Safety Network (NHSN)
NHSN-driven healthcare-associated infection surveillance, 141
NICE-SUGAR. *See* Normoglycemia in Intensive Care Evaluation-Survival Using Glucose Algorithm Regulation (NICE-SUGAR)
NICHSR. *See* National Information Center on Health Services Research and HealthCare Technology (NICHSR)
NIH. *See* National Institutes of Health (NIH)
95% confidence interval, 277
Node, 331, 364
Nondifferential misclassification, 236
Nonparametric analytic methods, 247–248, 330
Nonresponse bias, 306
Nontechnical skills for surgeons (NOTSS), 90, 93
Normal distribution, 247, 247f, 260
Normoglycemia in Intensive Care Evaluation-Survival Using Glucose Algorithm Regulation (NICE-SUGAR), 13, 219
NOTECHS. *See* Oxford nontechnical skills scale (NOTECHS)
NOTSS. *See* Nontechnical skills for surgeons (NOTSS)
Nudge units, 158
Null hypothesis
   chi-squared test, 279
   confidence interval (CI), 276
   P value, 270, 272
   t test, 278
Null value, 277
Nurse practitioners, 63. *See also* Primary care providers
NYC. *See* New York City (NYC)

O

Objective function, 348
Observable power and prestige order (OPPO), 88–89
Observable teamwork assessment for surgery (OTAS), 90
Odds ratio (OR), 276, 277
Off-policy evaluation, 369
Ohno, Taichii, 163, 167
OLAP. *See* Online analytics processing (OLAP)
Omission error, 83
Omnicell, 74
Oncology care, 61–62
Online analytics processing (OLAP), 211
Open-ended questions, 305
"Operation That Rated Hospitals Was a Success, but the Patience Died," 14
Operations research, 390. *See also* Modeling patient flow
Opioid epidemic, 16–17, 17f
OPPO. *See* Observable power and prestige order (OPPO)
Optimal value, 54
OR. *See* Odds ratio (OR)
Ordinal categorical data, 249
Organ dysfunction scores, 381
Organic food, 208
Organized protests, 427, 429
Osler, William, 5
OTAS. *See* Observable teamwork assessment for surgery (OTAS)
Outcome measures, 217t, 218
Outer setting, 126
Outliers, 32, 256, 258, 330
Output gate, 364
Overcrowding. *See* Modeling patient flow
Overfitting, 328

Overprocessing, 168
Overproduction, 168
Overutilization of healthcare system, 44
Own the idea of "we," 122
Oxford nontechnical skills scale (NOTECHS), 90

P

p-chart, 283t
P value, 13, 236, 270–272, 277
Padding, 359n
"Pain as the Fifth Vital Sign" program, 16
Pain management, 15–17
Parametric methods, 313
PARiHS. *See* Promoting action on research implementation in health services (PARiHS)
Partnering with community organizations, 178–199
  accountable care community (ACC), 181f
  advocacy groups, 184
  approaches to successful partnerships, 194–195
  community-based organizations (CBOs), 183–184
  essential public health services, 182b, 183f
  government entities, 185–186
  healthcare payers, 184–185
  NYC. *See* New York City (NYC)
  private industry, 185
  public health agencies. *See* Public health agencies
  social determinants of health, 179, 179f
  stakeholders, 181–186
Patient activism, 60–61
Patient-centered care, 60
Patient-centered medical home (PCMH), 74
Patient-Centered Outcomes Research Institute, 52
Patient-Centered Outcomes Research Trust Fund, 52
Patient experience surveys, 227
Patient flow. *See* Modeling patient flow
Patient Flow: Reducing Delay in Healthcare Delivery, 404

Patient portals, 74
Patient Protection and Affordable Care Act. *See* Affordable Care Act (ACA)
Patient-reported outcomes measurement information system (PROMIS), 218
Patient-reported outcomes (PROs), 218
Patient safety. *See* Quality and safety in healthcare
Patient safety events, 137, 139–141
Patient safety movement, 55
Pay-for-performance schemes, 52, 59, 227–229
Payment reform, 180–181, 180b
PCMH. *See* Patient-centered medical home (PCMH)
PDCA ("Plan, Do, Check, Act"), 157
PDSA ("Plan, Do, Study, Act"), 157–158
Pearl, Judea, 418–420
Pearson correlation coefficient (r), 315
Perceptron, 356–358
Percutaneous transluminal coronary angioplasty (PTCA), 6
Performance outputs, 89
Perioperative surgical home (PSH), 74
Personalized medicine, 61–62, 65, 67
PET scan. *See* Positron emission tomography (PET) scan
Petabyte, 346
Physician assistants, 63. *See also* Primary care providers
Pie chart, 265–267
Pioneer ACOs, 52
"Pioneer Project Publishes First Rankings of Cleveland Hospitals," 14
Planned change management, 132
Poisson distribution, 248, 407
Poisson model, 334n
Poisson process, 407
Political protests, 427, 429
Pooled variance, 278
Pooling, 360
Population health, 195
Porter, Michael, 54
Positive predictive value, 274
Positron emission tomography (PET) scan, 57

Postsafety era, 56
Potential predictor variable, 353
Power, 271
Power of "we," 122
Practical strategies for building an HDS network, 434–445
  centers and institutes, 436, 437t
  embedding HDS in your system. *See* Embedding HDS in your health system
  joining/building a community of healthcare delivery science, 434–438
  training programs in HDS, 436, 438t
Practice effect, 301
Prediction rule, 323–327
Predictive models, 58, 312–340
  classification and regression tree (CART), 330–332
  clustered data, 333
  collinearity, 329–330
  covariance structure, 336
  Cox regression, 314
  effect modification, 329
  generalized estimating equation (GEE) model, 337–338
  inaccurate and unstable models, 327
  interaction, 329
  linear fixed effects model, 336–337
  linear mixed effects model, 333–336
  multiple linear regression. *See* Multiple linear regression
  multiple logistic regression, 314, 322–323
  nonparametric tools, 330
  outliers, 330
  overfitting/underfitting, 328
  parametric tools, 313
  pitfalls, 327–330
  prediction rule, 323–327
  proportional hazards regression, 314
  random intercept model, 335
  random slope model, 335
Predictive validity, 302
Premature closure, 82
Prevalence, 275
Preventable adverse event, 138
Prevention and wellness activities, 59
Primary care providers
  burnout, 392
  role of physician, 62–63, 65
  workload, 392
Private industry, 185
PRO. *See* Patient-reported outcomes (PROs)
Probabilistic mental models, 80
Process mapping, 155–156, 170–171
Process measures, 217–218, 217t
Professional billing data, 212
Program evaluation, 416–433
  assumptions, 421, 431
  causal methods, 417–421
  collider, 420
  consistency, 421
  counterfactual, 418
  difference in differences (DiD), 424–426
  exchangeability, 420
  fork, 419–420
  ignorability, 421
  instrumental variable (IV) analysis, 427–430
  interrupted time series (ITS), 422–424
  quasi-experimental design, 421, 422–430
  regression discontinuity design (RDD), 426–427, 427f
  seeking the assistance of statisticians, 422
  stable unit treatment value assumption (SUTVA), 421
  wiggling a variable, 419
PROMIS. *See* Patient-reported outcomes measurement information system (PROMIS)
Promoting action on research implementation in health services (PARiHS), 127–128
Promoting wellness and health, 57–59
Pronovost, Peter, 165
Proportional hazards regression, 314
Prospective hindsight, 85
Protest size, 427, 429
Proton therapy, 57
PSH. *See* Perioperative surgical home (PSH)
PSI-90, 228
PTCA. *See* Percutaneous transluminal coronary angioplasty (PTCA)

Public health agencies
  access to population-level data, 187–192
  convening multiple parties around a common goal, 192–193
  federal agencies, 186
  insight into the community, 186–187
  policy development, 193–194
  principles of epidemiology, 192
Public health systems, 181–182
PubMed, 10
Pulmonary artery catheter, 292
Pyxis, 74

Q
Q function, 368
Q-learning, 367
Q-table, 368
QPS. *See* Quality Positioning System (QPS)
Quality and safety in healthcare, 37–50
  Crossing the Quality Chasm, 40–41, 41t
  deaths from medical error, 41–42
  effectiveness of safety improvements, 45–46
  To Err Is Human, 39–40
  Harvard Medical Practice Study, 37–38
  improvements in healthcare in last century, 46–48
  international comparisons, 42–45
  McGlynn study, 39
  measuring quality. *See* Measuring quality and safety
  patient flow, 391–392
  Six Aims of high-quality healthcare, 41t
  Utah-Colorado Study, 38–39
Quality and Safety Symposium, 442
Quality improvement tools. *See* Standard quality improvement tools
Quality of Dying and Death instrument, 303
Quality of Health Care Delivered to Adults in the United States (McGlynn study), 39
Quality Payment Program, 226
Quality Positioning System (QPS), 226

Quasi-experimental design, 421, 422–430
Questionnaire, 295–296, 304–305
Queuing theory, 319, 405–410

R
r. See Pearson correlation coefficient (r)
R^2, 250
R^2. *See* Coefficient of determination (R^2)
R03, 443
Random effects, 335, 379
Random forests, 351–353
Random intercept model, 335
Random sampling, 293
Random slope model, 335
Random survival forest, 352
Randomized control trial, 416
Range, 259–260
Rational mapping, 145
RCA. *See* Root cause analysis (RCA)
RCA^2, 145, 147, 148t, 149
R&D. *See* Research and development (R&D)
RDD. *See* Regression discontinuity design (RDD)
RE-AIM
  adoption, 129
  effectiveness/efficacy, 129
  family-on-rounds intervention, 130–131
  identifying outcomes of interest, 131f
  implementation, 129
  maintenance, 130
  reach, 128–129
Reason, James, 142
Rectified linear unit (ReLU) function, 357, 361f
Recurrent neural network (RNN), 362–365
"Reducing waste and error: piloting lean principles at IHC" (Jimmerson et al.), 175
Reflective thinking, 77
Regional health information organization (RHIO), 191
Regression discontinuity design (RDD), 426–427, 427f
Reinforcement learning, 343, 365–369
Relational database, 211

Relative frequency, 261, 263t, 264t
Relative risk (RR), 276
Reliability, 300–302
ReLU function. *See* Rectified linear unit (ReLU) function
Reluctant rationality, 79
Representativeness heuristic, 80, 82
Research and development (R&D), 3, 4f
Residual, 317, 318, 319f, 320f
Residual confounding, 241
Resilience engineering, 86
Rework, 167
Reynolds, Craig, 26
RHIO. *See* Regional health information organization (RHIO)
Right-skewed data, 401f
Right-skewed distribution, 247f, 259
Risk, 377
Risk adjustment, 222, 377–389
  calibration, 382–383
  comparing hospitals, 379–380
  comparing interventions, 380–381
  confounder, as, 385
  discrimination, 382
  effect modifier, as, 385–386
  generalizability, 383–384
  guiding interventions, 386
  how can using risk adjustments fail use?, 384, 386
  importance of, from insurance standpoint, 378–379
  insurers, 377–378
  risk, defined, 377
  scoring systems, 381–382
  selection bias, 378
  uses, 385–386
Risk priority number (RPN), 153
"Risks of Risk Adjustment, The" (Iezzoni), 381
RNN. *See* Recurrent neural network (RNN)
Robinson, Daniel, 15
Robotic surgery, 57
Rogers, Will, 237
Root cause analysis (RCA), 142–151
  blameworthy events, 147
  cause mapping, 145, 146f
  five rules of causation, 147, 149t
  5 Whys, 143, 144t
  focus on systems of care, not individuals, 143
  goals, 143
  intermediate actions, 150–151t
  Ishikawa diagram, 143–144, 145f
  prioritization, 147
  process mapping, 145. *See also* Process mapping
  RCA team, 143
  RCA^2, 145, 147, 148t, 149
  RCA^2 matrix for safety assessment codes, 148t
  RCA^2 severity and probability criteria, 148t
  stronger actions, 150t
  Swiss cheese model, 142–143, 142f
  weaker actions, 151t
  when not to use RCA, 143
Rose dyspnea scale, 218
Rowley, Coleen, 86
ROWS. *See* Rule out worst-case scenario (ROWS)
RPN. *See* Risk priority number (RPN)
RR. *See* Relative risk (RR)
Rubin, Donald, 418
Rule of three, 85
Rule out worst-case scenario (ROWS), 84
Run chart, 268–270
  astronomical point, 269
  runs, 269
  shift, 269, 269f
  trend, 269, 269f

S

Safety. *See* Quality and safety in healthcare
Safety attitudes questionnaire (SAQ), 90
Safety I, 154
Safety II, 154
Sample size, 294
Sampling, 293
Sampling frame, 293
Samuel, Arthur, 342
SAPS. *See* Simplified acute physiologic score (SAPS)
SAQ. *See* Safety attitudes questionnaire (SAQ)
Scatter plot, 264t

INDEX 465

SD. *See* Standard deviation (SD)
Seattle angina questionnaire, 218, 291
Selection bias, 236, 378
Seneca, Lucius Annaeus, 73
Sensitivity, 273
Sentinel events, 139
Sequential organ failure assessment (SOFA), 381
Serious reportable event (SRE), 139
Serious safety event (SSE), 139
SEU. *See* Subjective expected utility (SEU) theory
SF-36. *See* MOS 36-item short-form health survey (SF-36)
Shannon number, 342–343
Shared savings, 180b
Shewhart, Walter, 280
Shewhart cycle, 157
Shift (run chart), 269, 269f
Shock index, 249
Signal and the Noise, The (Silver), 328
Silver, Nate, 328
Silverman Symposium, 442
Simon, Herbert, 79
Simple covariance matrix, 336
Simplified acute physiologic score (SAPS), 381
Simulation methods, 408–412
Simultaneous efforts to improve care (too many interventions at once), 119–120
Six Aims of high-quality healthcare, 41t, 221t
Skilled nursing facility (SNF) admission, 30
SNF. *See* Skilled nursing facility (SNF) admission
Social care and healthcare spending, 44f
Social determinants of health, 179, 179f
Social hierarchy, 87
Socioecological model of health, 179f
SOFA. *See* Sequential organ failure assessment (SOFA)
Softmax regression, 362n
Southwest Airlines Flight 1380 explosion, 104
SPC chart. *See* Statistical process control (SPC) chart
Speaking time, 89

Spear, Steven, 165, 166
Special cause variation, 279, 281
Specific AI, 342
Specificity, 273
SQL. *See* Structured Query Language (SQL)
SRE. *See* Serious reportable event (SRE)
Stable unit treatment value assumption (SUTVA), 421
Stage migration, 238
Standard deviation (SD), 247, 260, 285–286
Standard error, 260–261
Standard quality improvement tools, 137–161
  choice architecture, 158
  definitions, 137–139
  failure mode effects analysis (FMEA and FMECA), 151–154
  identifying patient safety events, 139–141
  Model for Improvement, 156–158
  PDSA, 157–158
  process mapping, 155–156
  RCA. *See* Root cause analysis (RCA)
  Safety I/Safety II, 154
  voluntary patient safety reporting, 139–140
Standing teams, 107
Statistical process control (SPC) chart, 279–283
  c-chart, 283t
  common cause variation, 280
  one-/two-/three-sigma control limit, 280f
  p-chart, 283t
  special cause variation, 279, 281
  u-chart, 283t
  x-chart, 281
  X-mr-chart, 282f
Status, 87–88
Stride, 359
Strong AI, 341
Stronger actions, 150t
Structural measures, 216–217, 217t
Structure-Process-Outcome-(Balancing) framework, 216, 217t
Structured approach to CDM, 94
Structured data, 246

Structured Query Language (SQL), 211
Subjective expected utility (SEU)
   theory, 79, 80
Summative measures of data, 257–261
Supervised learning, 348
Supplier-induced demand, 45
Support vector, 355
Support vector machine (SVM),
   353–3356
Surgical Care Improvement Program,
   13
Surrogate end points, 219
Surveillance bias, 239
Survey-based data, 289–311
   administering the survey, 297–298,
      306
   analyzing the results, 299–302
   assessing attitudes, 291–292
   assessing knowledge, 292
   branching logic, 296
   cognitive testing, 296–297
   computer-adaptive test, 296
   convenience sample, 305–306
   deciding whom to survey, 293–294
   defining goal of survey, 293
   double-barreled questions, 295, 304
   epidemiological survey, 291
   free-text response, 296
   getting specialist's advice, 307
   increasing survey response rates,
      298–299t
   item nonresponse, 300
   key drivers, 307
   Likert-type response scales, 295–296,
      304
   nonresponse bias, 306
   open-ended vs. closed-ended
      questions, 305
   ordering of questions, 305
   pilot testing, 297
   pitfalls, 303–307
   purposes of surveys, 290–292
   question phrasing on survey
      responses, 304–305, 304t
   questionnaire, 295–296, 304–305
   random sampling, 293
   reliability, 300–302
   revising the survey, 296–297
   sample size, 294
   sampling frame, 293
   treating ordinal scales as continuous
      variables, 306–307
   two-stage sampling, 294
   using existing survey instruments
      whenever possible, 295
   validity, 302–303
SUTVA. *See* Stable unit treatment value
   assumption (SUTVA)
SVM. *See* Support vector machine
   (SVM)
Swiss cheese model of accidents,
   142–143, 142f
Symbolic AI, 343
System 1, 81
System 2, 81

T
t distribution, 278
T. rex, 234f, 235
t statistic, 278
t test, 248, 278
Table, 261, 262t, 263t. *See also*
   Displaying data
Target, 185
Task forces, 106–107
Tavistock Institute, 105
Team performance literature, 90
Team training, 55
Teams, 104–116
   crew resource management (CRM),
      110–112
   crews, 105–106
   defined, 105
   healthcare, in, 108–110
   organizational support, 108
   resources, 107–108
   standing, 107
   task forces, 106–107
   TeamSTEPPS, 112, 113f
Telemedicine, 65
TEM. *See* Threat and error
   management (TEM)
Ten essential public health services,
   182b, 183f
Terminal node, 331
Test-retest reliability, 301
ThedaCare Improvement System, 164
Theory of probabilistic mental models,
   80
Theropods, 234, 234f, 235

Thing Explainer: Complicated Stuff in Simple Words (Munroe), 303
Thinking Fast and Slow (Kahneman), 81
ThinkReliability, 145
Threat and error management (TEM), 111
3-day rule, 30–31
Three-dimensional graphics, 265, 266f
"Tight glycemic control" protocols, 13
Time-varying effects, 379
To Err Is Human, 39–40, 73, 74
Toledo, Alexander, 15
Too many interventions at once (simultaneous efforts to improve care), 119–120
Total-cost-of-care payment model, 181
Total knee arthroplasty, 30–31
Toyoda, Eiji, 163
Toyota Production System (TPS), 163. *See also* Lean improvement techniques
TPS. *See* Toyota Production System (TPS)
Training effect, 301
Training programs in healthcare delivery science, 436, 438t
Training-serving skew, 370–371
Transportation redundancies, 167–168
Trapping errors, 111
Travel grants, 442
Treatment-effect homogeneity, 430
Tree-based machine learning approaches, 349–353
Trend (run chart), 269, 269f
Tufte, Edward, 262, 265, 267
Tufte's principles of graphical excellence, 262–265
Turing, Alan, 344
Tversky, Amos, 80
Two-stage sampling, 294
Type I error, 271, 327
Type II error, 271, 327
Type III error, 327
Type 1 processes, 81
Type 2 processes, 81
Tyrannosaurus rex, 234f, 235

U
u-chart, 283t
Uncertainty, 67
Underfitting, 328
Understanding patient flow. *See* Modeling patient flow
Unified data platform, 210, 211
Univariate tests of association, 321
Univariate tests of difference, 270–279
University of Chicago Medicine, 442
Unnecessary motion, 168
Unnecessary movement of supplies or people, 167–168
Unpreventable adverse event, 138
Unstructured data, 246
Unsupervised learning, 348–349
U.S. Census, 291
U.S. News and World Report, 380
Usability testing, 74
USDA-certified organic food, 208
Use cases, 205
User-centered design, 74
Utah-Colorado Study, 38–39

V
VA Hospitals, 112
VA National Center for Patient Safety, 154
Validation data set, 324
Validity, 302–303
Value-added time, 172
Value-based payment, 180b
Value-based reimbursement, 57
Value in healthcare, 42, 43f, 53–54
Value stream mapping, 155, 171–173
Vanishing gradient, 364
Variance, 260, 285, 286
Ventilator-associated pneumonia, 292
Virginia Mason Production System, 164
Virtual visits, 65
Visual analog scale, 294
Visual display of data. *See* Displaying data
Volume-based contracting, 59
Voluntary attention, 79
Voluntary patient safety reporting, 139–140

W
Waiting time, 167
Walking the walk (leading by example), 441
Walmart, 185

"We," power of, 122
Weak AI, 342
Weak instruments, 430
Weaker actions, 151t
Wealth shocks, 43
Weekend effect, 239
Western Electric worker productivity study, 33
"What Makes an Effective Executive" (Drucker), 121
White, E. B., 263
Wiggling a variable, 419
Wikipedia, 29–30
Wilcoxon rank-sum test, 248
Wilcoxon signed rank test, 330
Will Rogers effect, 237, 238f
Wimmer, Roger, 294
Winship, Chris, 420
Within-subject variation, 334, 336, 337

X

x-chart, 281
X-mr-chart, 282f
XGBoost tool, 353

Z

Zettabyte, 346